AUDITORY DISORDERS
IN CHILDREN

a manual for differential diagnosis

AUDITORY DISORDERS
IN CHILDREN

a manual for differential diagnosis

HELMER R. MYKLEBUST

Professor of Audiology, School of Speech
Professor of Otolaryngology, School of Medicine
and
Director, Children's Hearing and Aphasia Clinic
Northwestern University

GRUNE & STRATTON   NEW YORK   1954

Library of Congress Catalog No. 54-7372

Printed and bound in U.S.A.

TO THE JUNIOR LEAGUE OF EVANSTON
for its vision and support
in behalf of children with
auditory disorders

Table of Contents

Preface

THIS MANUAL IS FOR THE PEDIATRICIAN AND
audiologist, for the psychologist and otolaryngologist and others who
are concerned with the complex problem of auditory disorders in
infants and young children. Its purpose is to suggest and describe
clinical procedures and techniques which have been found useful in
making a differential diagnosis. The method described is intended
primarily for children between the ages of one and six years. It has
been used with children not more than six months of age and at
times it has been necessary to employ these procedures with children
between six and fourteen years of age. This method, however, is
suggested chiefly for those occasions when formal hearing tests, such
as audiometric and tuning fork tests, are not applicable. Usually this
is with children below six years of age. Even when formal tests of
hearing can be used, it has often been advisable to use the techniques
suggested in this manual to secure corroborative information.

The plan of the book derives logically from the clinical procedures
required for making diagnoses of auditory disorders in children.
These procedures consist of three basic steps which constitute the
major divisions of the book. Part One includes the introduction, a
discussion of the problem and a consideration of auditory disorders
and language development. Part Two is a discussion of differential
history taking and interpretation of the history, which is the first step
toward making a diagnosis. Part Three is a discussion of the second
step, the evaluation of behavioral symptomatology. Part Four is a
presentation of the method, procedures and techniques for making
the examination. Part Five is a summary with suggestions for recommendations and training.

Throughout the book it is assumed that the child has no speech
and that he has inadequate ability to communicate to the extent that

verbal procedures are not applicable. Furthermore, auditory disorders are considered broadly. Children with psychic deafness, aphasic children and the mentally deficient who are presumed to have hearing impairment are included in the problem of auditory disorders. This seemed essential because if the evaluation of auditory capacity reveals that the lack of response to sound and the lack of speech are not due to deafness, it is necessary for the specialists to pursue the problem further and to make an appropriate diagnosis. It is the purpose of this manual, as stated, to suggest clinical methods which have been found useful to this end. Therefore, this book is not mainly an attempt to present conclusive experimental evidence. It is a manual for differential diagnosis intended for practitioners and students in training. The summaries at the end of each chapter have been included especially for those clinicians who are interested primarily in a brief description of how these clinical procedures can be used. It is possible to use these summaries as a guide without going through the more inclusive discussions throughout the manual. The author is hopeful that it will stimulate research in this challenging area of human behavior.

Many colleagues, students and friends have assisted me with the preparation of this book. Sincere appreciation is expressed to the Junior League of Evanston, Inc. for the part it has played in sponsoring the Children's Center for Hearing and Aphasia. Special recognition is due Mrs. George B. Milnor, Mrs. F. Edward Watermulder, Mrs. Raymond M. Galt, Mrs. Edward Wheeler, Mrs. Robert C. Barr and Mrs. H. Robert Harper for their untiring efforts in support of the Children's Center where most of the work has been in progress.

My graduate students have assisted with the development of the concepts and have made noteworthy criticisms. I am especially indebted to Robert Frisina, Graduate Clinical Assistant, who has supervised tabulation of the data and the statistical treatment. I also acknowledge my obligation to my former graduate assistants.

My colleagues, Dr. Harold Westlake, Chairman of the Department of Speech Correction and Audiology and Dr. Raymond Carhart, Professor of Audiology, read the manuscript and made many helpful criticisms. I am happy to acknowledge my indebtedness for this assistance and for their help in many other ways.

Appreciation is due Dr. George E. Shambaugh, Jr., Chairman of the Department of Otolaryngology, School of Medicine, Northwestern University for his suggestion to include summaries at the end of each chapter and for his assistance in preparing them. I am indebted to him also for opportunities for collaboration in the study of children with auditory disorders. Dr. William Nolan, Psychiatrist, has read parts of the manuscript and has made many other contributions to our work with children and their parents.

To Dr. Edgar A. Doll, formerly Director of the Psychological Laboratory, The Training School, Vineland, New Jersey I express appreciation for his criticisms of the manuscript and also for his stimulation and encouragement. It was from my association with him that I developed special interest in the problems of auditory behavior, language and brain injury. James H. McBurney, Dean, School of Speech, Northwestern University has provided me an unusual opportunity for working with children having auditory disorders. For this I am grateful. It is a pleasure to acknowledge my obligation to my secretary, Louise Bruns, for her diligent and painstaking typing of the manuscript and to Richard League for his generous assistance with the index. Finally, I wish to express gratitude to my wife for her patience and understanding.

HELMER R. MYKLEBUST

Northwestern University
Evanston, Illinois
November, 1953

PART ONE: INTRODUCTION

Chapter I

The Problem

THE IMPORTANCE OF THE CHILD'S EARLY LIFE to his later adjustment has been acknowledged in recent years. One of the outgrowths of this acknowledgement has been an intensified interest in handicapped children. For those who are predominantly interested in children with auditory disorders this has resulted in a need for clarification of early diagnosis and for more precise classification. Among those who emphasize the importance of early detection and accurate diagnoses of auditory disorders in children are pediatricians, otolaryngologists, neurologists, psychiatrists, clinical psychologists, speech pathologists, educators and audiologists. The enthusiastic interest shown by these various specialists during recent years suggests that in the future the divergent needs of these children will be determined at an early age. Such an accomplishment would minimize consequent psychological effects of auditory disorders. Positive remedial measures would be applied during that interim of life when the child is most amenable to corrective measures and management; secondary problems would not have developed to complicate the effects of the handicap and, thereby, initiate a condition which is relatively less remediable. A child with impaired hearing acuity who is erroneously diagnosed as mentally deficient, aphasic, or emotionally disturbed suffers greatly, not only from his deafness but from being misunderstood. Inadequate diagnoses, treatment and

I

psychological management in early life often cause problems of intense magnitude in later life.

One of the primary problems confronting specialists in auditory disorders of children is the development of reliable methods for determining auditory acuity. The methods most commonly used were designed for adults, but many diagnosticians have assumed that these methods were equally suitable for infants and young children. This assumption must be questioned. Evaluating the auditory capacity of adults who are emotionally, intellectually and physically mature is a different diagnostic problem from that of evaluating the auditory capacity of young children who are physically, emotionally and intellectually immature. It is necessary for all clinicians who examine the auditory capacities of children to consider whether the techniques and procedures are genetically suitable, whether the tests require mental, physical and emotional maturity beyond the child's capacity to respond.

Another assumption which has been made by many specialists is that lack of response to sound is an invariable indication of reduced auditory acuity. This assumption implies that overt responses will be made invariably. Thus, if a sound is presented and there is no overt response the inference is that the individual could not hear it and, therefore, has impaired acuity. This assumption, too, must be questioned. For example, an adult with psychogenic deafness does not respond to sound normally but his condition is not one of impaired acuity. This lack of a direct relationship between poor responsiveness to sound and peripheral deafness is encountered frequently in children. The younger the child the greater is the possibility of such a discrepancy being present. Therefore, the diagnostician of auditory disorders in young children is confronted with the obligation of ascertaining, not only whether impaired hearing acuity is present, but whether other types of auditory disorders which simulate deafness are present.

Parents often are not aware of the auditory disorders in their children until the symptom of lack of speech development appears. Many children manifesting a lack of speech development are taken to the family physician, a pediatrician or an otolaryngologist, because the parents make the common assumption that hearing acuity must be deficient. Moreover, some parents take their children to a psychologist or a psychiatrist because they become concerned about mental and emotional development. Still other parents take their children to a speech pathologist because they become concerned primarily about speech deficiencies. Significantly, lack of speech development may be due to any one of these conditions and to various combinations of them. Some children do not develop speech normally because of mental retardation, some because they are emotionally disturbed, others because they are aphasic and still others because they have impaired auditory acuity. However, because of the common presumption that lack of speech is due to peripheral deafness, and that lack of direct response to sound means that such deafness is present, many of these children are erroneously diagnosed and misunderstood. Children who do not develop speech frequently do present problems of auditory responsiveness and capacity. However, many of these children do not have reduced acuity. It is the responsibility of the clinician to determine which of the various conditions is present. This means that the diagnostic problem is one of differential diagnosis. Before a diagnosis is made the condition must be differentiated from others which may produce the common symptom of lack of response to sound. It is of genuine importance that the condition be differentially diagnosed early in life. The auditory disorders of the aphasic, mentally deficient and emotionally disturbed child should not be confused with those of the child who has peripheral deafness. Such confusion may seriously impede later development and adjustment.

The psychology and the psychopathology of hearing have been over-simplified as they pertain to both children and adults. Hearing has been studied and is currently understood chiefly as a physiological process. Consequently auditory capacities have been viewed separately and as something distinct from other capacities, rather than as an integral part of behavior. The relationship of hearing to genetic development in general and to mental and emotional development in particular has been largely overlooked. The emphasis in child audiology and differential diagnosis, however, is that hearing cannot be evaluated as something separate from other capacities. Hearing can be evaluated adequately only when it is considered in relation to the child's total development and behavior. This emphasis and rationale is the basis of the concept of auditory disorders in children. Auditory disorders is a more inclusive concept than that which emphasizes degrees and types of peripheral deafness. Auditory disorders include any incapacities relating to the reception or interpretation of sound, whether they be physical or psychological. This concept includes impaired auditory acuity as a type of auditory disorder, but it emphasizes that other types of auditory disorders are common and that these must be differentiated diagnostically. If all auditory incapacities were due to deficiencies of acuity the problem of diagnosis would be greatly simplified and the relationships between hearing and other attributes of the child would be unimportant. However, it is apparent that the diagnostician who over-simplifies auditory functioning and assumes a direct relationship between inadequate response to sound and impaired acuity will erroneously diagnose certain children as deaf. Such a diagnosis can be made with assurance only after other conditions which simulate deafness have been carefully considered and differentially eliminated. This process assumes a study of the child's total functioning. Likewise, it assumes that hearing is not evaluated only in terms of responses to intensity. Rather, auditory behavior is evaluated in relation to general behavior and specifically in relation to the child's physical, mental and emotional development.

This concept of auditory disorders and their evaluation in infants and young children stresses other related problems in auditory behavior. As stated previously, some children may not respond to sound although they have normal hearing acuity. In contrast, some children may respond normally to certain sound frequencies although they have a marked impairment of hearing for the speech frequencies. The diagnostician of auditory disorders in children is confronted with the paradox of children making no obvious response to sound although they have normal hearing, and of children responding normally to certain sounds although they have a significant loss of hearing relative to speech acquisition and development.

Another type of atypical response to sound is made by some children. A child may respond to sound both intermittently and inconsistently. Some children will respond to faint sounds instantaneously but otherwise do not respond although very intense sound levels are used. Some children are inconsistent in another way. They respond momentarily and fleetingly to a specific sound, especially the first time it is presented, but on repeated presentations of this sound they do not continue to give responses. The concept of auditory disorders in children includes the presumption that children's auditory responses may be variable. Moreover, that they may respond to faint sounds but not to loud sounds and that they may not respond to the same sound consistently. From the point of view of evaluating auditory behavior, lack of response to sound is not considered an invariable indication of peripheral deafness. Likewise, inconsistent responses to sound are not considered as deficiencies of acuity in the usual sense. Lack of, or inconsistent response to sound is considered only as a symptom. The child's auditory behavior is analyzed in relation to the total symptomatology. It may follow that the child has peripheral deafness but further study may reveal that his auditory functioning is disturbed for other reasons. The diagnostician does not rely wholly on the child's responses to sound. Diagnosis is made only after other symptomatology and clinical evidence has been used to corroborate and validate the child's auditory responses.

In addition to ascertaining which of various conditions is causing the auditory disorder, it is frequently necessary in a given child to establish how much of the disorder is due to a disability, such as impaired acuity, and how much is due to other causes. This is the problem of multiple handicap, of one handicap superimposed on another with concomitant need for multiple diagnosis and management.

In order to analyze the problem of differential diagnosis of auditory disorders in young children a special study was inaugurated. This study was an analysis of two hundred and twenty-eight children on whom a differential diagnosis had been established. This group represented a population seen during a period covering approximately one year.* These children were referred to a children's hearing clinic because of their lack of speech development and because of a presumption of impaired auditory acuity. With few exceptions they were referred by the family physician, pediatrician or otolaryngologist. The families were predominantly of middle class circumstances. The primary selective factor in the population was that they were referred for study and evaluation because they presented complex problems of auditory functioning. Thus, the number of children with auditory disorders other than peripheral deafness might be higher than that found in other centers. The incidence of the types of problem found in this group is given in table 1.

Table 1. — *The Diagnostic Distribution of 228 Children Seen for Differential Diagnosis of Their Auditory Disorder*

Diagnoses	No.	% of total	Males	% of total	Females	% of total
Peripheral deafness	104	45.6	59	25.9	45	19.7
Aphasic	67	29.4	44	19.3	23	10.1
Psychic deafness	36	15.8	25	11.0	11	4.8
Mentally deficient	21	9.2	13	5.7	8	3.5
Totals	228	100.0	141	61.9	87	38.1

Approximately forty-five per cent had problems of peripheral deafness; malfunctioning of the ear itself accounted for the auditory disorder. Speech was not heard because of the reduced auditory acuity and therefore speech was not acquired.

The second largest group consisted of children who were brain injured and as a result had an aphasia. These children could hear speech but they could not learn to interpret it and thereby could not acquire it. Their auditory disorder was due to a damage to the central nervous system. Although their problem was not due to reduced

* From the files of the Children's Hearing and Aphasia Clinic, Northwestern University, Evanston, Ill.

acuity they usually could not respond normally to commonly used hearing tests. Approximately twenty-nine per cent of the children were found to fall within this group.

The third group in order of size consisted of those children who were emotionally disturbed; their auditory disorder was due to psychic deafness. These children simulated impaired auditory acuity for psychological reasons. Approximately fifteen per cent of the group had an emotional disturbance with psychic deafness.

The remaining children were found to be mentally deficient. Due

Table 2. — *The Age Distribution in Years for 228 Children on the Basis of Their Type of Auditory Disorder*

	Peripheral deafness	Aphasic	Psychic deafness	Mentally deficient
No.	104	67	36	21
Mean	4.25	4.79	4.23	4.46
S.D.	1.59	1.03	1.84	2.01

to their mental retardation they were not acquiring speech normally and they could not respond adequately to the commonly used tests of hearing. Their auditory disorder was directly attributable to their mental deficiency. Nine per cent of the children were found to be in this group.

It is interesting to observe also from table 1 that the incidence of males exceeded females; approximately sixty-two per cent were males and thirty-eight per cent were females. As in some other areas of handicapped children, this suggests a higher incidence of problems in males. Perhaps the most noteworthy implication of the finding presented in table 1, however, is that children who do not acquire speech (the children in this study can be considered essentially as speechless) because of auditory disorders fall into four groups and many of them have auditory disorders other than reduced acuity.

The mean ages of the children in each of the diagnostic groups are given in table 2. The age range for the group was from six months to seven years and eleven months. The mean ages for the diagnostic groups are similar. The only statistically significant difference was between those with peripheral deafness and the aphasic; the aphasic were older. This suggests that children with aphasia are encountered by the diagnostician at a slightly later age than children with peripheral deafness.

It is apparent that there is a need to view the problem of auditory disorders in children as one requiring differential diagnosis. When the problem is approached from this point of view and when appropriate procedures are used, the children fall into four groups. The basic diagnostic problem is to determine which of these four conditions is present in a particular child. Methods and procedures for this purpose are discussed in the following chapters.

SUMMARY

During one year two hundred and twenty-eight children between the ages of six months and seven years, eleven months were seen in a children's center for auditory disorders. They were referred for lack of speech development and suspected deafness. Many of these children had been previously diagnosed as deaf. Utilizing the methods described in the following chapters, it was found that approximately forty-five per cent actually had deafness due to deficiencies in the ear. The remainder (fifty-five per cent of the total) had auditory disorders due to emotional disturbance, aphasia or mental deficiency, but they were shown to have essentially normal hearing acuity when special diagnostic methods were applied. The practical importance of making a correct diagnosis is that children having different types of auditory problems vary significantly in their needs and unless a differential diagnosis is made, their potentialities are lost.

Chapter II

Auditory Disorders and Language Development

THE PROBLEM OF AUDITORY DISORDERS IN young children and the need for differential diagnosis has been discussed in Chapter I. In this chapter the relationship between auditory disorders and language is considered. Young children with disturbed auditory behavior present problems primarily because of their inadequate language development. Therefore, the diagnostician needs to be oriented to the broad areas of language development and language disorders. Language incapacity is the common basis for all of the auditory disorders in infants and young children. All diagnosticians, regardless of their major specialization, should assume as their minimum obligation the ability to identify the type of language disorder which is present. They should be capable of exploring the various diagnostic possibilities to the extent that they determine the type of auditory disorder, and then infer the appropriate relationship to language development. Evaluation of the auditory disorder and the concomitant language disturbance proceed simultaneously. For example, if the problem is not simply impaired auditory acuity the diagnostician should be capable of determining the alternatives. Specialists in deafness in the past have assumed little responsibility for other areas of auditory disorders. There was no need for such specialists to be concerned about other auditory problems so long as the diagnostic work did not include young children. Likewise, it was not necessary to be concerned with the implications for language development until early diagnosis became essential. The various auditory disorders commonly overlap in infancy and childhood and they are directly related to language development. Thus, the area of auditory disorders in children entails background, experience and insight

9

into all phases of language, but especially it entails knowledge of the problems of receptive language.

An extensive discussion of language and language development will not be given, only basic concepts will be considered. Historically disorders in ability to communicate with one's fellow men have been considered as disorders of speech. Auditory disorders, broadly viewed, have been emphasized only in the recent past. Moreover, scientific study of the process of language acquisition in children has occurred principally during recent years [2, 7]; the study of language acquisition and symbolic behavior must be considered as being in its infancy [9, 10]. In fact, current knowledge regarding language development in children is limited essentially to information concerning speech and speech development [6]. Nevertheless, speech and language cannot be viewed as synonymous. Language is a more inclusive term than speech. Language is an intricate form of symbolization which is essentially unique with human beings. In language the signs or symbols are words, either written or spoken. Lower animal forms have language for signification but not for symbolization [5]. A chimpanzee can use language only in a highly restricted manner [13]. Language is one of man's most fundamental characteristics. It is regrettable that so little scientific knowledge is available regarding this basic function.

Symbolization is not limited to words, either written or spoken. Literature, folklore and music are replete with examples of symbolization which are non-verbal. Therefore, it is necessary to consider language as a part of symbolic behavior; symbolic behavior is more inclusive than language behavior [1]. However, from the point of view of auditory disorders our primary concern is with that aspect of symbolic behavior which entails verbalization; this is language. The human being can use written or spoken symbols to symbolize a tremendous variety of objects, places, experiences, feelings and ideas. This capacity for language makes it possible for him to refer to places, people, things and feelings, whether or not they are present. Psychologically this makes abstract behavior possible. Acquiring this intricate system of symbols called language is the task of every child.

In order for language to develop normally it is necessary for the child to have adequate integrity of the peripheral nervous system (sensory capacities), of the central nervous system, and adequate integrity psychologically. It has been assumed that if a child had adequate integrity physically, language would be acquired. It is now apparent that both physical and psychological processes must be functioning at a certain level in order for language to develop. This is shown diagrammatically in figure 1.

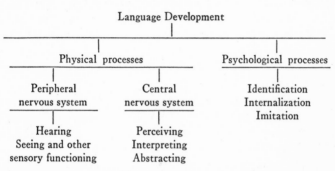

Fig. 1. — Function of physical and psychological processes in language development.

Certain disturbances of the peripheral nervous system (such as an impaired auditory nerve), of the central nervous system (such as a brain injury which causes aphasia) or of psychological development (such as occurs in childhood psychosis) will impede language development [8]. It must be emphasized that these conditions do not impede language in the same way. Thereby, part of the diagnostic problem is to ascertain in what manner language acquisition has been disrupted.

Hearing is a receptive sense. It is the sense through which spoken language is received. Speech is a form of expressive language. It is verbally expressed language and it is intended for a listener. Neither speech nor hearing should be viewed as the all of language; both speech and hearing are essential for normal language behavior. However, before a child can speak he must, first, be able to hear, then to interpret what he hears, and thirdly, he must be able to relate these interpreted verbal symbols to the speech motor system. This emphasizes the reciprocal relationship between hearing and speech, between receptive and expressive capacities.

Another way of describing the language process is to divide it functionally into three parts: receptive language, that which is used to understand what others say; expressive language, that which is used in talking to others; and inner language, that which is used for thinking, in "talking to ourselves." This classification of language function is shown diagrammatically in figure 2.

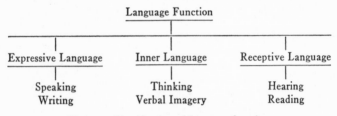

Fig. 2. — Classification of language function.

Perhaps the fundamental basis of symbolic behavior, and thereby a fundamental basis of human behavior, is inner language. Scientific data are meagre relative to the nature of inner language [3, 11]. Nevertheless, it is apparent clinically that children do not understand what is said to them until they have acquired a minimum of inner language. From the point of view of language development this indicates that an infant must first receive language for a certain period of time in order for the symbols to acquire their characteristic meanings. The infant then has the beginnings of inner language and he can comprehend certain spoken symbols. After hearing and comprehending these spoken symbols for another period of time, he begins to use them expressively, he begins to speak. The sequence of development is reception of language stimulation, development of inner language, and then development of speech, or expressive language. This concept emphasizes the importance of normal receptive processes; it emphasizes, further, that there is a normal process of reciprocation between reception and expression of language. A child who is impeded, irrespective of cause, from receiving auditory stimuli will be reciprocally impeded in verbal language expression. Without normal language reception there cannot be normal language expression. One way in which children are impeded in language reception is through impaired auditory acuity, by peripheral deafness. Aphasia is another such factor. Although auditory acuity is adequate, the child cannot make the association between the auditory sensation and the accepted meaning of the sensation. Verbal symbols remain meaningless, impeding the development of speech, expressive language. Likewise, emotionally disturbed children with normal auditory acuity, may find it impossible to accept (receive) and to use their auditory world. Because of psychic disturbances, including psychic deafness, they reject auditory language stimulation; they do not use language receptively or expressively.

As indicated previously, for purposes of diagnosis and study it is advantageous to categorize language into three areas, inner, receptive and expressive [3, 4, 12]. Disorders might occur in any of these areas and in combinations of them. However, the problem of auditory disorders is concerned directly only with the area of receptive language. But inasmuch as there are corresponding relationships between all of the areas of language function it is beneficial for the diagnostician to be familiar with all aspects of language development and language pathology.

Receptive language disorders can occur on three bases, and through various combinations of these three bases. These three bases are, damage to the peripheral nervous system, the central nervous system, and through disturbance of psychological processes. This is shown diagrammatically in figure 3. This diagram illustrates the relationship between auditory disorders and language development. Furthermore, it emphasizes the nature of the diagnostic problem. Some children having an auditory disorder will have impaired acuity, others will have sustained damage to the central nervous system and their problems will be different from those having impaired acuity. Still others will have auditory incapacities as a result of psychological involvements. All of these children will be impeded in language reception. Perhaps the problem of these various types of children with auditory disorders should be stated differently. The problem of the child with impaired acuity is that he is sensorially deprived; he does not receive the sensation because of a defective receiving mechanism, the ear. The aphasic's primary difficulty is an inability in using the sensation

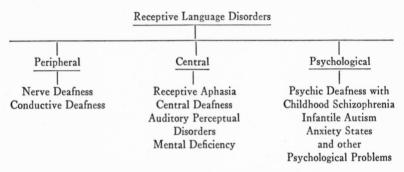

Fig. 3. — The three bases of receptive language disorders.

after receiving it auditorially. He cannot acquire the basic system of symbols which constitutes the language. His problem usually is substantially greater than that of the child with impaired acuity. The language problem of the emotionally disturbed child is not well understood, but it is apparent that the process of language acquisition may be arrested at various stages or levels. For example, some of these children cease to respond to language stimulation during the pre-verbal age so their language behavior is extremely limited. Some understand, at least intermittently, but do not speak. In the mentally deficient the language incapacity often is a direct reflection of the generalized amentia.

Auditory disorders are directly related to reception of language stimulation. The diagnostician therefore cannot avoid being concerned with the psychopathology of language. Language disturbances are an inherent outcome of auditory disorders in children and the type of language disturbance varies reciprocally with the type of auditory disorder which is present.

SUMMARY

The presenting symptom that prompts parents to bring their child for diagnosis of a suspected hearing loss usually is failure to acquire language. Language consists of symbols, either written, spoken or thought, which make it possible for the individual to refer to places, things or feelings, whether or not they are present. Symbolic behavior, of which language is a part, is essentially unique in human beings. In order for the child to acquire verbal language he must first hear it spoken; he must receive the sounds. Then he must learn the meaning of the words; he must interpret the sounds. Finally, he must learn to express the words meaningfully; he learns to speak. Therefore, to acquire language the child must have adequate hearing and intactness of the central nervous system. The child who is peripherally deaf and the child with brain damage that interferes with the interpretation of sound will both fail to acquire speech, but for different reasons. Furthermore, the child having a psychological disturbance including psychic deafness also fails to acquire speech because he rejects auditory language stimulation. The mentally deficient child fails to learn speech because of generalized mental incapacity. Thus the same symptom, failure to learn to speak, may be the result of any one of these four disorders. The main task of the diagnostician is to determine which of these four conditions is preventing a particular child from acquiring speech.

BIBLIOGRAPHY

1. Cassirer, Ernst: An Essay on Man. New Haven, Yale University Press, 1944.
2. Gesell, Arnold et al.: The First Five Years of Life. New York, Harpers, 1940.
3. Goldstein, Kurt: Language and Language Disturbances. New York, Grune & Stratton, 1948.

4. Head, Henry: Aphasia and Kindred Disorders of Speech. Cambridge, Cambridge University Press, 1926, vol. I.
5. Langer, Susanne K.: Philosophy in a New Key. New York, Penguin Books, 1942.
6. Lewis, M. M.: Infant Speech. London, Kegan Paul, Trench, Trubner & Co., 1936.
7. Mowrer, O. H.: The autism theory of speech development and some clinical applications. J. Speech & Hearing Disorders *17:* 263, 1952.
8. Myklebust, H. R.: Aphasia in children. J. Exceptional Child. *19:* 9, 1953.
9. Piaget, Jean: Language and Thought of the Child. New York, Harcourt, Brace, 1926.
10. ———: Play, Dreams and Imitation in Childhood. New York, W. W. Norton, 1951.
11. Vigotsky, L. S.: Thought and speech, Psychiatry *2:* 29, 1939.
12. Wepman, J. M.: Recovery from Aphasia. New York, Ronald Press, 1951.
13. Yerkes, Robert M.: Chimpanzees: a Laboratory Colony. New Haven, Yale University Press, 1943.

Chapter III

Professional Specialization and
Auditory Disorders in Young Children

THE EMPHASIS ON DIAGNOSIS OF AUDITORY disorders at the earliest possible age has added immensely to the complexity of the diagnostic problem. It is evident that the applicability of most types of formal diagnostic procedures increases with advancement in age. Furthermore, techniques and procedures for the study of auditory disorders in infants and young children have not been extensively developed. However, as the concept of auditory disorders in children has developed, the need for specialized training and cooperation between specialists has become evident [2]. It is apparent that various specializations are entailed in the area of differential diagnosis of auditory disorders in young children. This area will develop according to its importance largely on the basis of the integration and cooperation of these various professional specializations.

Some of the specializations most relevant to the problem of differential diagnosis of auditory disorders in children are otolaryngology, pediatrics, neurology, child psychiatry, clinical psychology, audiology, speech pathology and special education. The role and primary function of these specializations is considered briefly. The most adequate services, diagnostically and therapeutically, will be achieved for these children when various professional areas are integrated. Genuine integration might be fostered by changes in professional training, such as providing an orientation in clinical psychology for otolaryngologists, and an orientation in the psychopathology of language for child psychiatrists. Cooperative effort in auditory disorders, however, is progressing rapidly and can be expected to achieve unusual proportions in the future.

THE OTOLARYNGOLOGIST

Traditionally the otolaryngologist has had the final responsibility for diagnosis of deafness in both children and adults. Inasmuch as the otolaryngologist is trained especially for this work he will continue to be the primary specialist in this area. Even for him, however, the diagnostic problems are not the same as those which were encountered in the past. Current otolaryngological practice requires the otolaryngologist to make differential diagnoses of auditory disorders in very young children. This necessitates a more extensive knowledge of auditory incapacities and auditory behavior. It is necessary for the otolaryngologist to acquire additional proficiencies and background. For example, his practice now assumes understanding of the genetic development and the psychology of young children. Likewise, new clinical techniques and procedures must be incorporated and used. He cannot rely only on tuning fork tests and formal audiometry in evaluating the auditory disorders of young children. Such procedures are applicable mainly to children above pre-school age and to adults. The otolaryngologist must develop proficiency with the young child who does not respond to auditory tests in the same manner as older children or adults. He must have a working knowledge of children relative to mental, emotional, and genetic development. Deviate auditory behavior can be adequately evaluated only in terms of the child's total development.

The otolaryngologist, also, is now more dependent on other specialists than he was in the past. Often he will find it advisable to secure the assistance of a pediatrician, a neurologist, a child psychiatrist, a speech pathologist, or a clinical psychologist. This does not assume that the otolaryngologist will not become increasingly trained and experienced in the auditory disorders of young children. Rather, it suggests that he, like various other specialists, will find that specialization in the problems of adults is not necessarily synonymous with competence in diagnostic work with children. Different chronological age levels require a certain degree of specialization within the framework of any field. This has been recognized in medicine and psychology by the development of pediatrics, geriatrics, child psychiatry and child psychology. It is conceivable that coordination between pediatrics and otolaryngology will develop in the future to the extent that such specialization will be referred to as pediatric-otolaryngology. A similar emphasis has been indicated in Europe by the term Paedo-audiology. In any event, whatever changes occur, it is apparent from the sustained interest and contributions of the otolaryngologist that he will incorporate the unique demands of young children relative to the differential diagnosis of auditory disorders.

THE PEDIATRICIAN

The pediatrician has specialized in the medical problems of children and is in a strategic position to make a contribution to children with auditory disorders. Often he is the first specialist to encounter these children. He makes the initial diagnosis and then frequently refers the child to the otolaryngologist, the neurologist, or to other specialists. However, although the pediatrician has been trained in the medical problems of children, he has not had special orientation to the problem of auditory disorders. Perhaps, in the past, he has underestimated the importance of such symptoms as lack of response to sound and retardation of language development. Furthermore, the pediatrician, too, has assumed an invariable relationship between lack of response to sound and impaired auditory acuity. The concept of auditory disorders and the need for differential diagnosis has not been emphasized. However, the importance of the pediatrician in connection with children having auditory disorders is generally recognized [9].

In general, like the otolaryngologist, the pediatrician finds it necessary to be oriented to the genetic and developmental aspects of young children in order to appraise more fully the significance of disturbed auditory behavior. No one can be highly specialized in all of the types of deviation presented by children with auditory disorders. Because of his strategic position, however, it is necessary for the pediatrician to be keenly aware of the symptoms of impaired auditory acuity, of psychic deafness, of aphasia, and of mental deficiency. If the pediatrician is not aware of these symptoms, and if he does not pursue a differential diagnosis accordingly, clarification of the child's problem might be greatly delayed. Pediatricians can be expected to continue to make contributions to the understanding of these problems and to stimulate integration of professional services.

The pediatrician is directly engaged in treating childhood illnesses. He is aware of the significance of such diseases as rubella, meningitis and encephalitis, and their relationship to auditory disorders [19]. His treatment of childhood illnesses is a significant factor in the prevention of many auditory incapacities. Furthermore, he is the specialist who is in an opportune position to assist the parents in planning for the long range needs of children with auditory disorders. He can assist the parents by clarifying why the child has impaired acuity, or aphasia, and why psychotherapy, or a program of special education is necessary.

THE NEUROLOGIST

The neurologist, like many other specialists, traditionally has specialized in the problems of adults. Genetic neurology and the congenital neurological disturbances of infants and young children have been emphasized only in recent years. Nevertheless, neurological involvements are of considerable importance in the differential diagnosis of auditory disorders. As indicated in figure 1, auditory disorders occur because of impairment to the peripheral nervous system, the central nervous system or because of psychological disturbances. The neurological evaluation frequently is of primary importance in distinguishing between these various types of auditory incapacities. However, the neurologist, too, usually has assumed a direct relationship between lack of response to sound and impaired auditory acuity. The child neurologist in the future can be expected to be increasingly oriented to the broad problem of language pathology and to auditory disorders as they are encountered in young children.

Many neurologists have made unusual contributions to the study of aphasia [10, 20, 21]. However, this work has been limited largely to adults. Congenital aphasia with its broad implications for auditory disturbances in early life remains to be explored intensively. A major development in this area can be anticipated in the future. Other expected developments by the neurologist, from the point of view of auditory disorders in children, include the clarification of central deafness and auditory agnosia. Better understanding of the neurology of these conditions as they occur congenitally would greatly foster the differential diagnosis of auditory disorders in early life.

Another major way in which the neurologist will be of assistance is through clarifying the motor disturbances which are frequently associated with auditory disorders. These motor involvements include confused lateral dominance, incoordination, and disturbances of balance. It is not uncommon to encounter children with relatively gross incoordination, but in whom the neurological study does not manifest deficiencies. In the future, as child neurology continues to develop, such discrepancies might be clarified. It is apparent that the neurologist will make substantial contributions to the area of auditory disorders in children.

THE CHILD PSYCHIATRIST

Language development is peculiarly related to mental and emotional development. For example, language acquisition and the complexity of language are directly related to intellectual growth and capacity. This is illustrated by the mentally deficient [7]. In general the idiot, with a mental age of two years or less, does not acquire speech although he does comprehend some speech auditorially. The imbecile, with a mental age of two to seven, does learn to speak but he does not learn to read. The moron, with a mental age of eight to ten, learns to speak and he learns to read up to approximately the fourth grade level. Other evidence of the relationship between language and intellectual capacity is revealed by studies of gifted children. These studies show that gifted children not only acquire language more rapidly but they use language of greater complexity [14].

The relationship between intellectual capacity and language acquisition is well established and generally accepted. However, the relationships between emotional development and language acquisition are less well established and are not generally accepted. Progress is being made in child psychiatry in this connection. For example, the works of Bowlby [1] and Spitz [25] show a significant relationship between speech development and maternal deprivation. It remains for child psychiatry to explore carefully the associations between auditory disorders and early emotional disturbances. Such study and exploration can be expected to be especially productive, not only for children with auditory disorders but for all children.

Psychiatric workers during World War II significantly clarified the incidence and problem of psychogenic deafness in military personnel during war time [24]. Comparable work on children has not been achieved. Professional workers in clinics for children with auditory disorders are urgently aware of the need for such psychiatric work. The psychiatric implications of pre-verbal experiences seem especially pertinent and consequential on the basis of clinical findings. In a somewhat broader sense the development of symbolic behavior in general and its association with childhood schizophrenia and infantile autism is in need of study by child psychiatrists [12].

If a child has an auditory disorder caused by such conditions as impaired acuity or aphasia, he may develop emotional disturbances as a secondary problem. Many of these children do develop emotional problems concomitantly with their physical handicaps. The child psychiatrist has the major responsibility for evaluating the relationships between the child's various disabilities and his emotional problems. In order to provide such professional assistance the psychiatrist will find it necessary to become oriented to children without ability to comprehend auditorially and without ability to speak. At the present time the child psychiatrist's diagnostic and treatment methods usually are highly verbal. The child must be capable of good language reception and expression to profit from these procedures, whereas, this is the primary incapacity of children with auditory disorders from early life. Thus, many of the traditional diagnostic and treatment procedures of the child psychiatrist are not directly applicable to these children. Non-language techniques are essential for this purpose and must be developed more extensively.

The child psychiatrist's role includes working with the parents of children having all types of auditory disorders. However, it is especially necessary that he assist the parents of children whose emotional disturbances have caused psychic deafness. This covers a greater number of children than is generally recognized. To effectively contribute to this area, the child psychiatrist should be oriented to the psychology of language, to auditory behavior and to the auditory disorders of infants and young children.

THE CLINICAL PSYCHOLOGIST

The problem of differential diagnosis of auditory disorders in children has various implications for the clinical psychologist. These implications are both clinical and research in nature. Clinical psychologists have made noteworthy contributions to the understanding of mentally deficient and emotionally disturbed children. However, deaf, aphasic, and other auditorially disturbed children have not been studied extensively. The work of Pintner is an exception [23]. It should be emphasized that experimental psychologists, traditionally, have been interested in audition and have made far-reaching contributions to the psycho-physics and psycho-physiology of hearing [11, 26, 27]. More recently clinical psychologists have become interested in auditory disorders and language pathology. This is illustrated by Mowrer's work with talking birds [17]. Other psychologists have studied the normative aspects of language development in normal children [8, 15].

The clinical psychologist's responsibilities in the area of auditory disorders of children include both diagnosis and therapy. His contribution should include the development of objective clinical techniques for evaluating children with disturbed auditory behavior. He should study and determine the normal genetic pattern of auditory maturation, including auditory perceptual development in infancy and early childhood. Piaget's work is significant and revealing in this connection [22]. As the maturation of auditory capacities is more fully understood, the diagnosis of auditory disorders will be facilitated.

As in other areas of specialization, competence with adults does not necessarily qualify one to work with children. Clinical psychologists in general have little knowledge, or skill, relative to the use of hearing tests, especially with young children. Furthermore, the clinical psychologist, too, frequently has assumed a direct relationship between lack of response to sound and impaired acuity. The clinical psychologist primarily engaged in work with children should be oriented to the psychology of handicapped children. From the point of view of auditory disorders, he should be familiar with the psychology of deafness, aphasia and language development. The psychology of auditory disorders as it relates to both children and adults has been oversimplified. The clinical psychologist has major responsibility for ascertaining the behavioral effects of sensory deprivations and disturbances. Clarification of the behavioral concomitants of impaired auditory acuity, aphasia and psychic deafness would greatly facilitate differential diagnosis. Furthermore, such knowledge would contribute to the understanding of all children. The clinical psychologist with his broad training and orientation to the study of human beings is in a position to make a prominent contribution to the area of differential diagnosis of auditory disorders in children.

Tests of intelligence, motor ability, social maturity and personality are essential to the total evaluation of auditorially disturbed children. Magret [16] has emphasized that children with language handicaps should be evaluated in terms of their total functioning and behavior. In order for this to be accomplished more satisfactorily in early life it will be necessary to further develop appropriate clinical psychological techniques. Many psychological tests are not directly applicable to children with marked receptive and expressive language disorders.

Most of these tests require language facility and this is the primary incapacity of these children. Procedures which make it possible to objectively evaluate what the child does, rather than what he says, would be helpful in the differential diagnosis of non-speaking, non-hearing children. The Vineland Social Maturity Scale is an illustration of such procedures [6].

The clinical psychologist carries other responsibilities. He is by tradition and training in a position to suggest the most appropriate educational classification for children with auditory disorders. Differential educational placement is a primary requisite for these children. The clinical psychologist, also, should be expected to assist with devising and critically appraising the remedial educational procedures being used. History techniques, parental guidance and counseling, and psychotherapy are other areas in which the creative efforts of clinical psychologists are necessary.

THE AUDIOLOGIST

A new specialization called audiology has developed in recent years [4]. Audiology is a broad field including various sciences which emphasize the study of human beings relative to the normal and abnormal aspects of audition. The audiologist is particularly trained in the remedial and rehabilitative needs of those who are deaf or hard-of-hearing. This is an important specialization in terms of children with auditory disorders. Audiologists have contributed significantly to knowledge of the psycho-psysics and psycho-physiology of hearing. They have devised auditory testing techniques such as speech audiometry [3]. Other contributions include research on tests of bone conduction, tests for malingering, and techniques for fitting hearing aids. Audiologists are rigorous scientists; their work is noteworthy in view of the recency of the development of this type of specialization.

The audiologist has responsibility in regard to diagnosis and remedial training of children with auditory disorders. In cooperation with other specialists he should assist in determining the differential diagnosis. He should collaborate with the educator in planning and initiating remedial measures such as auditory training, speech reading and language development. The audiologist has primary responsibility for appraising the child's auditory acuity and residual hearing from the point of view of using amplification remedially. He should explore carefully the applicability and suitability of hearing aids for young children.

Currently the audiologist is oriented more to the problems of impaired auditory acuity and to adults than to the auditory disorders of infants and young children. However, interest and research in the area of young children is developing rapidly. As this work develops the audiologist will find it necessary to be more comprehensive and to become oriented to receptive language disorders in general. In terms of differential diagnosis of children, this entails a background in such problems as receptive aphasia and psychic deafness in children. The audiologist can be expected to devise differential tests of auditory acuity and tests for other types of auditory disorders. The Doerfler-Stewart test is an example of the audiologist's contribution in this area [5]. Comparable techniques and procedures for children are necessary and gradually are being developed. However, audiology, like otolaryngology, has been interested largely in the problems of impaired acuity. Interest in auditory disorders is developing and the audiologist can be expected to make significant contributions to this area in the future.

THE SPEECH PATHOLOGIST

The speech pathologist traditionally has been identified with the problems of speech disorders. More recently he has become interested in hearing. Through this interest the speech pathologist has greatly stimulated other professional groups to become interested in auditory disorders. However, like other specialists, the speech pathologist has not been particularly oriented to auditory dysfunctions in early life. Rather, he has been trained in the remedial aspects of defective speech. Language behavior, in contrast to speech, has not been stressed; normal symbolic functioning usually has been assumed. In the future speech pathologists may be expected to become more specialized in the broader area of language disorders. It may be expected, also, that receptive disorders will be given equal emphasis as compared to the current greater emphasis on expressive disorders. Comparable training will be given in both areas with scientifically appropriate distinctions made between the areas of expressive and receptive language. Concurrently language will be emphasized as the basic problem; symbolic development will not be assumed but studied as a critical aspect of both hearing and speaking. Peripheral, central and psychological aspects of language will be studied and stressed.

Relative to auditory disorders in young children, the speech pathologist has responsibilities for both diagnosis and therapy. This is especially true for children with multiple involvements, such as the cerebral palsied and those with maxillo facial deformities. The speech pathologist often functions in a university speech and hearing center which has equipment designed primarily for the appraisal of auditory disorders. Such a center provides many speech pathologists with excellent opportunities for both research and training. Accordingly, speech pathologists have responsibilities especially for pioneering remedial work in language development. Other responsibilities include work with the parents of children having auditory disorders.

THE EDUCATOR AND SPECIAL EDUCATION

In the past the educator's role was limited largely to work with school age children. This is no longer true, especially with respect to handicapped children. The educator's responsibility begins as soon as the differential diagnosis has been determined and includes remedial programs for the child and his parents. The educator, as well as other specialists, should be aware of the importance of the relationships between the child and his parents. Programs and remedial procedures should be planned in such a manner that good relationships are developed.

The educator is not traditionally oriented to the problems of infants and young children. As the diagnosis of auditory disorders has been made earlier and earlier in life, the educator has found it necessary to devise and to inaugurate appropriate remedial training programs. Much remains to be accomplished in this regard. Educational programs are available for young children with impaired auditory acuity, but programs for children with congenital receptive aphasia are virtually non-existent [18]. Special education can be expected to develop programs for these children in the future. Other areas in which the educator can be expected to contribute are socialization and personality development. The work of Kirk on training programs for the mentally deficient is illustrative of this type of program development [13].

The task of providing appropriate educational programs for handicapped children is tremendous. Perhaps one of the greatest dangers in developing these programs is over-generalization and over-simplification. All language impaired children are not alike; all children with auditory disorders are not alike. Classification for educational purposes is essential, however, and special education can be expected to develop appropriate criteria for young children with auditory disorders. Perhaps such programs will develop primarily on the basis of classifying those with peripheral deafness, those with central nervous system damage, and those who are emotionally disturbed into separate groups. Educationally, those with peripheral deafness have a non-symbolic type of disorder, whereas those with aphasia do have a basic language disorder; the emotionally disturbed may not be impaired sensorially or symbolically from the point of view of physical disability. Each of these groups has different learning and educational needs and the educator will find it most advantageous to develop programs according to these differences. His cooperation with other specialists will insure that the child's educational program is based on the psychology which is peculiar to each type of child with an auditory disorder. The educator's role is a salutary one. He has the long time task of providing the child with educational training which will make it possible for him to adjust to society according to his potentialities.

COORDINATION OF SPECIALISTS

The importance of ability to communicate is so consequential that when disorders occur it naturally entails many professional specializations. Only the most obvious, from the point of view of auditory disorders, have been included for discussion. Integrity of auditory capacity is an essential of normal ability to communicate. Auditory capacity might be disturbed in a number of ways. Auditory behavior has not been sufficiently emphasized in regard to its significance in human behavior and everyday living. Modern civilization places a premium on ability to verbalize, talk on telephones, respond to bells, buzzers, radios, television, traffic sirens and other sounds which are an integral part of our daily living. Hearing and ability to communicate are capitalized to an unusual degree.

The differential diagnosis of auditory disorders in infants and young children entails the cooperative efforts of various specialists. No one professional group is sufficiently comprehensive to encompass all of the problems presented by these children. Appropriate referrals and consultation with other specialists is the obligation of all workers. Cooperative diagnostic programs have developed rapidly during recent years. Hearing clinics are conducted through the mutual endeavors of otolaryngologists, pediatricians, audiologists, psychiatrists, and other specialists. Often these individuals meet and work as a team. However, the team approach is not always necessary, or desirable; this approach is too demanding in time for some children. Nevertheless, it is necessary that many of these children be examined by several specialists, but these examinations can be done at different times and at the discretion of the clinicians involved. This procedure frequently assures a more complete diagnosis. Such diagnostic work can be provided even for the indigent through clinics at medical schools and through university speech and hearing centers. The combined resources of these specialists will provide immeasurable benefits for children with auditory disorders.

Coordination and integration of knowledge and services involved in complex problems is not simple, or automatic. It is achieved largely through mutual respect, open-mindedness, and a minimum of defensiveness. This can be illustrated by the suggestion that the physician should know the importance of speech reading, or the use of hearing aids, but he should not presume to be the educator. The speech pathologist, or audiologist, should know the importance of intellectual and emotional factors, but he should not presume to be the clinical psychologist. Other illustrations could be given. It must be emphasized, however, that awareness, orientation, and background which give breadth and scope are not presumptions but result in better services for all people.

SUMMARY

The differential diagnosis of auditory disorders in infants and young children requires the cooperative efforts of various specialists. The otolaryngologist, pediatrician, audiologist, psychiatrist, psychologist, educator and other specialists may work cooperatively in a diagnostic center for auditory disorders, but it is not necessary for every child to be examined by these diagnosticians working together as a team. By appropriate referrals and consultations many of the children can be diagnosed more completely and satisfactorily when the various examinations are made at different times at the discretion and convenience of the clinicians involved. The important aspect is that each specialist maintain a respect and an open-mindedness toward those in related fields. It is especially important that the otolaryngologist, who frequently has the responsibility for directing the diagnostic program, be aware that the diagnosis of auditory disorders in infants and young children requires more than use of tuning forks and the audiometer. He should be familiar with the psychology and genetics of normal development. He should assume that auditory difficulties in the young child can be evaluated only in terms of the child's total behavior which necessitates assistance from the child psychiatrist, clinical psychologist, neurologist and other specialists.

BIBLIOGRAPHY

1. Bowlby, John: Maternal Care and Mental Health. New York, World Health Organization, Columbia University Press, 1952.
2. Canfield, Norton: Audiology, The Science of Hearing. Springfield, Ill., C. C Thomas, 1949.
3. Carhart, Raymond: Speech audiometry. Acta oto-laryng. *40, 41:* 18, 62, 313, 1953.
4. Davis, H. (ed.): Hearing and Deafness. New York, Murray Hill Books, 1947.
5. Doerfler, L. and Stewart, K.: Malingering and psychogenic deafness. J. Speech & Hearing Disorders *11:* 181, 1946.
6. Doll, E. A.: Vineland Social Maturity Scale. Minneapolis, Educational Test Bureau, 1947.
7. ———: The feebleminded child, in, Carmichael, L. (ed.): Manual of Child Psychology. New York, Wiley, 1946, pp. 845–885.
8. Eisenson, John: The Psychology of Speech. New York, Crofts, 1947.
9. Gesell, A. and Amatruda, C. S.: Developmental Diagnosis. New York, Paul B. Hoeber, 1948.
10. Goldstein, Kurt: Language and Language Disturbances. New York, Grune & Stratton, 1948.
11. Hirsch, I. J.: The Measurement of Hearing. New York, McGraw-Hill, 1952.
12. Kanner, Leo: Child Psychiatry. Springfield, Ill., C. C Thomas, 1948.
13. Kirk, S. and Johnson, G. O.: Educating the Retarded Child. New York, Houghton Mifflin, 1951.
14. Louttit, C. M.: Clinical Psychology. New York, Harpers, 1947.
15. McCarthy, Dorothea: Language development in children, in, Carmichael, L. (ed.): Manual of Child Psychology. New York, Wiley, 1946.
16. Magret, Ann: Psychological evaluation of language handicapped children. Symposium—Northwestern University, 1952. (Unpublished)
17. Mowrer, O. H.: Learning Theory and Personality Dynamics. New York, Ronald Press, 1950.
18. Myklebust, H. R.: Aphasia in children. J. Exceptional Child. *19:* 9, 1953.
19. Nelson, W. E.: Textbooks of Pediatrics. Philadelphia, Saunders, 1950.
20. Nielsen, J. N.: Agnosia, Apraxia, Aphasia, Ed. 2. New York, Paul B. Hoeber, 1946.
21. Orton, S. T.: Reading, Writing and Speech Problems in Children. New York, W. W. Norton, 1937.
22. Piaget, Jean: The Origins of Intelligence in Children. New York, International Universities Press, 1952.

23. Pintner, R., Eisenson, J. and Stanton, M.: The Psychology of the Physically Handicapped. New York, Crofts, 1946.
24. Ramsdell, D. A.: The psychology of the hard of hearing and the deafened adult, in, Davis, H. (ed.): Hearing and Deafness. New York, Murray Hill Books, 1947, pp. 392–418.
25. Spitz, R. A. and Wolf, K. M.: The smiling response: a contribution to the ontogenesis of social relations. Genet. Psychol. Monogr. *34:* 57, 1946.
26. Stevens, S. D. and Davis, H.: Hearing: Its Psychology and Physiology. New York, Wiley, 1938.
27. Wever, E. G.: Theory of Hearing. New York, Wiley, 1949.

PART TWO: THE HISTORY

Chapter IV

Differential History Taking

VARIOUS AREAS OF SPECIALIZATION REQUIRE different diagnostic approaches. All of the specializations involved in the diagnosis of auditory disorders in children will not use the same history. However, inasmuch as there is some uniformity in the information needed by all specialists who examine such children it seems pertinent to consider the history and its usefulness in some detail.

Considerable progress has been made in the refinement and standardization of diagnostic techniques and procedures as they pertain to adults with auditory problems. Comparatively, there has been less progress in devising and standardizing diagnostic procedures for infants and young children. Nevertheless, clinical experience with these children is becoming more extensive and diagnostic procedures are developing. Currently this type of clinical work is demanding in time. However, experience reveals that there are no short cuts. Diagnosticians will find it necessary to adhere to the time consuming methods until others can be devised, if accuracy of diagnosis is to be maintained.

Making a differential diagnosis of auditory disorders in young children consists essentially of three steps. The first step is differential history taking, the second is clinical observation and the third is the clinical examination. A fourth aspect of a complete diagnosis is determining the etiology. In practice these steps are not separated from each other. Usually they are accomplished simultaneously, but it is necessary for purposes of discussion and training of diagnosticians to consider the steps separately. Only by systematically evaluating each step in the diagnostic process can clinical skill and insight be acquired. This is true especially in an area such as auditory disorders in young children because this area is not well established clinically.

ESSENTIALS OF A DIAGNOSIS

Before discussing the first step, differential history taking, it is necessary to consider briefly the essentials of a complete diagnosis. There are certain requisites which must be fulfilled when making any diagnosis. Doll [1] has suggested that a complete diagnosis consists of making four basic determinations. These are, first, the past status; a determination of the onset and early development of the problem, and this determination is made chiefly through taking and interpreting the history. The second determination is referred to as the present status; the problem as it exists at the present time. Usually this is the diagnostic classification into which the child falls, such as impaired acuity or aphasic. The third determination is the future status; a statement regarding prognosis. The diagnostician should predict the outcome of the problem. For example, if the child has impaired hearing acuity, should it be expected to improve; if the child is aphasic, to what extent will he acquire language. The fourth essential is to determine the etiology; to ascertain the cause of the condition.

It is evident that these four essentials of a complete diagnosis are reciprocal in nature. Ascertainment of the past status is necessary for the determination of the present and future status, and for determining the etiology. Likewise, ascertainment of the present status is reciprocally related to determining the past and future status. This means that the diagnostic process consists of obtaining certain information and synthesizing it into a logical sequence. Diagnostic procedure consists of both analysis and synthesis. A common diagnostic error is that of not relating or synthesizing the present with the past status of the child. It is not possible to make accurate diagnoses, in general, without relating the present condition to early development and to the etiology. For example, if the child has a history of having heard and of having acquired speech and then ceasing to respond to sound, the diagnostician's task is to ascertain what caused the interruption of otherwise normal development. Subsequently it is his task to relate the total past status to the present condition and to the prognosis. Failure to synthesize these relationships causes the diagnosis to be relatively incomplete and unsatisfactory, if not erroneous.

In addition to the four essentials of past status, present status, future status and etiology, there is another significant factor in making a differential diagnosis in young children. This is ascertaining the age of onset of the condition. Determining the age of onset is directly related to determining the etiology and the past status, but it requires special emphasis. The child's present condition and symptomatology should be consistent with expectations according to the age at which the impairment was sustained. Failure to recognize this relationship, likewise, causes diagnostic errors. Diagnosticians often overlook obvious differences between children who sustain auditory disorders at different age levels. Often the child's verbal ability is the best key in this connection. Any ability to speak means that the child's receptive capacity was functioning within certain limits at a certain age; complete auditory dysfunction could not have occurred in the pre-verbal age. Therefore, a child who sustains peripheral deafness from meningitis at three years of age presents a different symptomatology than a child whose hearing impairment was caused by prenatal influences such as rubella.

One of the significant aspects of determining the past status and the etiology is establishing the time of the onset of the problem. The age of onset is influential in determining the symptomatology and it serves as a background against which the diagnostic possibilities can be evaluated.

HISTORY TAKING

The first step in making a diagnosis of deafness in young children is skilled and systematic differential history taking. Each specialist will take a history which covers especially those phases in which he carries major responsibility diagnostically. There are certain aspects of the history, however, which are common to all specialists working with young children. Furthermore, there are basic principles and methods for expert history taking which are preferable and useful to all who take histories regardless of their area of specialization. Louttit [3], Pearson [5], Kanner [2], Watson [6], and others have discussed these history taking methods in detail. Diagnosticians who are unfamiliar with these methods should read these sources for background information. Only brief consideration is given here to this important aspect of the total diagnostic process.

Parents who bring their child for examination usually are not familiar with what the diagnostican wants to know relative to the history, so he should not expect them to supply the exact information desired without direction and appropriate questioning. Moreover, all parents become emotionally involved in the problem which their child presents. The information they provide should be skillfully interpreted. Parents, inadvertently, not only are providing information on their child's auditory disorder, but they are incorporating their wishes, fears, apprehensions, misgivings and misunderstandings of the disorder. Frequently parents feel that they are at fault, that they have caused the disorder, so they unconsciously do their utmost to put their child in the best possible light. This emphasizes what some workers have referred to as the psychotherapeutic phases of history taking [4]. Considerable psychological benefit can be given the parent by diagnosticians skilled in interviewing and history taking. A parent's negative reply to a question often does not mean that the particular problem is absent. Rather, it might mean that the parent finds it impossible to recognize the problem because of its assumed reflection on him. The diagnostician who does not have background in the psychological aspects of human behavior should exercise caution in regard to securing and interpreting the history. Such clinicians might err in taking the parents' responses too literally. History information given by parents is highly useful diagnostically, but this information is accurate, spontaneous and pertinent mainly to the extent to which the clinician can relieve the parents of their defensiveness and anxieties. Parents often can and will give useful information if the skill and attitudes of the interviewer are appropriate.

A minimum amount of time is required for differential history taking if diagnostic accuracy is not to be sacrificed. This area of differential diagnosis entails a high degree of qualitative analysis and clinical judgment. Moreover, the complexity of the problem is such that there can be no abbreviated or condensed diagnostic approximations. Clinical judgments, observations and objective test findings must be corroborated by data obtained from the history. The history is a substantial and influential part of the total examination. Moreover, information obtained from the history often becomes a part of the total body of knowledge in this developing field of clinical work.

It is helpful for the diagnostician to see the child briefly before he begins taking the history. This gives him an impression of the child which helps him in taking the history, the child being discussed is more concrete. Furthermore, many symptoms are obvious to the trained clinician even from only brief observation, and after having seen the child the diagnostician can inquire expeditiously about such symptoms, or conditions. Another reason for the advisability of seeing the child before proceeding with the history is that rapport with the parent can be established more readily when this procedure is followed. The parents speak more freely and easily about their child if the clinician has first seen him. Whether the child is present throughout the taking of the history is determined by the facilities of the diagnostician, the behavior of the child and the emotional stability of the parents. If the child is highly disturbing and if he understands conversation through speech reading, or hearing, it is preferable that he not be present throughout the interview. Likewise, if the parents are so emotionally disturbed that anything he does causes them to interrupt the history taking, it is advisable not to have the child present. However, there are advantages to having the child present during the interview. It affords an excellent opportunity for obsering the inter-actions between the child and his parents, and the diagnostician can make clinical observations of behavioral symptomatology. Many diagnosticians will find that these advantages of having the child present outweigh the disadvantages.

History taking begins by establishing rapport with the child's parents. The most important single factor in establishing rapport is the attitude of the diagnostician. An attitude of impatience, indifference, blamefulness or criticalness is sensed immediately by the parents. Kanner refers to this as "nonverbal communication" [2]. It is essential that the parents sense acceptance and permissiveness. Rapport develops when the parents feel confident that the specialist is genuinely interested in their child and that he is considerate and understanding regarding their problem. Perhaps the most critical factor in establishing rapport is to alleviate their feelings of helplessness and blamefulness. The diagnostician must realize that the parents are unfamiliar with auditory disorders. The parents' fearfulness and apprehensiveness should be expected and accepted. Often their child's atypical development is the most critical problem they have encountered in life. Their concern for their child usually can be taken at face value; it is an indication that they will put forth effort to pursue the problem diagnostically and remedially. If rapport is not adequately established and managed, parents often are dissatisfied and seek further examination, advice and guidance from diagnosticians who are more insightful and understanding. Moreover, it is essential from the point of view of maximum benefit to the child, that the diagnostician take time to answer questions and to consult with the parents regarding the implications of their child's problem. Short, piece-meal, and hurried approaches to them and to their child are exceedingly unsatisfying to them. Some parents ask how a certain diagnostician could know what their child's problem was when only a few minutes had been spent with them and their child. These parents may state further that it is true that their child did not respond to sound while in the diagnostician's office but that he has responded to sound while at home. This situation may reflect inadequate history taking and caution on the part of the diagnostician. More cautious and complete differential diagnosis of such children may reveal that the diagnostician misinterpreted the child's responses.

The attitudes of the diagnostician are not consequential only in regard to establishing rapport. They are highly important in his management of the child during the examination (this is discussed further in Part Four) and while discussing his findings with the parents. An arbitrary manner is unwise while informing the parents that their child is deaf, aphasic, mentally deficient or emotionally disturbed. Parents who have been given the diagnosis in this manner often find it unacceptable and proceed to ask assistance elsewhere. A more satisfactory method of presenting the findings is to assume an attitude of cooperativeness with the parents. It is more tactful and prudent to refer to the information that the parents themselves have supplied. For example, the clinician might begin with the statement that the parents wisely were seeking assistance for their child, that he has a problem, but that it is possible to give them considerable information regarding it. The parents might be included again by indicating that their observations of failure to respond to sound are in agreement with the findings of the examination. An attitude of cooperativeness, not condescension, of sympathy but not indulgence, can be expected to be more acceptable to the parents. Frequently, the work of an excellent diagnostician has been of little value because of the manner in which he presented his findings to the parents. Some parents find the diagnosis unacceptable because of their own emotional difficulties. In such instances the diagnostician should be aware of the parents' problem and make efforts to advise and counsel them accordingly. This might mean that the parents should be encouraged to seek assistance from a psychiatrist or a clinical psychologist.

The case history interview should not be without a careful plan in all respects. A general question rather than a specific one is most satisfactory as a beginning point for the interview. Even the initial comment, or question, is part of the planned approach. To begin the interview with specific questions often causes the parents to become apprehensive and defensive. Furthermore, if the first question pertains to the birthdate or other routine information, the parents are not permitted to present their problem and observations in a manner which is more spontaneous and opportune for them. Usually this creates an artificial situation which is less productive of diagnostically useful information. The diagnostician is chiefly concerned with eliciting a description of the child's problem and of his major symptomatology. Therefore, a more efficacious beginning is to simply ask the parents why they have brought their child for an examination; what is it about their child that concerns them? This is done in a friendly way and then the parents are permitted to state their problem and main concern immediately. The parents' response to this general question is important and revealing diagnostically. They might respond by stating that they are concerned about their child's lack of speech development and that they fear he might be deaf. Generally such responses mean that the parents have been concerned about their child for some length of time; that they have observed him and tried to get his attention to sound. Such information is surprisingly accurate. A complete differential diagnosis frequently corroborates the parents' opinion that their child has seriously impaired hearing acuity.

Other parents, in response to the question relative to what it is about their child that concerns them, make a significantly different statement. They might state that they are puzzled and confused about their child. They are anxious about his lack of speech and infer that his difficulty may be deafness. However, they are confused because, according to their observations, he sometimes responds to sounds normally while at other times he does not respond even to loud sounds. These parents may state frankly that this inconsistency of response has left them completely bewildered. Such parental observations are revealing to the astute diagnostician. From this report he hypothesizes that this inconsistent response might occur if the child has moderately impaired acuity and when there are intermittent ambient noises producing a variable masking effect. Another, and perhaps more generally appropriate inference is that this inconsistent and intermittent response to sound is symptomatic of an auditory perceptual disorder and of receptive aphasia. Such an inference would become the basis for securing further history data to corroborate, or to vitiate this inference. If the inference was corroborated by clinical observation and further history data, then the examination would proceed by further exploring the possibility of central nervous system damage which had caused receptive aphasia or a disturbance of auditory perception.

A third parent, in response to the question regarding their concern for their child, might respond quite differently from the two characteristic responses discussed above. They might explain that their child has been difficult to manage from early life, that he has been a feeding problem, that he learned to walk at the usual age, that he is not toilet trained, that he lives in his own world, and that disciplinary measures have been ineffective. They might state further that he has been unusually "stubborn," that he "said a few words" but then talking ceased and now he seems willfully unaware of sound. Much clinical information is contained in such a report. The more understanding of young children with auditory disorders that the diagnostician has, the more such information will mean to him. From this parental report the diagnostician might hypothesize that this child's auditory disorder is due to an emotional disorder, one of the manifestations of which is psychic deafness. On the basis of this inference the specialist would proceed by emphasizing questions relative to parental attitudes and the emotional management of the child in the home. This type of history taking must be done cautiously and skillfully in order not to intensify parental emotional conflicts which frequently accompany emotional disturbances in children. Undue questioning and probing are undesirable. The necessary information can be secured without disturbing the parents further. Only those specialists who are especially oriented to emotional disorders should proceed with the deeper aspects of the emotional problems. If the history data and the clinical observations corroborate the inference that the child's auditory disorder is due to an emotional disturbance, then the examination would be conducted in such a manner as to further evaluate this possibility.

Another characteristic response is given by some parents when questioned regarding their concern for their child. They might express concern relative to his total development. They might state that he has been slow in learning to sit alone and to walk, that he has not learned to feed himself or to assist with his dressing, that it has not been possible to establish toilet training. These parents may be concerned about his lack of speech and his inadequate response to sound, but they emphasize the slowness of his development as compared to other children. From this report the diagnostician might hypothesize that the child's problem is generalized incapacity due to mental deficiency; the lack of speech and atypical auditory behavior are a part of the generalized retardation of central nervous system development. The diagnostician might pursue securing further history data pertinent to this inference. If the clinical observation and the history data corroborate the suggestion of mental deficiency, then a diagnosis of the auditory and language disorder should be deferred until a complete examination of mental capacity has been achieved.

These examples of characteristic statements by parents relative to their concern about their child have been over-simplified to illustrate the importance of their reports. The way in which they describe their child's problem is highly relevant diagnostically. The diagnostician should not minimize the importance of his initial contact with the child's parents. Although parents' responses to certain questions frequently cannot be taken literally, the type of auditory behavior they describe is of unusual importance to the diagnostician. The complete history provides information from which the specialist can check and recheck the parents' report and his own impressions. The significant factor diagnostically is that the clinician be mindful of the implications of the information presented. The astute diagnostician must be constantly attempting to integrate the history information with his own impressions and with the examination and test findings. The parents' initial statements serve as a tentative frame of reference for securing the most pertinent history information. Likewise, the parents' report, the total history data and the diagnostician's clinical impressions serve as a frame of reference, or as a hypothesis, for the examination which is to follow; the examination procedures and the referral possibilities should be planned on this basis. The diagnostician is continually raising a question in his own mind as to whether the child's auditory disorder is due to impaired acuity or whether other conditions, or combinations of other conditions, are present. He does not simply accept a parental report of lack of response to sound. Instead, throughout the history taking he looks for evidence which corroborates or denies a presumption of a type of auditory disorder and for a possible etiological explanation of it. Simultaneously he might observe the child in order to form a clinical impression regarding whether the child's behavior is consistent with the presumed type of auditory disorder, then he proceeds to examine the child. If the initial examination procedures reveal that the clinical impression is in error then other diagnostic possibilities must be explored; the examination serves as a further check, or "test," of the hypothesis which has been formulated. This is discussed further in Part Four.

Differential history taking is not a routine question asking procedure. It is a dynamic process of inter-relationship between individuals, the purpose of which is to secure data which can be integrated into a pattern. It is a process of matching the information given by the parents with the specialist's impression of the child, including his inferential, or presumed diagnosis. This means that differential history taking is part of the total diagnostic examination. Differential history taking includes securing identifying information and in this respect it is not unlike commonly used history taking techniques. It differs from these techniques in that it includes history taking as an essential aspect of the total examination. Furthermore, this implies that, ideally, the history should be taken by the diagnostician himself. If this is not done by the specialist who is preparing to examine the child, then the individual who does take the history should be trained in this method to assure the integration of the history data with the diagnostician's clinical impressions and with the findings of the examination.

The difference between differential history taking and more routine types of history taking should be emphasized. Differential history taking requires expert skill and training, it assumes clinical knowledge and insight. This is apparent because it requires that the diagnostician be continuously evaluating the information which is obtained. It is a process of constantly evaluating the history data and clinical impressions, formulating a hypothesis, making inferential diagnoses and relating them to the findings of the examination. To illustrate further, to the leading question regarding what it is about their child that concerns them, the diagnostician might get the report that the child hears certain sounds but seems to ignore other more intense sounds. After a brief discussion with the parents regarding their report, and after brief observation of the child, the specialist might infer that the child's problem is aphasia. The differential history would then emphasize securing information pertinent to central nervous system damage. Usually this includes a careful exploration of pre-natal conditions, birth and early disease history.

This illustrates the first step in making a differential diagnosis of auditory disorders in infants and young children. The findings of step one would be integrated with step two—behavioral symptomatology—and with step three—examination findings. Usually if the information from the three steps is discrepant and in disagreement, diagnosis would be deferred until further information can be secured. Significantly, differential history taking is not limited to exploring etiological, developmental, or disease aspects. This procedure emphasizes especially that other types of diagnostically pertinent information be secured. The diagnostician inquires regarding the child's eating and sleeping habits, his toilet training, his crying and laughing behavior, his walking, his vocalizing, and many other aspects of behavior according to the clinical involvements of a particular child.

A history which has been found useful in the differential diagnosis of auditory disorders in infants and young children is given below. It is presented in detail in order to illustrate the manner in which it can be used most completely and most quickly. As the various types of information are secured it is intended that the items be checked, with notations being made where necessary. Copies of the history are prepared in advance and at the completion of the diagnosis it is used as a permanent part of the child's record. Other sources of information, such as reports of previous examinations, agency, hospital, or clinic reports, should be obtained before the initial contact with the case. Such information should serve as background for securing additional history information, and for integration of all the data.

A CASE HISTORY FOR YOUNG CHILDREN WITH AUDITORY DISORDERS

I. Identifying Information

Name: _____ Date: _____

Address: _____ Telephone: _____

History taken by: _____ Informant: _____

Date of birth: _____ Referred by: _____

Father's name: _____ Age: _____

Occupation: _____

Parents' descent: _____

Siblings: _____ Ages: _____

Other persons in the home: _____

Family doctor: _____

Nature and onset of the problem:

II. Birth and Prenatal History

Conditions during pregnancy:

_____ Illnesses: (Rubella, etc.)

_____ False labor

_____ Rh incompatibility

_____ Other unusual conditions

Conditions during birth:

_____ Length of pregnancy

_____ Duration of labor

_____ Birth weight

_____ Breech birth

_____ Cesarean

_____ Anesthetics

_____ Forceps

_____ Anoxia

_____ Jaundice

_____ Other indications of damage

Conditions immediately following birth:

_____ Scars, bruises or deformations at birth
_____ Birth weight regained
_____ Seizures
_____ Swallowing and sucking
_____ Feeding difficulties
_____ Other

III. History of Illness:

(Specify the age at which child had any of the following illnesses. Specific information, such as degree of temperature and medical treatment, should be included.)

Childhood diseases:

_____ Measles   _____ Chicken pox
_____ Whooping cough   _____ Diphtheria
_____ Scarlet fever   _____ Mumps
_____ Influenza   _____ Other

Diseases of central nervous system:

_____ Meningitis   _____ Encephalitis
_____ Poliomyelitis   _____ Epilepsy

Diseases affecting the middle ear:

_____ Tonsillitis   _____ Sinusitis
_____ Otitis media   _____ Nasal allergy
_____ Colds   _____ Other

Conditions during illness:

_____ Degree of   _____ Rigidity
temperature
_____ Coma—Undue
sleepfulness
_____ Seizures   _____ Duration of illness

Inoculations: (Age at time of each inoculation and after-effects)

Surgery:

_____ Tonsillectomy and adenoidectomy
_____ Other

Familial deafness: (Give age of onset)

_____ Deaf parents
_____ Deaf siblings
_____ Other

Other conditions in the family:

_____ Alcoholism
_____ Epilepsy
_____ Mental illness

IV. Genetic Development:
At what age did the child: *

_____ Show response to mother
_____ Sit alone
_____ Walk alone
_____ Eat with spoon; fork
_____ Drink from glass
_____ Pull off socks
_____ Put on, button or take off coat
_____ Ask to go to toilet
_____ Care for his toilet needs

Does the child:

_____ Prefer the right or left hand
_____ Have a characteristic gait
_____ Fall, lose balance easily
_____ Seem awkward and uncoordinated
_____ Have difficulty in chewing; swallowing
_____ Grasp objects readily
_____ Other

V. Emotional Adjustment:
Is the child:

_____ Responsive to people
_____ Primarily responsive to objects
_____ Especially alert to movements
_____ Sensitive to vibratory sensations
_____ Sensitive to being touched
_____ Highly distractible, hyperactive
_____ Behaviorally consistent from day to day
_____ Retarded in social perception
_____ Playful with children, adults, pets
_____ Oblivious, withdrawn
_____ Easily managed in the home

Does the child:

_____ Eat well
_____ Sleep well
_____ Make his wants known
_____ Cry, sob, shed tears
_____ Show concern when separated from parents

* Adapted from Doll, E. A.: Vineland Social Maturity Scale, Ed. Test Bureau, 1946.

_____ Laugh, smile, seem happy
_____ Pick, pull, rub his ears
_____ "Rock" in crib, or while sitting, standing
_____ "Bang" his head on crib, chair, floor
_____ "Stare" at lights, objects, people, into space

VI. Auditory Behavior:
    Does the child:

_____ Respond to any sounds
_____ Respond to the sound of the human voice,
                        telephone bell, doorbell, auto horn or airplane
_____ Respond to loud sounds only
_____ Respond to sounds consistently
_____ Use his hearing projectively
_____ Unexpectedly respond to background sounds
_____ Seem to ignore sound willfully
_____ Respond to intense "pain level" sounds
_____ Respond to other than auditory stimuli
_____ Show fear of sound

VII. Language Behavior:
     Did, or does the child:

_____ Babble
_____ Use jargon
_____ Vocalize for pleasure
_____ Use gestures meaningfully
_____ Communicate by crying, laughing, smiling
_____ Unexpectedly understand speech
_____ Use echolalic speech
_____ Use vocalizations which are characteristic in
                        tonal quality
_____ Attempt to imitate speech
_____ Use vocalizations projectively
_____ Acquire speech and then stop talking
_____ Never use his voice

VIII. Educational History:

_____ Nursery school
_____ Public school
_____ Private school
_____ Individual tutoring

SUMMARY

The differential diagnosis of auditory disorders in young children proceeds in three steps: history taking, clinical evaluation of the child's behavior and the clinical examination. A complete diagnosis includes the onset and early development of the auditory problem, the present status of the problem, the prognosis and the etiology. The history is an important part of the diagnostic procedure but the diagnostician must weigh the information given by the parents in light of their wishes, fears and feelings of blamefulness. The skill and attitude of the interviewer are important in determining the usefulness of the information. To gain rapport with the parents they must feel that the interviewer is sympathetic and genuinely interested in their child. They must not feel that he is hurried, impatient or arbitrary. A good beginning is to simply ask the parents why they have brought their child for an examination; what is it about their child that concerns them? The response to such a question usually is revealing. If the parents say that they fear their child is deaf, often it means that they have been concerned about his hearing for some time and have observed his lack of response to sound. On the other hand they may state that they are puzzled and confused about their child's hearing because sometimes he responds to faint sounds but at other times he does not respond even to very loud sounds. Such a history suggests a central auditory disorder such as receptive aphasia. A third parent may say that the child has been difficult to manage from early life; that he has been stubborn, is a discipline problem, learned a few words and then ceased talking. Such a history suggests an emotional disturbance which has produced psychic deafness. A fourth parent might state that the child has been slow in all respects; learning to sit, walk, dress himself as well as in learning to talk. Such a history suggests generalized mental deficiency. The diagnostician follows the initial general question with specific questions to corroborate and develop his first impressions. It is helpful to see the child briefly before taking the history and there are advantages to having the child present during the interview since it affords an excellent opportunity to observe the child's behavior. This type of history taking by the skilled diagnostician is termed differential history taking to contrast it with a routine history taken by an untrained individual.

BIBLIOGRAPHY

1. Doll, E. A.: Some things we know in clinical psychology. J. Applied Psychol. *24:* 20, 1940.
2. Kanner, Leo: Child Psychiatry. Springfield, Ill., C. C Thomas, 1948.
3. Louttit, C. C.: Clinical Psychology, Revised Ed., New York, Harpers, 1947.
4. Menninger, Karl: A Manual for Psychiatric Case Study. New York, Grune & Stratton, 1952.
5. Pearson, G. H. J.: Emotional Disorders of Children. New York, W. W. Norton, 1949.
6. Watson, Robert: The Clinical Method in Psychology. New York, Harpers, 1951.

Chapter V

History Interpretation

INFORMATION SECURED FROM THE HISTORY must be evaluated and interpreted. The extensiveness of the background and clinical experience of the clinician largely determines his ability to interpret and integrate such information. Each specialization entailed in the area of auditory disorders in young children will develop interpretations which are peculiar to its needs. However, some interpretations apply generally to auditory behavior and to auditory disorders as they occur in young children. As such, certain interpretations are pertinent to all specialists encountering this problem diagnostically. Some of these general and basic interpretations are discussed in this chapter.

THE HISTORY AND ETIOLOGICAL DETERMINATION

As stated previously a complete differential diagnosis includes the determination of etiology. The history furnishes essential information for making this determination. The etiology has implications for the medical, educational and psychological management of children with auditory disorders. Moreover, etiological determination is essential for the inauguration of effective programs of prevention. For example, it has become urgent to prevent mothers from contracting rubella during pregnancy now that the disease is known to cause deafness, aphasia and other disorders prenatally [18]. Furthermore, determination of etiology is an essential step in the process of differential diagnosis because the etiology must be consistent with the eventual diagnosis. For example, if a diagnosis of peripheral deafness is made and the etiology is presumed to be meningitis, then the child's total syndrome should be similar to other children who have sustained deafness from this disease. Lacking such similarity of syndrome, the etiology of meningitis and sometimes the diagnosis must be questioned. Etiology also is reciprocally related to determining the prognosis.

Various types of classifications have been used with children having impaired auditory acuity. Comparable experience is lacking with children having other types of auditory disorders such as aphasia. The medical specialist has classified children with impaired acuity on the basis of the type of deafness; conductive or nerve. This classification is based on the site of the lesion; impairment of the middle ear is referred to as conductive deafness and impairment of the inner ear is referred to as nerve deafness. Another type of classification used by many workers is: deaf or hard of hearing. The basis of this classification is the degree of hearing impairment. If the child's hearing loss has not precluded his acquisition of language he is referred to as hard of hearing whereas, if special methods are necessary for developing language and if amplification is not effective, the child is referred to as deaf. There is another term which has been used in this connection; this term is deafened. It is used to refer to those children who sustained a severe loss of hearing after they had acquired speech normally. The implications for remedial programs according to the classification of deaf, deafened and hard of hearing are obvious.

Another etiological classification procedure used traditionally by many workers in the area of hearing impairment is congenital and acquired. The presumption has been that acquired conditions were those that were sustained after birth and therefore were non-hereditary. Congenital conditions were presumed to have occurred prior to birth and therefore were hereditary. These erroneous and unwarranted presumptions have caused confusion. The classification of congenital and acquired is dependent on the chronology or time of onset of the condition; not the cause. A time concept is useful for certain purposes clinically and scientifically, but to concomitantly infer causal factors leads to errors of classification. For example, conditions such as otosclerosis may not be sustained until long after birth but they might be considered hereditary. Likewise, conditions such as rubella may be sustained prior to birth but they are not hereditary. A time concept such as congenital and acquired has value etiologically when it is correctly applied. Acquired in this connection means that the condition was imposed on an otherwise developmentally normal organism and this occurred following birth. Congenital means only that the condition was present at the time of birth and a presumption of hereditary factors is unwarranted.

Terms of chronology should not be used for causal concepts. Doll [9], Strauss [38] and others who have emphasized causal factors in mental deficiency have used the classification of exogenous and endogenous for this purpose. Myklebust [26] suggested the use of these terms in etiological study of children with deafness. Endogenous means within the genes and includes all familial or hereditary conditions. Exogenous means outside the genes and includes all conditions which are not due to originally defective genes and are not transmittable genetically. This system of etiological classification is based on causal factors; the why of the condition rather than the when or the extent of the involvement. Continuing the example cited previously, it is possible to classify rubella as exogenous although it occurred prior to birth, and otosclerosis as endogenous although its actual occurrence is some time after birth. Such classifications are significant diagnostically and they are of importance to the child and to his family. Due to the traditional presumption regarding deafness that congenital means hereditary, parents frequently make this interpretation even if it is not stated for them. It is unfortunate that they assume hereditary involvement when it is not present. One of the purposes of differential history taking is to determine whether the auditory disorder is due to endogenous or exogenous causes. Such classification is necessary for all types of auditory disorders in children; not only for those who have impaired acuity.

In addition to determining the etiology it is necessary diagnostically to establish whether the condition has resulted in peripheral or central nervous system damage, and whether the condition is psychological. This was shown diagramatically in figure 3. It is necessary to determine the etiology and the type of disorder for children having primarily emotional disturbances as well as for those having primarily organic disturbances. The differential history is useful in determining the type of emotional involvement because it includes a careful exploration of the affectional relationships between the child and his parents.

There are several sources of damage to the organism prenatally, at the time of delivery and postnatally [14]. These include anoxia, birth damage due to other factors than deficient respiration, toxic conditions such as those produced by rubella, virus invasions such as those which derive from meningitis, and agenetic development. These conditions might cause either peripheral or central nervous system impairment, or both. The diagnostician of auditory problems in children traditionally has emphasized peripheral damage. It is desirable that he also include considerations of central damage. To summarize, the various determinations to be made include functional versus organic, endogenous versus exogenous and peripheral versus central. For these and other purposes it is essential to interpret carefully the history data and to synthesize it with other evidence from clinical observation and from the administration of tests.

INTERPRETATION OF HISTORY DATA

The case history for young children with auditory disorders presented in Chapter IV has been used by a number of specialists for several years. Furthermore, the work of Doll [10, 11], Gesell [16], Strauss [38] and others has made it possible to draw conclusions regarding many of the items used in this history. However, these conclusions generally should not be accepted as final because clinical and research evidence is being collected continuously. Some of the interpretations given should be considered as suggestive and illustrative. Each of the seven areas as given in the history in Chapter IV is considered briefly from the point of view of its importance to the total differential diagnosis.

Identifying Information

The meaning and significance of identifying information usually is apparent. However, such information should be stated definitely and clearly. It is an important part of the permanent record for the child. Dates of the initial contacts and examinations are of considerable value for future study. It is necessary to record the name of the individual taking the history and of the informant. The occupational status of the parents serves as an indication of their background educationally and of their socio-economic level. This information can

Table 3. — *A Comparison of Ages in Years of the Mothers of the First Born Children in Each of the Groups*

Group	No.	Mean	S.D.
Peripheral deafness	44	26.05	4.31
Aphasic	27	26.30	4.87
Psychic deafness	10	25.20	4.18
Mentally deficient	9	28.00	5.14

be evaluated according to the norms of the occupational schedules and it has both clinical and scientific implications [5]. Ages of the parents, especially the mother, should be included. Stander [37] states that labor is prolonged in mothers over thirty-five years as compared to those under thirty-five. Clinical experience suggests that a higher incidence of defects is related to age of conception, especially in first born children. A comparison of the ages of the mothers of the first born children according to the auditory disorder of the child is given in table 3. The mean ages for the groups were not significantly different according to statistical tests. Unfortunately, norms for first born normal children are not available but on the basis of observation, these ages seem to be above the average. It is interesting to note, however, that if increased age at the time of the first pregnancy is related to auditory disorders it is equally related to all types.

A comparison of the mean ages for the multipara mothers is given in table 4. These means and standard deviations are very similar but statistical tests revealed a difference at the five per cent level of confidence between mothers of children with peripheral deafness and mothers of the aphasic; the mothers of aphasic children were significantly younger. None of the means exceeded the age of thirty-five years which is given by Stander as the age at which labor can be expected to become prolonged. In general, these data suggest that the age of the mother is not a contributing factor to the incidence of

Table 4. — *A Comparison of Ages in Years of the Mothers of the Later Born Children in Each of the Groups*

Group	No.	Mean	S.D.
Peripheral deafness	38	30.84	5.92
Aphasic	23	27.70	5.07
Psychic deafness	11	30.82	5.32
Mentally deficient	12	31.00	5.72

auditory disorders. This implication, however, requires further study with larger samples.

Names and ages of the siblings should be recorded. Whether the child is the first born, whether he is the youngest, and the relationship of the child to his brothers, sisters and to his parents is pertinent. Other persons living in the home also have importance to the child clinically. The name of the referring specialist or agency and of the family physician are necessary for securing additional information and for purposes of sending reports of the findings. Identifying information includes a statement of the nature and onset of the problem. As indicated in Chapter IV this information is usually elicited first. Some specialists refer to this as the chief complaint. In general it is a statement of the parents relative to why they are concerned about their child. This statement often serves as a point of departure and as a frame of reference for taking the history.

BIRTH AND PRENATAL HISTORY

Conditions During Pregnancy

Because of the relationship between conditions during pregnancy and auditory disorders in children, the mother's prenatal illnesses should be ascertained. Rubella is an outstanding example of the importance of illnesses during pregnancy. It has been generally concluded that if the mother contracts rubella during the third month of pregnancy, it might cause impaired auditory acuity in the child and if rubella is contracted before or after the third month, the presumption is that other defects might occur [18]. Other conditions reportedly deriving from rubella are blindness, cardiac disorders and mental deficiency. Such conditions might accompany auditory disorders. For example, clinical experience suggests that some rubella children have a mild impairment of auditory acuity superimposed on an aphasia or a general mental retardation. Such children might have been considered as having only impaired acuity until further differential diagnosis revealed the multiple involvements. Presumably if the toxicity accompanying rubella is of sufficient intensity to damage the auditory nerve, it might also cause damage to other nerve tissues.

The history of prenatal influences should include other explorations. Information regarding marked emotional disturbance, accidents and Rh incompatibility should be secured. Biochemical and physiological changes might accompany emotional disturbances during pregnancy and impede normal fetal development. Accidents might cause injury to the fetus; the most obvious etiology for an aphasic child was injury sustained from a plane crash during the mother's fifth month of pregnancy. Rh incompatibility might cause brain damage due to anoxia, which in turn might result in aphasia or mental deficiency [18]. This occurs most often in the second and succeeding born child; rarely in the first born.

False labor is the circumstance of the mother behaving as though delivery is imminent but the birth does not materialize. In such instances the mother might be hospitalized for a few days with various symptoms of labor and after the episode has subsided, she might return home. The actual birth might not take place for a few days or a few weeks. False alarms occur with some frequency in the histories of children with auditory disorders. The significance of false labor is obscure but several factors might be operative. Because of actual labor the placental blood supply might be disturbed during the false alarm causing deprivation. Toxic conditions also might be present at this time. False alarms might be indicative of undue anxiety in the mother with concomitant physiological implications. Moreover, undue anxiety might cause increased tensions when the birth does occur.

Conditions During Birth

Diverse occurrences during birth can be related to auditory disorders in infants and young children. Disorders due to birth injury have been studied extensively, especially during the last two decades. Noteworthy are the studies of Doll [13], Bender [3], Strauss [39], Benton [4] and others. These studies, however, do not specifically consider auditory disorders and such research efforts are needed. Perhaps the most obvious relationship between auditory disorders and birth damage is that encountered through injury to the central nervous system, thereby causing aphasia. However, there are other possibilities. A number of children with peripheral hearing impairment have no other etiology except that of presumed damage at birth. It is conceivable that research will reveal that birth damage can affect the blood supply to the inner ear, causing either deprivation or hemorrhage with resultant deterioration of the organ of Corti or other cochlear and auditory nerve functioning. Another possible relationship between birth difficulties and auditory disorders is that of the child with emotional disturbances. Frequently children presenting marked emotional disturbances with accompanying psychic deafness have a history of difficult delivery. Although no organic symptoms have been determinable, it seems possible that a mild central damage has occurred making adjustment precarious and opening avenues for the imposition of emotional trauma in early life.

Duration of pregnancy has been found to be related to central nervous system damage at the time of birth [*13, 16*]. The probabilities of such damage are greater if the child is either premature or post term. The premature infant is less capable of withstanding the rigors of birth in general; his physical immaturity predisposes him to injury. Windle [*40*] has shown a relationship between anoxia in premature and post term infants. Gesell [*16*] suggests that prematurity is associated with malformations and intracranial hemorrhage. The total sample of two hundred and twenty-eight children seen for differential diagnosis of auditory disorders was studied to determine the number of premature births. Because of the small number in each group these findings could not be treated for statistical significance. However, when both time and weight are used for identifying these children, approximately twenty per cent of the population was found to be premature. For a sample of fifty normal children the number of premature births was under five per cent. This suggests that prematurity is a contributing factor in the incidence of auditory disorder.

Post term infants likewise seem to be susceptible to injury at the time of birth. They usually are larger than infants born in term and the additional size may increase the birth pressures which result in damage to the organism [*8, 19*]. Unfortunately, extensive experimental data showing the incidence of premature and post term births in the normal population have not been achieved. The significance of these concepts will be greatly enhanced when such data are available. It is of significance also to know the gestation age of the child in order to adequately evaluate his genetic development. The infant whose gestation age was seven months is not directly comparable to the infant whose gestation period was nine months. Forty weeks is considered as term, or the average gestation period. For clinical purposes a child whose gestation period is less than thirty-seven weeks can be considered premature and a child whose gestation period exceeds forty-three weeks can be considered as a post term infant [*16*].

The birth weight and duration of pregnancy are closely related. The gestation period is a time concept relative to prematurity or post term deliveries but the birth weight may be a more direct measure of physiological maturity. Thorough history taking requires that both the gestation period and the birth weight be ascertained. Some normal term children deviate significantly from the accepted birth weight. Spock [36] suggests, for example, that a child be considered premature if his weight is less than five and one-half pounds regardless of the gestation period. As with the duration of pregnancy a relationship has been found between birth weight and injury at the time of birth [19]. An unduly small child is more susceptible to birth

Table 5. — *A Comparison of the Birth Weights in Pounds for the First Born Children in Each of the Groups*

Group	No.	Mean	S.D.
Peripheral deafness	47	6.60	1.41
Aphasics	31	7.02	1.18
Psychic deafness	13	6.71	1.43
Mentally deficient	13	6.39	1.30

damage because of his physical immaturity, while an infant who is unduly large experiences increased pressures during the birth process, which might result in injury. Birth weights exceeding eight and one-half pounds or which are less than five and one-half pounds can be considered significant clinically.

Table 5 shows the mean birth weights for the first born children in each of the groups. Tests for statistical significance revealed no difference between the groups. Furthermore, from the point of view of group trends, none of the means deviated from the average. The samples are small and may be in error inasmuch as these findings seem not to agree with clinical experience.

A comparison of the mean birth weights for the later born children is given in table 6. As with the first born group, tests of statistical significance revealed no difference between the groups and the means for each of the groups are within the expected range. Again the samples are small but it suggests that as a group children with auditory disorders are not different from the normal or from each other

relative to average birth weight. This does not preclude the significance of deviations in birth weight in specific cases.

The duration of labor is another important factor in connection
with possible injury at the time of birth. Intracranial hemorrhage
might be associated with long and difficult labor. Anoxia too might
be present as a result of prolonged labor. Apparently after delivery
has commenced, the normal placental blood supply is disturbed and
inasmuch as normal extra-uterine respiration is delayed, the fetus

Table 6. — *A Comparison of the Birth Weights in Pounds
for the Later Born Children in Each of the Groups*

Group	No.	Mean	S.D.
Peripheral deafness	47	7.29	1.33
Aphasics	31	7.51	1.59
Psychic deafness	15	7.15	1.15
Mentally deficient	14	7.26	1.50

suffers oxygen deprivation. Presumably other birth dangers are increased when delivery is prolonged and it is significant that in the
past some fetuses have been held back to prevent delivery until the
obstetrician arrived. Clinical experience suggests that this practice
might increase the possibilities of anoxia and other damage during
delivery. Long duration of labor has been accepted clinically as a
cause of injury at the time of birth. Precipitate or very rapid births
have not been as generally recognized as being dangerous. However,
again clinical experience with young children having auditory disorders, as with children having other types of defects, suggests that
a rapid expulsion at birth is equally significant etiologically. It seems
that the fetus needs a certain amount of time to adjust to extra-
uterine life. This adjustment normally occurs as it passes through the
birth canal. For example, the fetus must adjust to air pressure as contrasted with the pressures present in utero. Some obstetricians have
observed that a rapid expulsion causes the fetus to react markedly
until adjustment to air pressure has been achieved. Precipitate de-

liveries also might cause more acute pressures with resultant deformations and hemorrhage.

The incidence of average, precipitate and prolonged births for each of the groups with auditory disorders is given in table 7. Although the numbers are small, some significance might be attached to these results. For example, the aphasic has the highest precentage of pro-

Table 7. — *The Number of Children in Each Group Born with Average, Precipitate or Prolonged Labor and the Median Duration of Labor in Hours* *

| Group | Type of Labor | | | | | | | | | Total No. |
| | Natural | | | Precipitate | | | Prolonged | | | |
	No.	Median	%	No.	Median	%	No.	Median	%	
Peripheral deafness	67	8.0	77.0	12	1.0	13.7	8	25.0	9.1	87
Aphasic	43	9.5	70.4	6	1.0	9.8	12	34.5	19.6	61
Psychic deafness	23	7.0	76.6	5	1.5	16.6	2	24.0	6.6	30
Mentally deficient	19	8.0	76.0	3	2.0	12.0	3	38.0	12.0	25
Totals	152			26			25			203

* Average — 2 to 24 hrs.; precipitate — 0 to 2 hrs.; prolonged — 25 hrs. or more.

longed labor while those with psychic deafness have the highest percentage of precipitate deliveries. These findings are inconclusive but warrant further study from the point of view of possible organismic effects. The higher incidence of prolonged, difficult labor in the aphasic group as compared to those with peripheral deafness is in agreement with clinical experience.

Difficulties during delivery cannot be evaluated only in terms of time, the duration of labor. However, determining the number of hours of labor is helpful in ascertaining the possibility of birth damage retrospectively. The average duration of labor for the first born child has been reported to be between fourteen and eighteen hours, and between eight and twelve hours for succeeding births [37]. Windle [40] has emphasized the significance of fetal circulation and respiration at the time of delivery. He found that early clamping of the umbilical cord increased the incidence of anoxia because this practice reduced the placental blood supply and deprived the fetus of oxygen before respiration was adequately established. Further research of this type would be enlightening relative to birth damage.

A comparison of the hours of labor for the first born children in

Table 8. — *A Comparison of the Hours of Labor for First Born Children in Each of the Groups*

Group	No.	Mean	S.D.
Peripheral deafness	40	14.32	13.43
Aphasic	32	15.27	11.74
Psychic deafness	17	8.91	6.29
Mentally deficient	10	11.0	10.87

each of the groups is given in table 8. The means for the children with peripheral deafness and for the aphasic are close to those reported for the normal. The mean for the mentally deficient is slightly below the average and the mean for those with psychic deafness is considerably less than the average of fourteen to eighteen hours. This suggests a relationship between rapid delivery and psychic factors in early life but this suggestion must be studied further. Tests for statistical significance revealed a significant difference at the five per cent level of confidence between those with peripheral and psychic deafness and the same difference was found between the aphasic and those with psychic deafness. These data indicate that those with psychic deafness are different from the aphasic and those with peripheral deafness relative to hours of labor in first born children. Prolonged labor by groups was not indicated by these data. However, the standard deviations for all of the groups are large and indicate considerable variation within each group. Therefore, it is evident that individual cases deviate markedly from the means. This is apparent also from clinical experience.

A comparison of the hours of labor for the later born children in each of the groups is given in table 9. The means for the aphasic and the mentally deficient are close to those reported for normal children [37]. The means for children with peripheral and psychic deafness are below those norms. The standard deviation for all groups are large and reveal considerable variation within each group. Statistical tests for significance between the groups were not significant, indicating that later born children with various types of auditory dis-

Table 9. — *A Comparison of the Hours of Labor for Later Born Children in Each of the Groups*

Group	No.	Mean	S.D.
Peripheral deafness	37	6.38	6.95
Aphasic	23	7.96	7.39
Psychic deafness	10	5.85	9.75
Mentally deficient	12	9.75	10.67

order did not differ relative to the number of hours of labor. Rapid and delayed births apparently were equally distributed throughout the four groups.

Dry birth is another type of deviation found in the birth histories of some children. This is the condition of the amniotic fluid having been discharged prematurely as a result of rupture of the amniotic sac; therefore, the fetus is born "dry". As a result the possibility of injury might be greater because of the lack of natural protection which the amniotic fluid affords, and because rupture of the amniotic sac might disturb normal fetal temperature.

Cesarean deliveries seem to be related to injuries sustained at the time of birth, so apparently delivery by cesarean section subjects the fetus to certain dangers. It is possible that this type of delivery requires the fetus to make an immediate and more drastic adjustment to extra-uterine conditions, including respiration and air pressure.

Another possibility is that cesarean delivery might disturb the normal placental blood equilibrium with resultant circulatory and anoxic effects.

Breech births and other atypical fetal presentations are encountered in birth histories of children with auditory disorders. Such atypical presentations often accompany a history of prolonged, difficult birth. A breech birth is described as a buttocks presentation in contrast to the normal fetal presentation of head first; it may be necessary to turn the fetus in utero before delivery. Breech births, like all unusual or difficult deliveries, apparently increase the probability of injury and furthermore, the atypical position in utero might cause damage prenatally.

It is not uncommon to find a history of instrument delivery, which means that forceps were used to expedite delivery. Use of forceps is common in obstetrics and should not be considered dangerous per se. However, if instruments were used in a difficult birth and if forceps were intense, there is evidence suggesting injury at birth. In retrospect, after it is apparent that the child has a defect such as an auditory disorder, it is necessary to evaluate this evidence in light of the child's atypicality.

Asphyxia neonatorum, or anoxia at the time of birth, has received considerable attention in recent years [40]. This condition results when there is deprivation of oxygen for any cause, prenatally or postnatally. Deprivation of oxygen postnatally creates an excess of carbon dioxide in the blood which apparently tends to paralyze the respiratory center in the brain. Oxygen deprivation prenatally results whenever normal fetal blood supply is impaired. This causes cellular deterioration to which brain tissue apparently is peculiarly susceptible. Cyanosis is a well known symptom of asphyxia neonatorum and should be included in the exploration of possible anoxia. Gesell [16] considers asphyxia as a symptom of wide clinical consequence. The use of anesthetics during pregnancy or during delivery, might be related to this condition because anesthesia of the mother might result in reduction in function of the central respiratory center of the fetus immediately following birth [40]. Courville [7] has demonstrated that complete anoxia of nervous tissue for only a brief period will cause permanent change of the tissue. Anoxia seems to be a common cause of congenital aphasia as determined by the birth histories of these children; this has important implications for the diagnostician of auditory disorders in young children. A relationship between anoxia and peripheral impairment auditorially has not been established clinically but such relationships might exist.

Conditions Immediately Following Birth

The child's condition and general behavior immediately following birth often is suggestive relative to whether injury has occurred. If the child was unduly phlegmatic, if he could not swallow or suckle normally and if convulsions occurred, there is retrospective evidence for central damage at birth. Gesell [16] and others have shown that convulsions in early life are highly influential in the later development of children. Such a relationship seems to exist for some children having auditory disorders, especially the aphasic and mentally deficient. A history of malformation of the head is consequential because marked skull deformation, even if not readily apparent at the time of examining the child, is suggestive of intracranial damage and therefore of considerable importance in the history. Moreover, the child's organismic well-being in very early life is indicated by the time he required to regain his birth weight. Some children having auditory disorders have not regained their birth weight normally; one such child had not regained his birth weight at six months of age. Problems of dehydration, fluid equilibrium, illness and central nervous system damage seem to be associated with incapacity of the infant to regain his birth weight.

All history information requires interpretation in light of the child's order of birth. First born children seem to sustain injury at birth more frequently than those born later. This suggests that the natural rigors of birth are greater for the first born child. Doll [13] has found this apparently greater incidence of disorders in the first born. However, comparative data are difficult to secure because of the unavailability of experience with first born children who are normal. However, for purposes of diagnosis and research it is advantageous to note the child's order of birth.

Parents frequently are aware of the possibility that their child was damaged prenatally or at the time of birth and they are apprehensive regarding this prospect. Their apprehensions might be well founded and realistic or they might not. Nevertheless, wise clinical procedures allow them to talk about such apprehensions because additional information frequently can be gained from such discussion. If their apprehensions are illogical and unwarranted, they should be so informed in a sympathetic manner.

Often it is possible to make a diagnosis of central nervous system damage at the time of birth. Such diagnoses can be made at the time of delivery only when the injury is severe and thereby clinically determinable. More frequently the diagnosis of birth injury must be made in retrospect; the symptomatology becomes obvious only in terms of the later development of the child. This is true especially of auditory disorders because atypical auditory behavior is not readily apparent until it is associated with reciprocal symptomatology. It is now apparent clinically that conditions related to central damage at the time of birth are influential and significant in differential diagnosis of auditory disorders in infants and young children. Differential history taking emphasizes that appropriate information be obtained in this connection.

HISTORY OF ILLNESS

Diseases are a common cause of permanent defects in children and therefore it is essential diagnostically that a careful appraisal be made of the child's background relative to illness. Many diseases contracted by children in early life might be etiologically associated with an auditory disorder.

Childhood Diseases

There is a relationship between etiology and the type of auditory disorder sustained. Childhood illnesses are frequently related to peripheral nervous system impairment. Characteristically, impaired auditory acuity which is sustained during the pre-speech age and in early childhood is due to such illnesses. Such deafness usually is of the nerve type. This means that the diagnostician should be aware that the diagnosis of peripheral deafness usually entails ascertaining whether inner ear dysfunctioning is present because conductive deafness is considerably less common. Apparently middle ear infections are successfully treated by the physician as far as most young children are concerned. It should be emphasized that this situation seems to be reversed for children above six years of age as there is a considerably greater incidence of otitis media in this group. Inasmuch as peripheral deafness of the nerve type is the most common in young children, it is apparent that their deafness should be expected to be severe. Nerve deafness typically causes greater hearing impairment than does conductive deafness in children. Another reason for the apparent greater incidence of nerve deafness in infants and young children is that most prenatal conditions, such as rubella, also result in damaging the inner rather than the middle ear. Likewise, endogenous deafness usually is of the nerve type. Thus it is evident that ascertaining the etiology of the peripheral deafness is reciprocally associated with the accuracy of such diagnoses.

Diseases of the Central Nervous System

Diseases or injuries which affect the central nervous system might cause a variety of auditory disorders. Diseases such as meningitis might destroy all inner ear functioning, auditory and vestibular. This is a common cause of exogenous deafness in early life. Children sustaining deafness from meningitis often require special consideration psychologically [26]. Meningitis is an inflammation of the outer membrane of the brain, the meninges. Damage specifically to brain tissues does not necessarily occur but apparently it is difficult to determine at the time of the illness the exact extent of the damage which occurred. While many children who have become deafened by meningitis do not have complications of brain damage, such damage does occur in a certain number. Encephalographic, neurological, psychiatric and psychological study of these children reveals that central damage has occurred so the illness in such instances might be referred to retrospectively as meningitis-encephalitis. Encephalitis is an inflammation of the brain or the encephalon. It is not uncommon to encounter children with auditory disorders who have a history of encephalitis and such a history has far-reaching significance. This disease often destroys the lower or mid-brain tissues and, therefore, typical aphasias usually do not follow. Rather, auditory or other agnosias are more commonly found in these children. If the encephalitis were severe, all areas of the brain might have been damaged resulting in mental deficiency.

The most common diseases of the central nervous system found by the diagnostician of auditory disorders in children are meningitis, encephalitis and epilepsy. Epilepsy is commonly associated with central nervous system disturbances. These diseases frequently are complications resulting from childhood illnesses such as measles and mumps and the disease might then be referred to as measles-meningitis or mumps-encephalitis. Such illnesses might cause peripheral deafness, aphasia, mental deficiency or multiple involvements such as hearing impairment and mental retardation. Diseases of the central nervous system are common contributors to all types of handicaps in children.

One of the significant findings revealed by the differential histories of children with auditory disorders is that meningitis and encephalitis frequently are undiagnosed at the time of the illness. This indicates the subtle manner in which these diseases might accompany other diseases and thus be masked by other symptomatology. The diagnosis then must be made in retrospect in terms of the total behavioral deviation and later development of the child. Clinical experience suggests that there is an increase in the number of children with auditory disorders resulting from meningitis and encephalitis. If this is true it might be due to improved medical treatments, such as the antibiotics, which save the child's life but do not always prevent permanent injury to the organism.

Diseases Affecting the Middle Ear

It has been suggested that conductive deafness is not as common as perceptive deafness in young children. A history of illnesses which are especially associated with middle ear disorder, however, is essential diagnostically. As stated above, illnesses such as rubella, influenza, mumps, whooping cough and meningitis are associated with impairment of the inner ear and of the central nervous system. Diseases such as tonsillitis, sinusitis, otitis media, otosclerosis and allergy are related etiologically to impairment of the middle ear. A history of earaches, discharge from the ear, frequent colds and nasal drainage is an indication that the child might have a conductive hearing impairment. Usually such hearing impairment is mild or moderate because profound or complete loss of hearing cannot result from impairment of the middle ear only. Nevertheless, otitis media, during the pre-speech age which results in a hearing loss of more than forty decibels, will cause a marked retardation in language acquisition. Inasmuch as conductive hearing impairment is reversible medically it is the obligation of all workers to emphasize treatment of this condition.

The history should include ascertaining the possibility of otosclerosis being present. Otosclerosis is a disease of the middle ear which causes a bone-like tissue to grow around the stapes and the oval window [35]. As a result the stapes becomes inflexible and rigid, thus reducing the conduction of sound to the inner ear. This disease commonly is encountered in young adults, although it does occur in children. It can be inferred diagnostically in very young children on the basis of history information. Characteristically otosclerosis is present in more than one member of the family but whether it is specifically endogenous or due to other factors has not been determined finally. If the history reveals that members of the child's family have otosclerosis the diagnostician should pursue the possibility of this type of conductive impairment in the child; it is referred to as congenital fixation of the stapes. If this condition is suspected the child should be seen for diagnostic purposes over a sufficient length of time in order to accomplish the diagnosis. Ordinarily this should be done by an otolaryngologist who is a specialist in otosclerosis and fenestration surgery. This surgery relieves the effects of the otosclerosis. It has been performed successfully on children seven years of age.*

Inoculations

The history of the child's inoculations occasionally is pertinent to the etiology. If there is a severe reaction to the inoculation it is tantamount to having severe illness and such reactions might have been permanently damaging. Complications with marked reactions might follow any of the inoculations such as those for mumps and whooping cough.

Familial Deafness

The history relative to endogenous conditions should be determined and this possibility is most readily explored under the history of illness. Parents and other family members frequently are reluctant to accept or to consider these factors but they must be evaluated because they are influential in the conclusiveness of the diagnosis. Likewise, many parents are apprehensive regarding endogenous factors when these are not present. The child and the parents are greatly benefited psychologically when endogeny is eliminated. The possibility of endogeny should be discussed sympathetically and with understanding. Some peripheral deafness obviously is endogenous. If the history reveals that deafness is present in a member of the child's family, specific information regarding the nature and onset of this condition is necessary. A relationship between the child's and the relative's deafness should not be assumed if such a relationship does not exist. For example, endogenous deafness should not be confused with presbycusia, otitis media or acoustic trauma. As knowledge of prenatal influences, such as Rh incompatibility and rubella, is increased, the number of children erroneously classified

* Personal communication from George E. Shambaugh, Jr., M.D., Northwestern University, School of Medicine, Chicago, Ill.

as endogenous is decreasing. Perhaps the most definitive information pertinent to ascertaining the presence of endogenous deafness is reliable information concerning deafness in other family members. This information usually extends to the parents, siblings, aunts, uncles and first cousins. Furthermore, endogenous classification assumes that a history of exogenous factors is lacking; if both endogenous and exogenous factors are present, the etiology is stated as being of mixed causality. It is not known whether auditory disorders other than peripheral deafness derive from endogenous causes. For example, endogenous receptive aphasia has not been clinically established. However, more than one child in a family has been found to have highly similar pathology and exogenous factors could not be established. Orton [30] and Barger [1] indicate that endogenous causes are related to pathology of language. The diagnostician of auditory disorders in children should be alert to this possibility and accumulate etiological information which might further clarify the problem. Likewise, it is diagnostically important to procure information on other types of disorders in the family members. For example, the history should explore the presence of mental deficiency, epilepsy, alcoholism, mental illnesses and others which are indicated in the child's problem. Psychosomatic disease might be especially pertinent to children having emotional disorders.

It has been assumed that marked pathology or permanent defects did not result in the child unless the illness was severe. This is not in complete agreement with clinical experience. In some children the history reveals that the illness was moderate, even mild, but the consequences have been far-reaching. Perhaps the severity of the illness is only one of the factors which determine the extent of the involvement or the outcome. Other influential factors seem to be the individual differences of children in withstanding certain diseases. Apparently children differ considerably relative to their toleration of certain diseases without suffering complications. Another possibility is that some diseases produce injurious toxicities without producing symptoms of severe illness. This is true of rubella during pregnancy and similar conditions might occur in young children. The age of the child at the time of the illness is another factor which clinically is related to the after-effects of the disease. In general, it seems that the younger the child the greater is the danger of more inclusive as well as permanent damage. Benton [4] suggests that selective brain damage is more common as the child becomes older but that in infancy generalized brain injury occurs more frequently. This perhaps explains some of the differences which occur in children whose auditory disorders derive from prenatal influences, as compared to those with an etiology of birth injury or postnatal causes. The involvements of the prenatal cases seem to be more diffuse and qualitatively different.

The history of illness contributes substantially to the diagnostic process. It is essential for research on etiology and it has implications for preventive medicine, psychological adjustment and remedial training. It is the responsibility of all specialists in auditory disorders of children to secure this information.

HISTORY OF GENETIC DEVELOPMENT

The history of the child's genetic development provides unusually relevant information for the differential diagnosis of auditory disorders in infants and young children. The child's pattern of genetic development is indicative of the type of auditory disorder which is present. Therefore, children with peripheral deafness, receptive aphasia, psychic deafness or mental deficiency can be expected to differ in the pattern of their genetic maturation. These differences should be explored in the history of genetic development.

Doll [10] and Gesell [17] have provided data relative to the genetic maturation of normal children. Furthermore, they have shown the relationship which exists between various abnormalities and developmental maturation. This work emphasizes that the child develops as a unitary organism. There is a reciprocal affiliation between the various phases of his development. The child grows and matures simultaneously in three ways; physically, mentally and emotionally. A retardation or disturbance in any one of these three areas might affect either or both of the other two. For example, an emotional disturbance might cause inability to use native intelligence and thereby produce pseudo-mental deficiency with concomitant inability to acquire language. Furthermore, an emotional disorder might cause deviations such as enuresis and consequently cause specific aspects of genetic development to be disturbed. Similarly defects in physical growth and development, especially mild deviations of central nervous system development, might cause disturbances of genetic maturation pertinent to auditory functioning and behavior.

A common diagnostic error in the differential diagnosis of auditory disorders in young children is not to recognize the reciprocal affiliation which exists between the various aspects of the child's development. The diagnostician considers language acquisition to be developmentally unrelated to physical, mental and emotional development. Specifically many specialists proceed to evaluate the child's auditory capacities without regard to his genetic development; auditory behavior is considered as being something apart and separate from other aspects of the child's functioning. The interdependence of ability to respond to auditory tests and ability to respond in other ways is overlooked. If a child's mind is maturing at one half of the normal rate, he will be reciprocally retarded in other aspects of his genetic development. Such a child will not be using words at one year of age because although he is one year chronologically, he has a mental age of only six months. Children do not use words meaningfully until they have a mental age of approximately one year [22]. A child who is making one half of normal progress mentally should not be expected to use words until he is two years of age chronologically. Auditory behavior has not been studied maturationally; this is an urgent research need. However, clinically, auditory behavior might be expected to be retarded in a like manner as compared to verbal behavior. A child whose chronological age is three years but who has a mental age of two years, should be evaluated in terms of a maximum of two year capability auditorially. Retarded mental development causes retardations in genetic development, including all aspects of language behavior.

Sitting and Walking

The ages at which a child first sits without support and walks without assistance have been found useful as indicators of genetic development, especially in terms of general motor maturation. Because as stated previously, the children having different types of auditory disorders seemed to present different patterns of genetic development, a comparison was made of the groups relative to the age of sitting and walking. Moreover to further clarify these developmental

Table 10. — *A Comparison of Each of the Groups with the Normal in Mean Age (Months) of Sitting Unsupported*

	Normal	Peripheral deafness	Aphasic	Psychic deafness	Mentally deficient
No.	50	73	60	27	27
Mean	6.41	7.03	8.81	7.56	10.33
S.D.	1.52	2.43	5.12	2.00	5.31
t		1.76	2.01	2.60	3.76
Req.t		2.00 *	2.00 *	2.04 *	2.77 †

* for 5% level of significance.
† for 1% level of significance.

factors each of the groups was compared to a sample of normal children. These comparisons are given in tables 10 and 11. The children comprising each of the groups in these comparisons are from the total sample as shown in tables 1 and 2 and represent the total number for whom this information was obtained. The normal children were from families in a midwestern metropolitan community of upper middle class socio-economic level.

Deviate patterns of genetic development must be interpreted in accordance with other history data, the behavioral symptomatology and test findings. It is apparent from the results in table 10, however, that deviations from the normal can be expected. Children with peripheral deafness are not significantly different from the normal sample used in this study, although there is a trend toward being slightly retarded. The aphasic, emotionally disturbed and mentally deficient are significantly different from the normal in the age of sitting alone. It is interesting to note that the mean age for children

Table 11. — *A Comparison Between Each of the Groups in Mean Age (Months) for Sitting Unsupported*

	Peripheral deafness	Aphasic	Psychic deafness	Mentally deficient
No.	73	60	27	27
Mean	7.03	8.81	7.56	10.33
S.D.	2.43	5.12	2.00	5.31
t		2.47	1.11	3.12
Req.t		2.00 *	2.03 *	2.76 †

	Aphasic	Psychic deafness	Mentally deficient
No.	60	27	27
Mean	8.81	7.56	10.33
S.D.	5.12	2.00	5.31
t		1.64	1.25
Req.t		2.01 *	2.04 *

	Psychic deafness	Mentally deficient
No.	27	27
Mean	7.56	10.33
S.D.	2.00	5.31
t		2.54
Req.t		2.05 *

* for 5% level of significance.
† for 1% level of significance.

with impaired auditory acuity is most like the mean for the normal and that the means become increasingly more deviate for the emotionally disturbed, the aphasic and the mentally deficient. This is in agreement with clinical experience and highlights the organismic differences of these various types of children with auditory disorders as discussed in Part Three: Behavioral Symptomatology. Nevertheless the number of children in each group is small so these results should be considered suggestive rather than conclusive.

The inter-group comparisons for ages of sitting alone are given in table 11. Children with peripheral deafness are significantly different from the aphasic (five per cent level) and the mentally deficient (one per cent level) in mean age of sitting; no difference was found between those with impaired acuity and the emotionally disturbed. The aphasic and the mentally deficient were significantly more delayed in learning to sit unsupported as compared to the group with peripheral deafness. This indicates that from the point of view of maturation of motor factors, such as sitting, the conditions of aphasia and mental deficiency are more generally disturbing. This too is in agreement with clinical experience and emphasizes the different organismic effects of the different types of auditory disorders. Many specialists do not take advantage of this type of information because they are unfamiliar with normal patterns of development and thus do not have ready, precise criteria for establishing the presence of genetic deviation. As indicated previously, Doll [10] and Gesell [17] have provided normative data for a number of maturational factors. Gesell states that children learn to sit upright by approximately seven months of age; the mean age for the normal sample in this study is 6.41 months. Therefore, from the point of view of differential diagnosis if a child has not learned to sit unsupported by the age of eight to ten months, developmental delay should be inferred. This inference might include that the child's lack of language is more likely to be caused by aphasia or mental deficiency rather than peripheral or psychic deafness. However, it must be emphasized that statistically significant differences in mean age of sitting were not found between the mentally deficient and the aphasic or between the aphasic and the emotionally disturbed. The difference between the mentally deficient and the emotionally disturbed was significant. These data support the point of view of reciprocal relationships between various maturational factors and they emphasize the importance of securing a history of genetic development.

The age of learning to walk has been used by many workers as an indication of genetic maturation. Studies reveal that the average normal child begins to walk by approximately thirteen months of age. They learn to walk without assistance and without falling by approximately eighteen months of age [2]. Furthermore, studies indicate that the average child learns to run at two years, to stand on one

Table 12. — *A Comparison of Each of the Groups with the Normal in Mean Age (Months) of Beginning to Walk*

	Normal	Peripheral deafness	Aphasic	Psychic deafness	Mentally deficient
No.	50	78	66	33	24
Mean	13.50	14.09	16.20	15.86	21.15
S.D.	2.07	3.48	5.08	4.22	9.07
t		1.20	3.91	2.98	4.08
Req.t		2.00 *	2.66 †	2.73 †	2.80 †

* for 5% level of significance.
† for 1% level of significance.

foot at three years, to skip on one foot at four years and to skip on alternate feet at five years [16]. Such indications of motor development are useful diagnostically and are discussed further in Chapter XII. The various types of children presenting problems in the differential diagnosis of auditory disorders were compared relative to the mean age of walking and each group was compared with the sample of normal children. These comparisons are given in tables 12 and 13. The mean age of beginning walking for the normals was 13.50 months which is in close agreement with that found by other workers [2, 20]. There were no statistically significant differences between the sexes for the normals or for the groups with auditory disorders.

The comparisons given in table 12 reveal that the only group which is not significantly delayed in beginning to walk is the group with peripheral deafness. The aphasic, emotionally disturbed and mentally deficient are different from the normal at the one per cent level of significance. Again it is important to note the order into which the groups fall. Those with peripheral deafness are near the normal, the emotionally disturbed are next in similarity followed by the aphasic and the mentally deficient are the most deviate group. Peripheral deafness impedes the maturation of walking less than any of the other factors. Apparently it is less organismically influential in connection with walking, even as compared to emotional factors. When central nervous system involvements are present, such as in aphasia and mental deficiency, the organismic influences exceed those found in peripheral damage and in emotional disorders.

The inter-group comparisons for mean age of walking are given in table 13. The children with peripheral deafness were significantly different from the aphasic and the mentally deficient at the one per cent level of significance, and different from the emotionally disturbed at the five per cent level. Children having auditory disorders due to other factors than impaired acuity were significantly delayed in walking. There was not a significant difference between the aphasic and emotionally disturbed. However, significant differences were present between the aphasic and mentally deficient and between the emotionally disturbed and the mentally deficient. It is important to note that both the aphasic and the emotionally disturbed differ significantly from the mentally deficient. Although these groups of children have marked disorders, especially in audition and language development, apparently they cannot be considered as markedly handicapped as the mentally deficient, at least with regard to certain maturational factors. As in the mean age of sitting, there were no significant differences between the sexes for any of the experimental groups or for the normal group.

From the point of view of differential diagnosis age of beginning walking must be considered as being related to certain types of auditory disorders. On the basis of these findings failure to learn to walk until after sixteen months should be evaluated in terms of possible relationship to aphasia, psychic deafness or mental retardation. The importance of central nervous system damage such as encountered in the aphasic and mentally deficient has been generally acknowl-

Table 13. — *A Comparison of Each of the Groups in Mean Age for Beginning Walking*

	Peripheral deafness	Aphasic	Psychic deafness	Mentally deficient
No.	78	66	33	24
Mean	14.09	16.20	15.86	21.15
S.D.	3.48	5.08	4.22	9.07
t		2.86	2.13	3.73
Req.t		2.65 †	2.03 *	2.80 †

	Aphasic	Psychic deafness	Mentally deficient
No.	66	33	24
Mean	16.20	15.86	21.15
S.D.	5.08	4.22	9.07
t		0.35	2.53
Req.t		2.02 *	2.06 *

	Psychic deafness	Mentally deficient
No.	33	24
Mean	15.86	21.15
S.D.	4.22	9.07
t		2.65
Req.t		2.06 *

* for 5% level of significance.
† for 1% level of significance.

edged. The importance of early emotional disturbance in maturation has not been emphasized. Apparently when an emotional disturbance is of sufficient intensity to cause the child to relinquish hearing, it effects developmental factors such as sitting and walking. There is a possibility also that these children had sub-clinical motor involvements super-imposed on emotional factors. In view of their more rapid births too, it seems most satisfactory to consider these children as presenting organismic disorders but that these disorders are different in general from those presented by the other groups. The history of beginning walking is an important aspect of the genetic history as it provides evidence which should be evaluated in terms of differential diagnosis of auditory disorders in early life.

Laterality

As indicated by the data on sitting and walking motor maturation is one of the most advantageous avenues through which to assess the maturation of young children. Neurological integrity and motor functioning are directly related. Another area of motor capacity which can be advantageously explored through the history is laterality. Normally individuals are right or left sided; the right hand, leg and eye or the left hand, leg and eye are dominant. Injury to the central nervous system might be manifested in dominance being delayed or mixed. On the average children begin to show a hand preference between six and twelve months of age. This preference does not become strong, however, until after eighteen months of age. If a child shows a preference for a right hand but a left leg or vice versa, it is referred to as mixed laterality. Nice [29], Gesell [16] and Orton [30] have stressed the relationship between laterality deviations and language retardation. In general, laterality disturbances are significant indicators of motor disorder. Such disturbances are common in various types of handicapped children and clinical experience indicates that a significant proportion of children with auditory disorders have delayed or mixed laterality. Therefore the history information should include ascertaining whether laterality has been established and whether parents have attempted to influence the child's laterality. Information should be secured concerning unusual awkwardness and falling. Unusual awkwardness is common in aphasic children and falling is associated with some types of inner ear disturbances and might be present with peripheral deafness. Inability to button clothes, to grasp objects and to manipulate eating utensils are other indications of motor involvements and such possibilities should be explored in detail.

Dressing

The Vineland Social Maturity Scale [*12*] provides a means of evaluating the child's maturation in several ways. This is a diagnostic instrument and it is discussed in Chapter XII. However, use of this scale requires special training. All diagnosticians will not use the scale as a diagnostic procedure but all specialists can use it as indicated here in the history of learning to dress oneself. A few items from this scale have been used to explore the child's maturational development in terms of learning to dress himself.

Doll [*10*] has shown that the average child tries to pull off his socks at approximately eighteen months of age. He learns to take off and to put on his coat between two and three years of age; he first learns to take off his coat and about six months later learns to put it on, but without buttoning or unbuttoning it. He learns to do simple buttoning of his coat at about three and one half years and to dress himself, except for tying his shoes, at about four and one half years. For clinical diagnostic purposes, if the child is four years of age but has not learned to take off or put on his coat, factors causing maturational delay should be suspected. Likewise such factors should be suspected if the child has not learned to dress himself (except for tying) by the age of five and one half years.

The importance of general social competence is revealed by the differences between the groups with auditory disorders. These data are presented in Chapter XII and they highlight the importance of all genetic development in differential diagnosis.

Toilet Control

It is not uncommon to encounter children who are retarded in toilet control. Children with any type of auditory disorder might show retardation in acquisition of toilet habits. The average child of two years indicates his need to go to the toilet [*12*]. The mean age for each group with auditory disorder and for the normal sample is given in table 14. These data are presented for illustrative purposes primarily because many of the children studied were not toilet trained and therefore could not be included in the data. This was especially true of the mentally deficient group. In an attempt to correct for the small samples, the Mann-Whitney Non-Parametric

Table 14. — *The Mean Age in Years for Indicating Toilet Needs for Each of the Groups as Compared to the Normal*

	Normal	Peripheral deafness	Aphasic	Psychic deafness	Mentally deficient
No.	50	56	36	18	8
Mean	2.43	2.27	3.24	2.57	3.21
S.D.	.70	1.05	1.67	1.02	1.46
t		0.94	2.74	0.54	2.46 ‡
Req.t		2.01 *	2.72 †	2.09 *	1.96 *

* for 5% level of significance.
† for 1% level of significance.
‡ for Mann-Whitney Test

Statistics Test of Significance [*23*] was used as indicated in tables 14 and 15.

The normal sample used in this study indicated their toilet needs at a mean age of slightly less than two and one half years. This is in close agreement with the results of other workers. There was a difference at the five per cent level of significance between the sexes for the normal group; the females indicated their toilet needs earlier than the boys. There was not a sex difference for any of the groups having auditory disorders. The children with peripheral deafness and those with emotional disturbance were not significantly different from the normal. However, those with auditory disorders due to aphasia and mental deficiency were significantly delayed as compared to the normal. This is in agreement with clinical experience and suggests the importance of the history of toilet training. This history requires careful interpretation because frequently complex factors seem to be present. For example, there is an indication clinically that aphasic children have difficulty in learning to interpret the internal signals which normally become associated with the need to go to the toilet. These children might be limited in interpreting and comprehending such signals in the same manner as they are lacking in ability to interpret auditory stimuli. Special consideration and training would then be indicated.

Emotionally disturbed children frequently acquire toilet control at the usual age but later regress and do not maintain control. This is not characteristic of the infantile autistic child because his toilet habits usually are established early and remain controlled. The history of toilet training is of considerable interest irrespective of the child's type of auditory disorder because it is not uncommon for parents to overemphasize toilet training with these children. It seems that unconscious factors motivate parents to overcompensate for their child's lack of ability to speak so they attach unusual significance to toilet training. Frequently parents need assistance with this problem and should be given explanations of the child's readiness for such training. Even an explanation to the effect that some delay is common in these children will relieve their anxieties and benefit both the parent and the child. From the point of view of differential diagnosis if toilet control has not begun by three years of age, it can be considered as an indication of maturational retardation. Furthermore, such delay should not be viewed as being typical of children with peripheral deafness. Likewise, children with psychic deafness do not show a typical delay in toilet control but they may show marked regressions after such training has been established.

Comparison between the groups in mean age of acquiring toilet control is shown in table 15. Because of the small samples these data too are presented chiefly for illustrative purposes. The trends indicated by these findings, however, are in the expected direction and in agreement with the findings in connection with sitting and walking. The children with peripheral deafness learned to indicate their toilet needs earlier than the aphasic but significant differences between the other groups did not appear. These data emphasize the organismic integrity of children with impaired acuity as compared to those with auditory disorders due to other causes.

Table 15. — *Comparison Between the Groups in Mean Age (Years) of Indicating Toilet Needs*

	Peripheral deafness	Aphasic	Psychic deafness	Mentally deficient
No.	56	36	18	8
Mean	2.27	3.24	2.57	3.21
S.D.	1.05	1.67	1.02	1.46
t		3.12	1.30	1.89 ‡
Req.t		2.71 †	1.96 *	1.96 *

	Aphasic	Psychic deafness	Mentally deficient
No.	36	18	8
Mean	3.24	2.57	3.21
S.D.	1.67	1.02	1.46
t		1.18 ‡	0.23 ‡
Req. t		1.96 *	1.96 *

	Psychic deafness	Mentally deficient
No.	18	8
Mean	2.57	3.21
S.D.	1.02	1.46
t		1.11 ‡
Req.t		1.96 *

* for 5% level of significance.
† for 1% level of significance.
‡ Mann-Whitney Test of significance.

Feeding

Children vary in the age at which they learn to feed themselves just as they vary in other areas of genetic development. Feeding habits, like toilet habits and dressing, are influenced by motor coordination, mental development, emotional status and methods of training used by the parents. Therefore, the history should include information relative to feeding difficulties because of their diagnostic value in these several respects. Doll [10] has established the genetic stages of learning to eat. At one year the child masticates food; he drinks from a glass without assistance at eighteen months of age; he uses a spoon to feed himself and learns to discriminate between edible and nonedible substances between eighteen months and two years of age. The child learns to eat with a fork between two and two and one half years of age. He learns to get a drink without assistance between the age of two and three years. Not until the child is at least seven years of age does he learn to use a table knife for purposes of cutting meat. For clinical purposes the diagnostician may conclude that genetic delay is present if the child is not using a spoon to feed himself by two and one half years of age and if he is above three years of age and has not learned to use a fork. Likewise, if the child is above three and one half years of age and is not capable of getting a drink without assistance under ordinary environmental and training routines, it is suggestive of genetic delay. Retardation in learning to feed themselves appropriately is common in young children seen by the diagnostician of auditory disorders. Children with peripheral deafness most often are more like the normal in this respect than are the aphasic, emotionally disturbed and mentally deficient. It is more difficult to train all children with marked limitations in ability to communicate and their ability to care for themselves should be expected to be delayed. This delay varies both in quality and extent on the basis of the total·problem which the child presents, not only on the basis of his ability to communicate, and this history information is highly relevant to differential diagnosis.

Children having auditory disorders have in common the lack of normal language development and the inability to profit experientially from their auditory environment. Nevertheless, this common problem should not obscure genuine differences genetically. In general, children with impaired acuity have a pattern of genetic development which is most like the normal. Their primary retardation is in verbal development and they present a pattern of discrepant delay in the acquisition of verbal language as compared to other aspects of their genetic development. Children with psychic deafness apparently will be slightly delayed in sitting and walking but not in initial toilet control. They are characteristically disturbed in the development of interpersonal relationships (see Chapter VIII). Aphasic children are retarded in most aspects of genetic development but not to the same extent as the mentally deficient, and in terms of differential diagnosis their deviations also are qualitatively different. Unusually marked, generalized genetic retardation is indicative of mental deficiency. An essential aspect of evaluating the auditory behavior of such children is a complete psychological examination. The history of genetic development is one of the most consequential parts of the total history for children having auditory disorders.

HISTORY OF EMOTIONAL ADJUSTMENT

Emotional factors are highly important in the differential diagnosis of auditory disorders in infants and young children and should be included in the history. Currently scientific study of human behavior does not include a normative standardization of the development or growth of feelings and attitudes but that children mature emotionally is apparent from observation. Furthermore, factors related to emotional growth are being ascertained and progress is being made even in relation to the emotional aspects of language development; the association between language acquisition and emotional development is being revealed by scientific study [6, 25]. The relationship between auditory behavior and emotional factors in children is apparent clinically but remains to be studied extensively.

For purposes of the differential diagnosis of auditory disorders the history of emotional adjustment provides an opportunity to explore expected patterns of behavior. Certain patterns of behavior are discussed in Chapter VIII because they are directly related to clinical observations and diagnosis of psychic deafness. The items on the history of emotional adjustment have been selected because they provide information specifically on this problem. Clinically, the child with peripheral deafness, the aphasic, the child with psychic deafness and the mentally deficient child present characteristically different syndromes of emotional adjustment. The history should elicit descriptions which are diagnostically significant in view of these syndromes. For example, the infantile autistic child is not responsive to people; he does engross himself with objects; he is not alert to movements nor is he highly distractible. The child with peripheral deafness is responsive to people; he is unduly alert to movements and sensitive to vibrations. He is reticent but playful with adults and pets; he is not oblivious or severely withdrawn. The receptive aphasic child is highly distractible, hyperactive, not sensitive to vibrations, not primarily responsive to objects, not oblivious and responds inconsistently from one situation to another. Obviously these syndromes of emotional adjustment are not dichotomous and the behavioral pattern in a particular child might be extremely varied and complex. However, it is beneficial in all cases to secure information on emotional adjustment and behavior. Such information most often assists in clarifying other history information and the test findings.

Some children having auditory disorders, especially the emotionally disturbed, present problems of eating and sleeping. Although eating has been included in the genetic history, eating habits might be explored again in the emotional history; if the child seems to be emotionally disturbed additional evaluation of feeding difficulties often is desirable. Information such as refusal to eat, extreme meticulosity in respect to cleanliness while eating, marked food preferences and aggressiveness while eating are indicative of emotional factors. Likewise sleeping habits are significant indicators of emotional well-being. Parents frequently inquire about unusual sleep habits in their children and when they do not, such information should be elicited. Extreme or unusual wakefulness, night terrors, sleep-walking and other difficulties in sleeping should be considered as pertinent diagnostic information. Such behavior indicates emotional involvements whether or not the child's auditory disorder is due to psychic disturbances. For example, a child might have peripheral deafness with superimposed emotional problems. Such children present a mixed behavior symptomatology which increases the difficulty of diagnosis. In this connection it is not valid to assume that because a child cannot be awakened by loud sounds, his deafness is not emotional because severe emotional disturbances do not disappear when the child is asleep. Emotional factors causing psychic deafness must be expected to be operative at all times and the child's symptomatology should be appraised accordingly.

Symptoms such as rocking, head banging and staring are not uncommon in children having auditory disorders, especially in those whose history and symptomatology are suggestive of emotional trauma. Rocking means that the child while sitting or standing sways himself from side to side. He might engage in this activity for long periods of time with little awareness of his environment. While this behavior is highly indicative of emotional disturbance, its significance has not been clearly determined but it seems that this behavior might be partially explained by the child's receiving autistic gratification from stimulating his vestibular mechanism. This explanation is in agreement with Schilder's [34] emphasis on emotional significance of sensations deriving from the balance mechanism. In general, children who rock themselves in this manner are highly withdrawn and might be more aware of sensations from within themselves than from stimuli deriving from their environment. This is discussed further in Chapter VIII. Some children who rock themselves also fixate visually and appear to be staring. Frequently they stare at lights but they might stare into space. Head banging also is a rather common symptom. The child bangs his head against his crib, the floor or against other objects. Such banging is not playful; rather, it is highly compulsive and severe to the extent that it is sometimes injurious. This behavior suggests emotional disturbance and the diagnostician should differentially consider the presence of psychic deafness. However, as stated above, emotional problems might be superimposed on other conditions such as peripheral deafness. But psychic deafness should not be minimized because it is a significant contributor to auditory disorders in young children. The history of emotional adjustment should not be treated in an isolated manner but as with all of the other information, it is continuously appraised in terms of other history data, clinical observation and examination findings.

HISTORY OF AUDITORY BEHAVIOR

The history of auditory behavior provides valuable information for the differential diagnosis of auditory disorders in young children. As in the other areas of the history it is assumed that children presenting various types of auditory disorders will have histories which are differentially suggestive. Auditory behavior is an integral aspect of total behavior. Therefore a child whose auditory disorder is due to brain injury might be expected to manifest a different syndrome auditorially than a child whose auditory disorder is due to peripheral deafness or emotional disturbance. The items on the history have been selected because they provide an opportunity for the diagnostician to elicit specific information regarding these expected differences. Such information should not be expected to be dichotomous but clinical experience reveals that it is useful in determining the diagnosis.

Unfortunately research evidence is meager concerning the genetic development of hearing and comparative difficulty of sounds perceptually is unknown. Likewise, the capacity of the hearing mechanism to respond to various intensities and frequencies during early infancy has not been established. However, children are known to respond to sound in an indirect and gross manner at the time of birth [32]. Gesell [17] found that the four week old child heeds sound because when a bell was rung while he was engaged in postural activity, the activity ceased. Piaget [33] has ascertained that the child relates hearing and vision between two and three months of age; when he hears a sound he attempts to locate the source visually by turning his head to see where the sound is coming from. Piaget [33] and Gesell [16] are in agreement that one of the earliest reactions to sound genetically is cessation of an activity. Gesell refers to this as "auditory staring". This means that the child is momentarily halted in play, crying, in motor activity or in other aspects of his behavior as a direct result of his response to sound. This type of reaction is of utmost importance in evaluating young children with auditory disorders and it is discussed further in Chapter XI.

Another significant factor in auditory behavior in very early life is that the child responds to vocal sounds most readily when they are imitations of his own vocalizations. Piaget [33] found that such imitation could be elicited by two months of age. It is significant that the child responded to imitations of his own vocalizations but did not respond to other vocal stimuli or to other sounds such as whistles. This too is highly consequential in connection with auditory testing of young children. One of the common errors of auditory testing is that it is applied without due regard for the child's genetic level of maturation. Many children do not respond to intense auditory stimuli of a certain type only to respond readily to imitations of their own vocalizations. Such clinical findings are in agreement with the reported reactions of normal children in early life. This raises an interesting speculation diagnostically. Perhaps some children are genetically immature relative to their ability to respond auditorially. For example, at twelve months of age they might be capable of auditory responses only at the six month level because of selective delay in the maturation of auditory behavior. This is in agreement with the clinical findings of a number of children but usually such retardation in auditory maturation is accompanied by delays in lateral dominance or in locomotor behavior such as walking. However, mental retardation with generalized deficiency is not present. Such children do not respond to auditory tests like other children of their age and as a result seem to be peripherally deaf. Through the history of auditory behavior other information usually can be secured to further explore the auditory capacities of such children.

The history of auditory behavior usually reveals that the child responds to certain sounds repeatedly, that he is inconsistent in his responses or that he gives no obvious response to sound. A history of no response to any sound is rare and might be suggestive of emotional involvements. Even children with marked peripheral deafness usually respond to intense environmental sounds such as an auto horn at close proximity. The history should include inquiry relative to the type of sounds to which the child responds. For example, inquiry might be made regarding the child's responses to the telephone, vocal calls or to sounds from the radio and television. If the parents report that he responds consistently to intense sounds such as an auto horn, the suggestion is that the child has marked peripheral deafness. If they report that he responds to more moderate sounds such as vocal calls or hand claps and that he does so consistently, the suggestion is moderate peripheral deafness but all such speculations are tentative and require appropriate corroboration.

The quality of the child's auditory behavior is equally revealing as compared to the intensity levels at which the child responds. For example, it is desirable to inquire whether the child has shown fear of sound, whether he seems to willfully ignore sound, whether he attempts to visually locate sound and whether his auditory responses are consistent. Children with peripheral deafness tend to respond consistently to those sounds which are genetically appropriate and which are above their thresholds. Consistency of response is not characteristic of children whose auditory incapacities are due to factors other than impaired acuity. Emotionally disturbed children at times might not respond to sounds even at the pain level of intensity while at other times they respond to sounds of normal intensities. Likewise, aphasic children characteristically respond inconsistently because they might respond to a sound of moderate intensity but not when this same sound is presented at a higher intensity. It seems possible that as a result of their brain injury some aphasic children have disturbed auditory perception relative to loudness; their experience is meaningless in regard to loudness and softness. Other clinical evidence of such auditory perceptual disturbances is seen in these children; they might not respond consistently to loud foreground sounds but unexpectedly respond to background sounds of mild intensities. In such instances the parents might report that the child responds inconsistently to their attempts to attract his attention with sounds, but that at times it is obvious that he is distracted by minor sounds in his environment which normally would be ignored. This might be an indication of an inability to structure the world of sound; meaningful selection of sound is impaired. Such disintegration of auditory perception is far-reaching in its consequences and can be compared to the visual perceptual disorders in brain injured children described by Strauss and Lehtinen [38]. This is discussed further in Chapter XI under auditory perception.

Other deviations in the manner in which young children respond can be included in the history. These deviations might be considered in terms of the distinction between hearing and listening. Doll [13] first suggested the importance of this distinction. The diagnostician might infer peripheral deafness in a child who has hearing but who finds it impossible to use his hearing integratively because he cannot listen. Such disturbed auditory behavior is found most frequently in those children who are brain injured. Interestingly children with reduced auditory acuity learn to use their hearing projectively in that they learn that auditory sensations occur only through external stimulation. Therefore, they tend to respond integratively to sounds above their threshold. They attempt to localize the sound visually and make meaningful responses in terms of listening. In this respect the child with peripheral deafness behaves like the normal child. Brain injured children, emotionally disturbed and mentally deficient children might have hearing but be unable to give listening type responses. This is pertinent to auditory testing because most such tests asume integrative listening ability.

The history of auditory behavior provides an opportunity to explore the child's responsiveness to other than auditory stimuli. This might include inquiry relative to his responses to pain, vision and to being touched as well as to vibratory sensations. Some children who do not respond normally to auditory stimuli do not respond to other stimuli any more adequately. Such generalized lack of normal responsiveness is indicative of marked emotional disturbance or of mental deficiency but not of impaired auditory acuity. All information secured from the history of auditory behavior must be integrated with the other history data, with the clinical observations and with the findings of the examination itself. Only through such synthesis can the full meaning and significance of the information be realized.

HISTORY OF LANGUAGE BEHAVIOR

As indicated in Chapter II there is a direct relationship between auditory disorders and normal language development. The problem of differential diagnosis of auditory disorders is essentially differentiating between various types of language disorders because hearing is the basic sensory avenue for language reception. The history of language behavior provides a means of exploring the child's specific problem of language acquisition. This information is not difficult to elicit from the parents because their child's inability to communicate is their primary concern. The items on the history of language behavior have been selected because of their value in eliciting information which assists in differentiating between types of language disorders. Basically the language disorders of children with peripheral deafness, receptive aphasia, emotional disturbance and mental deficiency are dissimilar in nature and in symptomatology. The aphasic child has a disorder in symbolic functioning and this inability characterizes his behavior. This is not true of the other three primary types. The hearing impaired child does develop symbolic behavior because his disorder typically does not include injury to the brain. Thus the sensations he receives tactually, visually and from the gustatory and olfactory senses are integrated experientially to form inner language. He behaves symbolically; he internalizes his environment and becomes capable of separating himself from it. It has been demonstrated that an object which is seen, felt, tasted, smelled and heard is different experientially from one which is seen, felt, smelled and tasted but not heard [28]. Therefore, the perceptual and conceptual development of the child with deafness is different from the normal; however, this difference is not analogous to the symbolic disorder of the aphasic child [27]. The aphasic child's damage causes him to have marked difficulty in integrating and interpreting his sensory impressions. Symbolization is disturbed and thereby receptive, expressive and inner language are impaired. Likewise the language disorders of the aphasic and the hearing impaired differ from those of the emotionally disturbed. Most emotionally disturbed children presenting atypical auditory behavior have unusually complex inner language and symbolic functioning. This is especially true of those with childhood schizophrenia. Characteristically, the basic atypicality of the language behavior of these children is that it relates only to their inner life. Therefore, it is unnecessary for them to use receptive or expressive language. They use language for inner life purposes only and as a result it is distorted and lacking in contact with other human beings. The history of such children frequently reveals that they acquired and used language rather normally until a certain age, then ceased to acquire it normally and began using what language they had for phantasy and autistic purposes. Usually at the same time, receptive and expressive language ceased to be used or was greatly reduced. In general the language of the mentally deficient child is at the level of his mental capacity. As indicated previously, mental ability and language acquisition are directly related and therefore a history of retarded language development should be expected in connection with generalized mental retardation.

It is necessary diagnostically to compare the language development of the child with auditory disorders genetically with that of the normal. A number of workers have established norms for the development of expressive language. A survey of this work is given by McCarthy [22]. Gesell [17] states that the average child uses one or two words at one year of age, which is in general agreement with the findings of other workers. For the diagnostician of auditory disorders it is significant that reception or comprehension of language precedes the expressive use of language. The child comprehends gestures, facial expressions and vocal intonations before he comprehends or uses words. Hurlock [20] suggests that there are three pre-speech forms expressively: crying, babbling and gesture. The gesture includes body expression such as squirming and holding out the arms to indicate desire to be picked up. As expressive language increases verbally, crying and non-verbal body gestures decrease proportionately. The history should explore this crying and body gesture behavior because of its significance in the diagnosis of language pathology. The lack of verbal language might be accompanied by a highly developed use of gestures. Such a history is indicative of peripheral deafness whereas the lack of verbal language with concomitant lack of gesture is indicative of aphasia or emotional disorder. Gesture is used only after a minimum of inner language has been established and when minimum inter-personal relationships are present. The critical age for lack of speech development is approximately two years. A child who has not developed ability to communicate verbally by then usually is suspected of having deafness or of being otherwise atypical. Frequently, however, parents suspect atypicality much earlier and seek diagnostic assistance relative to their child's lack of speech.

The history of language behavior might begin by inquiring whether the child babbled in infancy. The psychology of babbling is obscure but progress is being made in understanding the relationship between babbling and language development [21, 25]. Babbling, apparently, is directly associated with language development. Careful exploration therefore in regard to the child's babbling behavior is rewarding diagnostically. Babbling is defined as a pleasurable use of vocalizations; utilitarian use of the voice is not included. It occurs mainly in the absence of parents or siblings while the child is lying in his crib or after feeding. Although there is disagreement regarding the age at which babbling begins, it is engaged in freely by the average child between five and six months of age [22, 24]. This is the most satisfactory age to use when inquiring from parents in regard to their child's babbling. Ewing and Ewing [15] state that children with peripheral deafness babble normally for a period and then become increasingly mute. Clinical experience is not in complete agreement with this statement. If babbling is defined as a pleasurable use of the voice for autistic purposes only, then children with congenital peripheral deafness apparently do not babble. If the history reveals that the child babbled at the age of five or six months it might be considered as evidence that the child could hear within normal limits at that time. This suggests that normal auditory capacity is a requisite for typical babbling to occur. Pleasurable use of the voice at this age assumes autistic gratification, which in turn assumes capacity to respond auditorially to the self-produced vocalizations. Although evidence is meager, clinical experience suggests further that children with congenital receptive aphasia likewise do not babble. Their receptive disorder, perhaps as with the hearing impaired child, precludes the possibility of enjoying self-produced vocalization. Children with emotional disorders might have babbled normally but this behavior was interrupted so that imitation of the speech of others did not follow. Children with mental deficiency frequently have babbled but at a later age than the normal. The degree and type of mental deficiency may be significant in this connection. It is obvious that presence or absence of babbling must be interpreted in light of the total findings. Research on the psychology of babbling can be expected to add substantially to knowledge of the psychology of language development.

Children with peripheral deafness who are otherwise normal are not mute; the term deaf-mute is erroneous. They learn early in life, at least by the age of two years, that they can attract others by using their voice. This projective use of their voice is highly symptomatic. Aphasic and emotionally disturbed children are especially deficient in the utilitarian aspects of vocal production. Frequently they do not use their voices for communication even to the extent of using vocalizations to attract others. Furthermore, they may be mute. The tonal quality of the vocalizations also should be explored in the history. Likewise the unexpected understanding or use of speech are revealing diagnostically. Parents might report that their child at times understands or uses a word but that a moment later he seems incapable of doing either. Such experiences are exasperating to parents but should be considered as characteristic of some children with receptive aphasia. Echolalia, the automatic imitation of heard speech, is another revealing symptom diagnostically. Children with peripheral deafness are not echolalic. This symptom is commonly found in aphasia and might be present in certain forms in emotionally disturbed children [31]. The significance of these symptoms is discussed further in Part Three under Behavioral Symptomatology. All of the history data concerning language behavior must be interpreted in association with the total findings of the examination.

EDUCATIONAL HISTORY

Ordinarily the diagnostician of auditory disorders in young children does not encounter children who have been in school; they most often are too young to have had formal school experience or their auditory disorder and language retardation has precluded school entrance. However, if the child has had nursery or other school experience it should be included in the history. This information should cover the success of such school experience. A report from the school usually is desirable and differences of behavior in the home and in the school should be evaluated. Some children respond auditorially and use language expressively more effectively in the school than in the home and such information has obvious diagnostic importance.

SUMMARY

The history is one of the chief means for determining the etiology. A prenatal history of rubella in the mother, for example, may explain a cochlear lesion causing severe deafness. Other etiological possibilities explored in the history include Rh incompatibility, accidents to the mother, emotional disturbances and use of drugs during pregnancy. The type of birth may be important. For example, a difficult delivery, prematurity, prolonged labor, use of forceps, precipitous delivery seem related to asphyxia neonatorum and other conditions causing brain damage. The condition of the child immediately after birth is a significant indicator of whether damage has occurred. Jaundice, convulsions, apathy, difficulty in nursing and swallowing might suggest central nervous system damage. The history of illness may explain a nerve deafness. An example is meningitis which invades and destroys the inner ear, or measles, whooping cough, influenza, pneumonia and severe reactions to inoculations. Such illnesses may cause peripheral deafness or in some cases encephalitis. The family history is important in determining the presence of inherited deafness. The development of the child as compared to the average gives valuable clues as to his type of deafness. Thus the normal and the peripherally deaf child both sit unsupported at about seven months, the child with psychic deafness achieves sitting by seven and one half months, the aphasic is more delayed because his average age for sitting is eight and three fourths months, and the mentally deficient are still more delayed, not learning to sit unsupported until ten months of age. The ages for learning to walk, for learning to dress himself, and for learning toilet control show similar relationships between the groups with auditory disorders as compared to the average normal child. The history of emotional adjustment is indicative for children with peripheral deafness, aphasia, psychic deafness or mental deficiency. For example, a history of lack of response to people may indicate psychic deafness, while good responsiveness socially and extreme alertness to movement is characteristic of children with peripheral deafness. A history of distractibility and inconsistency characterizes aphasic children. Eating and sleeping habits, head banging and rocking are other important clues of emotional adjustment. The history of responses to sound also is revealing. One of the earliest reactions to sound in the normal infant is momentary cessation of activity when the sound first occurs. This may be observed as early as four weeks of age. Between two and three months of age the child learns to turn his head toward the source of the sound. Normal children seem to respond to imitations of their own vocal utterances before they respond to other sounds even though these sounds are very loud. In the history the sounds to which the child responds are important because a history of responding to only very loud sounds suggests peripheral deafness. Furthermore, the history of language behavior is important because of the direct relationship between auditory disorders and language development. The language disorders of the child with peripheral deafness, aphasia, psychic deafness or mental deficiency will differ. Before the child acquires speech he expresses himself by crying, then by babbling, followed by gestures. A highly developed gesture language with lack of verbal language suggests peripheral deafness. Lack of verbal language with lack of gesture language suggests aphasia or psychic deafness. The child's use of verbal language must be compared to the average normal child who uses one to two words at one year and has acquired ability to communicate in short sentences by two years. Babbling is a forerunner of language development and consists of the use of vocalization by the child for his own pleasure. It is engaged in mainly when he is alone and between five to six months of age by the child with normal auditory capacities. Present evidence indicates that the peripherally deaf child and the aphasic child do not babble, whereas the child with psychic deafness babbles and then fails to imitate speech, while the mentally deficient babble at a later age than the normal.

BIBLIOGRAPHY

1. Barger, W. C.: An experimental approach to aphasia and non-reading children. Am. J. Orthopsychiat. *23*: 159, 1953.
2. Bayley, Nancy: The Development of Motor Abilities During the First Three Years. Washington, Society for Research in Child Development, National Research Council, Mono. I, 1935.
3. Bender, L.: Organic brain conditions producing behavior disturbances, in, Lewis, N. and Pascella, B. (eds.): Modern Trends in Child Psychiatry. New York, International Universities Press, 1945, pp. 155–192.
4. Benton, Arthur: Development of Perception and Sensory Functions in the Child. Symposium: Language Development and Language Learning in Children, Northwestern University, 1952. (Unpublished.)
5. Bingham, W.: Aptitudes and Aptitude Testing. New York, Harpers, 1942.
6. Bowlby, John: Maternal Care and Mental Health. New York, World Health Organization, Columbia University Press, 1952.
7. Courville, C. B.: Asphyxia as a consequence of nitrous oxide anesthesia. Medicine *15*: 129, 1936.

8. Davis, D.: Comparative study of the growth and development of premature and full term children with special reference to oral communication. Unpublished dissertation, Northwestern University, 1951.

9. Doll, E. A.: Practical implications of the endogenous-exogenous classification of mental defectives. Am. J. Ment. Defect. *40*: 503, 1946.

10. ——: Measurement of Social Competence. Minneapolis, Educational Test Bureau, 1953.

11. ——: The feebleminded child, in, Carmichael, L. (ed.): Manual of Child Psychology. New York, Wiley, 1946, pp. 845–855.

12. ——: Vineland Social Maturity Scale. Minneapolis, Educational Test Bureau, 1947.

13. ——: Neurophrenia. Am. J. Psychiat. *108*: 50, 1951.

14. ——: Phelphs, W. M. and Melcher, R. T.: Mental Deficiency Due to Birth Injuries. New York, Macmillan, 1932.

15. Ewing, I. and Ewing, A.: Opportunity and the Deaf Child. London, University of London Press, 1947.

16. Gesell, A. and Amatruda, C.: Developmental Diagnosis, Ed. 2. New York, Paul B. Hoeber, 1947.

17. —— et al: The First Five Years of Life. New York, Harpers, 1940.

18. Goodhill, Victor: The nerve deaf child: Significance of rh, maternal rubella and other etiologic factors. Ann. Otol. Rhin. & Laryng. *59*: 1123, 1950.

19. Hood, P.: A study on the relationship of unilateral brain damage on speech and language functioning. Unpublished dissertation, Northwestern University, 1952.

20. Hurlock, E. B.: Child Development. New York, McGraw-Hill, 1942.

21. Langer, S. K.: Philosophy in a New Key. New York, Penguin Books, 1948.

22. McCarthy, D.: Language development in children, in, Carmichael, L. (ed.): Manual of Child Psychology. New York, Wiley, 1946, pp. 476–581.

23. Mann, H. B. and Whitney, D. R.: On a test of whether one of two random variables is stochastically larger than the other. Ann. Math. Statist. *18*: 50, 1947.

24. Morgan, J.: Child Psychology. New York, Rinehart, 1942.

25. Mowrer, O. H.: Learning Theory and Personality Dynamics. New York, The Ronald Press, 1950.

26. Myklebust, H. R.: Significance of etiology in motor performance of deaf children with special reference to meningitis. Am. J. Psychol. *59*: 249, 1946.

27. —— and Brutten, M.: A study of the visual perception of deaf children. Acta oto-laryngol. Suppl. 105, 1953.

28. ——: Aphasia in children. J. Exceptional Child. *19*: 9, 1952.

29. Nice, M. M.: Ambidexterity and delayed speech development. Ped. Sem. *25*: 141, 1918.

30. Orton, S. T.: Reading, Writing and Speech Problems in Children. New York, W. W. Norton, 1937.

31. Pearson, G.: Emotional Disorders of Children. New York, W. W. Norton, 1949.

32. Piaget, Jean: The Origins of Intelligence in Children. New York, International Universities Press, 1952.

33. ———: Play, Dreams and Imitation in Childhood. New York, W. W. Norton, 1951.

34. Schilder, Paul: Mind: Perception and Thought in Their Constructive Aspects. New York, Columbia University Press, 1942.

35. Shambaugh, George E. Jr.: Fenestration Operation for Otosclerosis. Acta oto-laryngol. Suppl. LXXIX, 1949.

36. Spock, Benjamin: The Common Sense Book of Baby and Child Care. New York, Duel, Sloan & Pearce, 1945.

37. Stander, H. J.: Textbook of Obstetrics. New York, Appleton-Century-Crofts, 1945.

38. Strauss, A. and Lehtinen, L.: Psychopathology and Education of the Brain-Injured Child. New York, Grune & Stratton, 1947.

39. ——— and Werner, H.: Comparative psychopathology of the brain-injured child and the traumatic brain-injured adult. Am. J. Psychiat. *99*: 835, 1943.

40. Windle, W. F.: Asphyxia Neonatorum. Springfield, Ill., C. C Thomas, 1950.

PART THREE: BEHAVIORAL SYMPTOMATOLOGY

Chapter VI

Auditory Disorders Due to Peripheral Deafness

ANALYSIS OF THE CHILD'S BEHAVIOR IS A significant step in the process of making a differential diagnosis of auditory disorders in young children. As stated previously the entire diagnostic process consists of three steps, differential history taking, evaluation of behavioral symptomatology and the clinical examination. Part Three is a consideration of the second step, clinical observation and evaluation of behavior. This process of differentially analyzing the child's behavior assumes that the diagnostician has clinical training and experience on which to base his evaluations. All specialists will not be comparable in this respect. Each specialization has its own frame of reference and will view the child accordingly. However, behavioral symptomatology can be used to some extent by all specialists. Furthermore, clinical observation of behavior affords information which is useful, not only in making a differential diagnosis, but in counseling the parents and in making recommendations for remedial programs.

Behavioral manifestations are a significant source of diagnostic information and the diagnostician is accumulating this information continuously as he observes the child. This observation begins immediately with his initial contact and usually continues throughout the history taking and the examination, until the diagnosis has been established. Through clinical observation the diagnostician attempts to answer the question of whether the child's behavior is characteristic of children with peripheral deafness, aphasia, emotional disturbance or mental deficiency. It is apparent that behavioral symptomatology should not be expected to provide a dichotomy between children with auditory disorders. All children who do not have normal auditory behavior have certain behavioral symptoms in common. Furthermore, there are children with multiple disorders with resultant behavioral characteristics of more than one type of handicap. A child might have impaired auditory acuity with superimposed emotional disturbance and thereby present a mixed type of behavioral symptomatology. Moreover, the behavioral manifestations of one handicap might be pronounced and mask, or obscure the behavioral symptoms of a second disorder. For example, the behavioral characteristics of aphasia might mask the symptoms of hearing impairment. However, there are characteristic behavioral sequelae which are concomitant with peripheral deafness, aphasia, emotional disturbance and mental deficiency, when an auditory disorder is common to them all. These behavioral syndromes have not been studied extensively and research is urgently needed for both diagnostic and therapeutic purposes.

Qualitative clinical evaluation is a necessary aspect of the differential diagnosis of auditory disorders in infants and young children. Objective procedures, such as psychometric and audiometric techniques are not highly definitive with children who do not speak and who are disturbed auditorially. The importance of behavioral symptomatology and qualitative analysis can be illustrated by the example of children with peripheral deafness, with aphasia, emotional disturbance, or mental retardation, all responding as if auditory acuity were deficient. Literal interpretation of auditory acuity tests would thus be in error with certain children. Such test findings require corroboration from behavioral symptomatology. Most quantitative, or objective, measurements assume certain normalcy of cooperation and response. These assumptions ordinarily cannot be made by the diagnostician of auditory disorders in infants and young children. These children by the nature of their disorders usually cannot be expected to cooperate and to perform according to predetermined standards. Thus, the incorporation of behavioral symptomatology as part of the total evidence for the differential diagnosis is consistent with rigorous scientific attitude. Moreover, in this area of diagnosis undue reliance on objective techniques and procedures without corroboration leads to erroneous diagnoses. This is discussed further in Chapter XII. It is apparent clinically that systematic evaluation of behavioral symptomatology adds substantially to accuracy of diagnosis and to knowledge of the psychology of language and auditory disorders.

NONVERBAL COMMUNICATION

Most of the children seen by the diagnostician of auditory disorders in early life have no verbal language. This is the primary concern of the parents and the predominant reason for their consulting the specialist, but this does not mean that these children do not communicate nonverbally. As shown by Allport and Vernon [1] everyone expresses inner feelings and meanings by body movements, not only by gesticulation. Hurlock [12] considers body gesture as a preliminary to speaking in normal infants. The infant shows fear, enjoyment, anger, hunger and other feelings through his expressive behavior bodily. Such nonverbal communication precedes speech both phylogenetically and ontogenetically. Therefore, it is interesting to note Yerkes' [28] finding that chimpanzees communicate effectively with "gestures, facial and bodily expression, postures and visible attitudes which function as meaningful signs." Kanner [13] emphasizes the importance of nonverbal communication in infants and young children. In general, young children have unusual ability to interpret and to communicate nonverbal meanings. Unless the facial expressions and general body behavior of the speaker is in agreement with what he is saying the child might ignore the verbal content and react mainly according to the nonverbal content. Perhaps this is because the child learns to interpret his environment by nonverbal communication before verbal communication. Further-

more, gestures, including facial expressions and body posture, continue to have significant communicative value throughout life. However, nonverbal expressive behavior has not been studied extensively.
This is unfortunate because its value psychologically and psychiatri-
cally seems to be especially great. Inasmuch as infants and young
children with auditory disorders usually do not have verbal language
it is necessary to carefully evaluate their nonverbal communication.
Frequently, their bodily expressiveness is highly revealing, and the
adage that "actions speak louder than words" is a necessary corollary
of the diagnostician's other procedures and findings.

The concept that auditory disorders of different types will be
manifested in the child's behavior assumes that a specific auditory
disorder changes behavior in a typical manner; each type of auditory
disorder will result in a characteristic behavioral syndrome. This
seems logical if auditory disorders are not viewed as being something
apart from the rest of the organism. Over-simplification in this respect has been common with resultant errors of diagnosis and classification. That peripheral deafness in early life results in organismic
changes which can be referred to as a syndrome cannot be denied.
Gesell [9], and Myklebust and Brutten [19] have studied some of
the behavioral changes to be expected. A sensory deprivation such as
peripheral deafness has far-reaching consequences organismically.
One of the intriguing aspects of the relationships between such deafness and behavior is the relatively normal adjustment which is
achieved by many deaf children and adults. Nevertheless, this should
not prevent critical evaluation of the limitations imposed on the
organism by peripheral deafness, because only by intensive study of
these behavioral effects can its diagnostic and therapeutic significance
be understood. For this reason the behavioral syndrome associated
with peripheral deafness is presented in some detail in Part Three,
and it is compared with the behavioral symptomatology associated
with other types of auditory disorders.

Gesell [9] describes hearing as the social sense, which emphasizes
the importance of hearing in establishing social relationships. The
psychological development of the child with marked impairment of

auditory acuity is different from the normal from very early life. Such deafness immediately imposes a restricting factor relative to the child's ability to relate to his mother and other family members. The human voice is capable of an undetermined variety of inflections, intonations and modulations. Children with normal hearing are continuously reacting to these vocal productions of their parents; not only what is said, but how it is said, is meaningful to the process of interaction psychologically. Inflections, modulations and intonations are profoundly significant in structuring and ascribing meaning to social situations. It is reasonable to assume that cultural stereotypes are maintained from father to son partially on the basis of the nonverbalized meanings of what is said to children. Clinical experience with young children with marked peripheral deafness suggests that much of this type of cultural impact is lacking in their personality organization and development. They are remote, isolated, and undeveloped in this respect, with a corresponding effect on their early behavior.

Perhaps all children learn and make adjustments primarily through the process of identifying with their parents, and later with siblings, teachers and other community members [17]. The process of identification is much more difficult for the child who does not hear and who does not find it possible to communicate normally with his parents. The period of trial and error experimentation through which all children must go while gradually harmonizing their subjective needs with their environment, is longer for the child with such sensory deprivation. Thus, he is retarded in his ego development, more time is required for him to make a distinction between himself and his world. He is retarded in his attitudinal and emotional development and the process of normal symbolic development and internalization is impeded. He is more immature in ability to make his wants known and, thereby, he is more diffusely and randomly subject to impulsiveness with associated misunderstanding on the part of his peers. Because his mental life lacks the normal structuring effect of audition he remains more concrete. He is less capable of abstract behavior which is highly dependent on auditory symbolism and ability to verbalize. His experience is undifferentiated and less integrated as compared to the normal and his personality is lacking in structure.

In addition to his inability to hear vocal sounds and to use verbal language, the child with impaired hearing acuity is deprived of basic contact with his environment in other ways. He is deprived of hearing all sounds, not only speech. He does not hear the sounds made in preparation to feed him, or any of the other sounds which are so common in the environment of the normal infant. He is dependent on seeing what is taking place because vision is his only distance sense. But vision is directional, while hearing is essentially non-directional. Hearing serves the individual in all directions simultaneously, including into other rooms of the home, around corners and into the dark. Children with normal hearing learn to recognize their auditory environment and to use it for purposes of adjustment. Although some sounds are frightening to them, all sounds serve to put the individual into realistic contact with his environment throughout the life span of the individual, including the time when he is asleep. Hearing is essentially mandatory because the individual cannot close his ears as he can his eyes; this is of considerable importance when contrasting the psychology of seeing and hearing. Hearing, apparently, more than any other sense, serves as a means of resolving subjective needs and external circumstances. Through hearing, the organism is in continuous contact with the outer world. Deafness results in a world which is more subjective and unrealistic, more fearful and less understood. Children with such deafness are deprived of one of man's primary signaling, or warning senses. Hearing more continuously than vision alerts man to the friendliness or to the danger of his environment. The young child with deafness is significantly isolated from other people and from his environment in general. His is a world which is essentially visual and tactual, not a world which is auditory, visual and tactual, and his behavior and adjustment must vary and compensate accordingly. Being largely limited to a seen and a felt world means that his world remains more unreal and unexplored experientially. This has profound implications for his development perceptually, conceptually and emotionally. We can infer with assurance that sensory deprivation which changes the child's world so extensively is observable in his behavior. It is surprising that these differences in behavior are not greater. Only the most observable characteristics of young peripherally deaf children are included in this discussion. Close association with such children will reveal many more subtle behavioral characteristics to the careful observer.

The diagnostician who understands the nonverbal communication of young children with this type of deafness will find it a significant source of diagnostic information. In making a differential diagnosis of auditory disorders in infants and young children the data from one source should be evaluated and validated against the data from the other sources. Therefore, the history information, the behavioral symptomatology and the examination test findings should be reciprocally corroborative. When these three types of data are not in agreement, but are discrepant, it is cautious procedure to defer diagnosis until further study can be made. This cautious procedure of deferring diagnosis unless the pattern of results is in agreement is followed even when the findings of the auditory tests suggest profound peripheral deafness. Such deafness is a syndrome and usually cannot be diagnosed by auditory tests alone. In this area of diagnosis the test findings ordinarily are not of more importance than the history data or the behavioral symptomatology. This means that when a diagnosis of peripheral deafness is made the child not only shows deficient acuity on auditory tests, but the history and his behavior also show this deafness.

Behavioral symptomatology as discussed here is most apparent in young children whose deafness is rather severe. However, these behavioral characteristics are manifested to some degree by all children whose impaired acuity precluded their acquiring language normally. Marked differences between the behavioral symptomatology of children whose hearing acuity is just below the conversational level of intensity (fifty to sixty decibels) and those with a profound loss of hearing is not apparent in early life. The remedial problems entailed in connection with moderate and severe losses are vastly different;

however, the different prognosis remedially is relatively unrelated to the problem of differential symptomatology in infancy. In early life, children with moderate or severe deafness are confronted with the comparable circumstance of not being able to acquire verbal language at the usual age and of inability to profit normally from other types of auditory experiences. Therefore, while the behavior of the child with a moderate impairment differs in some details from that of the child with a profound loss of hearing, all of these children present a behavioral syndrome which is characteristic of peripheral deafness. Likewise, the type of deafness does not substantially affect the behavioral symptomatology as discussed for purposes of diagnosis. As indicated in Chapter V, perceptive deafness is predominant in young children; however, conductive deafness is also encountered and usually is of a more moderate degree. Compensatory behavior as observed in behavioral symptomatology derives primarily from the sensory deprivation rather than from the type or the extent of the impairment, but this assumes that deficiency of auditory acuity precludes language acquisition and otherwise normal auditory experience, and therefore necessitates differential adjustment on the part of the organism. This does not include central deafness and auditory agnosia because these conditions are not considered under peripheral deafness; they result from damage to the central nervous system and are discussed under auditory disorders relating to aphasia in Chapter VII. Children who lose their hearing after having acquired language, also, have similarly characteristic behavior in terms of deafness. Usually, however, the problem of differential diagnosis is less complex in these children. The history of illness ordinarily is definitive, their speech is highly symptomatic and other factors are equally revealing.

Behavioral symptomatology is nonverbal communication in both a direct and indirect manner. The child might use gestures, which is a direct form of nonverbal communication, or he might use his vision in a compensatory manner and this is indirect nonverbal communication. This nonverbal communication, which is referred to as behavioral symptomatology, is highly useful diagnostically. A number of the most obvious behavioral symptoms of children with peripheral deafness are considered in this chapter. In Chapters VII, VIII and IX these behavioral symptoms are compared with those of children having other types of auditory disorders.

BEHAVIORAL SYMPTOMS OF PERIPHERAL DEAFNESS IN YOUNG CHILDREN

He Does Not Acquire Speech

One of the most obvious symptoms of this type of deafness, if it is present from the pre-speech age, is lack of speech development. The average normal child begins to use words at approximately one year of age. Furthermore, the normal child learns to speak according to the patterns of speech which he hears. The various geographic areas of the United States and of the world, have characteristic speech patterns and verbal symbols. These variations include a number of basic languages and many dialects. The normal child acquires the speech pattern used by his particular social group, which illustrates the close reciprocal relationship between hearing and speech. This relationship is further revealed by the study of peripheral deafness and its effect on speech behavior. If a child has partial hearing for speech, his speech will be comprised of that part of the speech pattern which he hears. For example, if he cannot hear the high frequency consonants but can hear the low frequency vowels, his voice will be low in pitch, and he will not include high frequency consonants in his speech pattern. Those speech sounds which are not heard will not be included in his articulated speech.

A more drastic example of the reciprocal relationship between speaking and hearing is revealed by the child who hears no speech and, therefore, does not acquire speech. A child whose hearing impairment precludes hearing speech does not acquire speech naturally, but such a child's lack of speech is not due to a defective speech mechanism. Rather, he does not acquire speech because he cannot hear it and, thereby, acquire it normally. This does not mean that the child with deafness has no language and is devoid of symbolic behavior; it means that he does not acquire verbal language. However, as indicated previously lack of speech is not an infallible indication of deafness. It is a noteworthy symptom of deafness in early life but, like all symptoms, it must be appraised in accordance with the total symptom complex manifested by the child.

Some children seen by the diagnostician of auditory disorders are not speechless. For example, the child with partial hearing for speech acquires a speech pattern consistent with his capacity to hear. Various other types of speech behavior frequently are met with clinically and must be carefully evaluated. Some children have jargon speech, others have isolated words which they use intermittently, and still others have ability to name certain objects but cannot use words sequentially. Some have a few words or phrases which they use indiscriminately for all situations and some have only echolalic speech; they automatically repeat the word, phrase or sentence which they have just heard. It is noteworthy diagnostically that such attempts to use speech are not characteristic of children with peripheral deafness. A child having such deafness from infancy does not use jargon, or isolated words, and he is not echolalic. These are manifestations of children who can hear speech but for other reasons are not developing verbal language in the normal manner. The child who has deafness from the age of one year, or earlier, does not have defective speech or speech which is otherwise identifiable. He lacks speech; he vocalizes and uses his voice for control of his environment, but he has no speech which can precisely be referred to as defective. The presence of speech, regardless of the type or its meagerness, means that the child can hear the spoken word, or that deafness was sustained after having acquired speech. This direct reciprocal relationship between the presence of speech and the ability to hear frequently is overlooked by diagnosticians. Children with ability to use speech intermittently, or who are echolalic, have been diagnosed as having severe peripheral deafness from infancy. The presence of this type of speech should be considered as being symptomatic of conditions other than impaired acuity. This is with the exception of those children who sustained deafness after having acquired speech. Such children have characteristic speech patterns acoustically. Their speech is lacking in inflection, intonation and melody; it may be described as monotonous. This speech pattern usually can be identified and differentiated diagnostically from other types of speech manifested by children having auditory disorders other than deafness.

His Vocalizations Have a Characteristic Tonal Quality

The child with peripheral deafness does not improvise vocalizations for pleasure but he does use vocalizations for other purposes. He learns to use his voice to call attention to himself. For example, he might use his voice in a calling, or screaming, manner to get the attention of his mother. This use of his voice is in itself highly diagnostic. He uses his voice to stress and express his feelings and needs; he frequently expresses fear, anger and discomfort by vocalizing. It is apparent that many such children cannot hear their own vocalizations so presumably they learn to associate the kinesthetic sensation accompanying vocalization with the environmental changes they desire; to get attention from mother they must produce a sensation which is felt in the throat. Such use of vocalization usually occurs by two years of age and it is differentially symptomatic in two ways. The meaningfulness of the vocalizations is significant, and the tonal quality of the vocalizations is characteristic.

Hearing not only is the sensory avenue for acquiring verbal language, but it serves, also, as a monitor of the speech which is produced. When hearing is deficient this normal monitory process is lacking, or is only partially adequate, and the vocal quality is symptomatically impaired accordingly. In general, the greater the loss of hearing the more vocal quality becomes distorted. This reveals that the normal child automatically and unconsciously learns to modulate his voice. His vocal patterns have inflectional, intonational and melodious qualities which derive directly from his unconscious imitation of those speech patterns which he hears. Moreover, similarly he adopts an intensity level which is characteristic of individuals with normal hearing. This is another monitorial function of hearing; it regulates the intensity of vocal production, causing it to be raised and lowered according to the demands of the situation. Because the child with deafness lacks monitoring auditorially, his vocalizations are monotonous, guttural and highly fluctuating in pitch range. His inflection, intonation and melody are unlike those of children with normal hearing even if they have auditory disorders other than deafness. Furthermore, the intensity of his vocalizations frequently vary spasmodically and atypically. Often his vocalizations are unduly loud as compared to the normal. Diagnosticians and teachers coming into close daily contact with children with deafness become expert at identifying the tonal quality which typifies hearing impairment. Often they state that a particular child's vocalizations are unlike those of children with deafness. Such an observation implies that the child's auditory disorder is due to aphasia, emotional disturbance or mental deficiency. Many electronic recordings have been made of the vocalizations produced by children presenting problems of auditory disorder. This procedure clarifies and objectifies the evaluation of vocal tonal quality. Also, it provides research material which is useful diagnostically and therapeutically.

He Does Not Improvise Sound for Pleasure but Uses Vocalizations Meaningfully and Projectively

Normal children typically improvise sound to add to their play activities. While engaging in play with a doll, a toy gun or a toy car, they hum, make a sound like a gun or like the motor of a car. Moreover, the normal child not only vocalizes by producing sounds associated with his toys, but he also verbalizes freely while at play. Piaget [21] and Vigotsky [27] have analyzed this verbalization psychologically. Piaget referred to it as egocentric speech, while Vigotsky considered it a manifestation of inner language. This autistic type of language behavior, which is typical of children especially between the ages of two and five, warrants further study psychologically. From the point of view of differential diagnosis of auditory disorders it is the absence of sound improvisation, vocalization and verbalization which is behaviorally symptomatic. Ideally the diagnostician should encourage the child being diagnosed to engage in play activities. Frequently observations of the child while he is engaging himself, relatively unaware that he is being observed, adds greatly to diagnostic information. This is especially true if the play materials have been carefully and appropriately selected. Pertinent play materials for this purpose are suggested in Chapter XI.

Children with peripheral deafness do not improvise sounds to add feeling and realism to their play activities; they do not say "choo-choo" while playing with a train. They do not hum or jabber to themselves. Likewise, deaf adults do not sing or whistle to themselves, nor do they engage in other production of sound for purposes of pleasure. Individuals with such deafness do not produce sounds simply for the purpose of hearing them. Anyone who engages in musical activities may be said to be pursuing sound primarily for purposes of enjoyment and such activity may be described as autistic in the same manner as babbling and vocalizing are autistic in the child. The child with peripheral deafness does not produce sound autistically for purposes of enjoyment. While he is not mute, he does not produce sound in a playful manner. Production of sound vocally, or in other ways, assumes capacity to hear such sounds. Some children with moderate losses of hearing do learn to engage in playful vocal production under certain circumstances and then the sounds used are characteristic in tonal quality and are considerably less variable and generalized than those used by the child without loss of hearing.

It is noteworthy and highly significant diagnostically that even the child with profound peripheral deafness learns to use his voice meaningfully. This is in marked contrast with children having other types of auditory disorders. The child with impaired acuity does not learn to use the conventional sounds which are designated as speech, but he does use vocalizations which have intent and meaning. Typically he learns early, between one and two years of age, that he can produce a vocal stimulus which attracts the attention of those around him. He readily "calls" to his mother and other family members in order to get their attention. This means that he projects himself into his environment and makes continuous integrated attempts to relate to it. He learns to manipulate his environment within the limits of his capacities and he is not a victim of environmental stimuli in the manner which typifies the brain injured child with aphasia.

The diagnostician's clinical observations should include careful evaluation of the child's vocalizations. If the child vocalizes freely and spontaneously the suggestion of peripheral deafness should be questioned. If the child does not use vocalizations for pleasure, but uses his voice to attract attention from others, the behavioral symptomatology is in agreement with a presumption of impaired acuity. Nevertheless, it must be emphasized that the total psychological behavior which accompanies and forms the background of the vocal behavior is as meaningful diagnostically as the vocal behavior itself. The child with peripheral deafness, irrespective of the limitations imposed by his lack of normal auditory experience, behaves in an integrated manner. He does not improvise sound for pleasure, but he uses his voice with intent and purpose, in a logical manner. This is unlike the emotionally disturbed child whose vocalizations might be without intent, without relationship to other people. Likewise, it is unlike the aphasic child who might use his voice playfully, or indiscriminately, without meaningful intent. The child with deafness usually is not mute, and, therefore, muteness must be carefully noted and analyzed in relation to other symptomatology; frequently it is found in association with psychic deafness. The differential diagnosis includes evaluation of all aspects of vocal behavior, relating it to the total problem which the child presents, and to all of the data secured from the examination.

He Uses Gestures

Gestures are an integral part of all communication. For diagnostic purposes gesture includes all nonverbal body expression. For example, shyness and reticence are communicated nonverbally. Likewise, haste, aggression, fear, resentment, hyperactivity and phlegm are all communicated nonverbally, especially by young children who cannot communicate verbally. Such nonverbal communication is natural for all infants prior to acquiring speech [*12*]. Gesture, also, includes more formalized and more symbolized expression, such as shaking the head for "no", turning the palms up and shrugging the shoulders for "all gone", and moving the forefinger back and forth for "come over to me". The most intricate system of symbolized gestures is the language of signs used by many individuals having deafness from early life. Gesture is a significant aspect of language behavior [*10*]. Frequently it is a form of symbolic behavior in that the gesture is a symbol in the same manner that a word is a symbol. In this respect it is a form of expressive language. As a means of expression it preceded verbal language both phylogenetically and ontogenetically [*13*]. However, gesture cannot be considered as comparable to verbalization as a means of expression because verbalization is vastly more flexible, subtle, and capable of more abstractness. Gestures are limited in time and space to a greater degree than words. Gestures are more concrete, but this does not preclude the study of them as a behavioral symptom. The diagnostician must be concerned with the question of why some children with auditory disorders use gestures fluently but others seem to be incapable of them, or indisposed to their use.

Gesticulation is a form of symbolic behavior. In this regard, like other forms of expressive language (speaking-writing) it assumes a minimum of inner language. Only those children who have internalized their world symbolically can use gesture as language. A child cannot use expressive language in any form without first having been capable of receiving sensory impressions and integrating these into meaningful experience; he must have had a minimum of perceptual and conceptual integration and development. Therefore, gestures reveal organismic functioning and constitute nonverbal behavior with far reaching implications for diagnosis. The child with peripheral deafness differs from other types of auditorially disturbed children in this respect. He uses gesture in a complex and natural manner. Through gesticulation he can communicate such thoughts as: "Where is daddy?"; "Give me the ball"; "It is my cap"; "I am going home"; and "Give me a drink". Ordinarily he uses gesticulation readily by the age of two years. In contrast, children with receptive aphasia characteristically do not gesture. Likewise, emotionally disturbed children often do not gesture because of their inability to relate adequately to other people. Mentally deficient children might use gestures but only at the level of their ability to function mentally.

Gesticulation is typical of children with peripheral deafness. Furthermore, it is of diagnostic importance that he not only uses gestures, he understands the gestures of others. A number of children with auditory disorders other than impaired acuity cannot understand the meaning of even simple gestures, such as the examiner holding a ball and gesturing that he wants the child to catch it. Such inability to comprehend gesture is not characteristic of children with peripheral deafness. This means that such children who are otherwise normal, acquire symbolic behavior (inner language) through their senses which are functioning normally, principally through vision, but, also, through tactile sensitivity, olfaction and gustation. To the extent that sensory capacities permit, experiences become structured, integrated and symbolized. Although sensory experience does not include audition and, therefore, is qualitatively different from the normal, it does serve as a basis for the development of symbolic behavior. This child can both use and interpret nonverbal symbols. Unlike the aphasic child in particular, he acquires symbolic behavior although he lacks auditory symbolization. He develops language although his language is not identical to the normal child. Moreover, his language expression is characteristic and distinctive when compared with the expressive language of other children with auditory disorders. The child with peripheral deafness is characterized by his adeptness in the use of gesture and his use of gesture is revealing and has implications in various other ways. Perhaps most importantly it reveals organismic integrative capacity, adjustment to other people, and it discloses attempts to relate to the environment. This behavioral symptomatology is a significant factor in the differential diagnosis because all children with auditory disorders do not gesture. Through gesture the child's normalcy in other respects can be evaluated. The presence of gesture must be related to the various symptoms constituting the child's syndrome. It serves as a basis of comparison with other children having auditory disorders and should be observed and analyzed accordingly.

He Responds to Sound Consistently and Uses Residual Hearing Projectively

The diagnostician of auditory disorders in young children receives many reports of inconsistent responses to sound. This inconsistency of response has been interpreted as being caused by intermittent peripheral deafness. Clinical evidence, however, suggests other interpretations. It seems unlikely that the child's auditory acuity varies momentarily; however, some otitis media conditions might be expected to vary, with associated variation in auditory acuity. Such variations seem to be gradual and relatively stable and peripheral deafness due to inner ear disorder is not known to fluctuate. Parental reports and clinical observation reveal that some children respond to auditory stimuli in a markedly inconsistent manner. They are inconsistent in respect to threshold of intensity, responding to mild, or moderate, loudness but not to very loud sounds. Furthermore, they might respond to a sound once, especially at the first presentation, but not respond to repeated stimulation even though the intensity is raised. However, not all children with auditory disorders are inconsistent in their responses. Therefore, the diagnostician continuously observes the child's auditory behavior and evaluates it in various ways. One of the ways in which he evaluates this behavior is the ability to respond consistently to sounds.

The diagnostician attempts to answer the question of why some children with auditory disorders respond consistently to sounds and some do not. Children with peripheral deafness characteristically respond consistently to sounds which are loud enough to reach their threshold, providing the sounds are suitable to their genetic level and appropriately presented. The type of response expected varies with the level of genetic maturation. Children at different age levels, from less than one year to six years, will respond differently to an auditory stimulus. However, even when appropriate allowance has been made

for age and maturational differences the child with peripheral deafness responds more consistently than other children with auditory
disorders. Repeatedly, as the sound reaches his threshold, he responds
by momentarily ceasing an activity (playing, crying, etc.) and
"staring," as described by Gesell [8], or by scanning the environment
visually in an attempt to locate the source of the sound. This type of
response is typical from children with peripheral deafness even if
their deafness is severe, because if they have no residual hearing they
respond similarly when the sound reaches the pain threshold. Children who do not respond when sounds reach the intensity of pain
usually should be suspected of presenting problems other than peripheral deafness because such children are more frequently found to be
emotionally disturbed. In clinical parlance such children are referred
to as "being too deaf to be deaf." This means that a child who gives
no response to sound, irrespective of intensity level, must be considered in terms of other symptomatology with the intention of
comparing his total syndrome with that of children with peripheral
deafness. The history and other sensory responsiveness are pertinent
in such comparisons.

The child with deafness, although he hears only loud stimuli, is
capable of integrating his auditory sensations. He uses his residual
hearing in a normal manner behaviorally; he responds consistently and
assumes a listening type of behavior. His response includes awareness
that auditory sensation is directly related to environmental stimulation. Moreover, listening assumes ability to respond organismically
and integratively to environmental stimulation and children with
peripheral deafness do respond to auditory stimuli in this manner.
In contrast, ability to hear does not necessarily assure ability to use
audition integratively, nor to respond consistently. Children with
receptive aphasia, because of the nature of their disorder, typically
cannot use their hearing integratively and, therefore, they respond
inconsistently in general to auditory stimuli. They do not associate
auditory sensations with environmental stimulation; their ability to
listen is characteristically reduced although hearing acuity might be
normal. The child with impaired acuity uses his hearing projectively.

In this respect he behaves like normal children. When sounds reach his threshold of audibility he responds projectively, with awareness that the stimulation has meaning and derives from the environment. He might search for the stimulation visually, or become fearful and cling to his mother. Although he does not know the meaning of the auditory stimulus he recognizes the relationship between auditory sensation and the outer world. His ability to respond consistently and to use hearing projectively is another behavioral symptom in the syndrome of peripheral deafness. The diagnostician evaluates this symptomatology and relates it to the total syndrome which the child presents.

His Laughing, Smiling and Crying Are Characteristic

Laughing, smiling and crying are significant aspects of behavior. Inappropriate and atypical laughing, smiling or crying are clinical symptoms of far-reaching importance. However, the laughing, smiling and crying behavior of young children has not been studied extensively. Gesell [8] has shown that the sixteen week old child laughs and smiles. Hurlock [12] states that the crying of babies has differentiated meanings by the third week of life. She found, further, that from the second month of life the baby's cry ceased to be a monotone and varied in intensity, tonal quality and rhythm. Cries of pain, discomfort, fatigue and hunger could be differentiated. Children with auditory disorders vary considerably in their laughing, smiling and crying behavior. It is apparent clinically that this variation in certain respects is related to the type of auditory disorder which the child has sustained. This is logical and comprehensible because laughing, smiling and crying are methods of communication and in certain usages are forms of symbolic functioning. Laughing and smiling are means of expressing pleasant and enjoyable relationships with others; they are means of expressing appreciation and friendliness and reveal social perceptual awareness and responsiveness [25]. In young children laughter and smiles are significant indications that the child feels assured, accepted and has a stable equilibrium with the situation and with the world. Such normal laughing and smiling are forms of behavior which occur only when the child has become responsive to external meanings as expressed verbally or nonverbally by others. However, as the child matures he might laugh or smile to himself, just as he talks to himself, because he has internalized situations in the form of inner language. Similarly, crying is a means of communication and precedes the use of speech. It is a form of nonverbal expression. The infant learns very early that by crying he receives help from others, and otherwise pleasant attention. In crying the child is communicating displeasure, discomfort, pain or frustration [4]. Frequently, crying becomes a means of expressing highly specific needs and in this respect is not unlike words.

Diagnostically laughing, smiling and crying are noteworthy behavioral symptoms because children with various types of auditory disorders differ significantly in these areas. Relative to the child with peripheral deafness, it is necessary to emphasize that laughing and crying are vocalizations, therefore, they are characterized, identified and interpreted essentially on an auditory basis. If they are not heard it can be assumed that much of their meaning and communicative value is lost. For example, much of the pleasure expressed in laughter is auditory in nature, and hearing laughter in others is a primary source of stimulation for laughter in those who hear it. Likewise, much of the meaning in crying is derived qualitatively and nonverbally from the acoustic aspects of the cry. It might be a whining cry, a cry of severe pain, or a cry demanding immediate attention such as frequently accompanies a tantrum. Such meanings and interpretations of laughing and crying assume normal auditory functioning. The child with peripheral deafness does not hear his own laughing and crying, nor the laughing and crying of others. Therefore, as Gesell [9] has indicated, his laughter is deficient. He laughs less than normal children and some young children with impaired acuity rarely laugh. Developing normal spontaneous laughter apparently is difficult when it is not heard. Learning to express oneself normally in laughter presumably is not only dependent on hearing, but is dependent on social contacts and relationships which, also, are more difficult when one does not hear. Certainly much of the enjoyment and stimulation of laughter is lacking when it is not heard. It is apparent that one of the differentiating aspects of laughter in children with peripheral deafness is that it is deficient in extent and spontaneity. Some such children even when stimulated and encouraged by the diagnostician will not laugh. However, laughter usually occurs in the home but the history reveals that it is notable in its infrequency.

The laughter of the child with impaired acuity is characteristic in another way. It has an atypical tonal quality for the same reason that his other vocalizations are acoustically identifiable. He does not hear himself laugh, or cry, because auditory monitoring is lacking, or deficient. His laughter and crying, thereby, are atypical in inflection, pitch range and acoustic quality. Like his other vocalizations, they are flat in tonal pattern and intensity variations might be unusually great. His laughter and his crying lack the acoustic differentiation of the normal child.

Smiling is not dependent on hearing. It has no acoustic aspect or quality. However, like laughter, it is an expression of happiness, pleasantness and general acceptance of those in a given situation. Smiling is dependent on awareness of others and on ability to participate in a situation with a minimum of meaningfulness. The child who smiles is projecting himself to a certain extent and presumably feels identified with the situation or with some person. This type of social behavior and adaptation is more difficult for the child with deafness. The mother's smiling at her baby usually is accompanied by endearing vocalizations and the child who does not both hear and see the mother as she smiles and vocalizes is missing significant intersensory stimulation and reinforcement. Therefore, smiling is less readily established and less meaningful as a means of expression. This might explain the deficiency of smiling in children with peripheral deafness. Other factors, too, might be operative. When parents become aware of their child's deafness they might project their feelings of despair and sorrow onto the child. They might look at him with doleful expressions and approach him with feelings of blamefulness and remorse rather than with feelings and expressions of happiness. Such an atmosphere might inhibit the child from developing feelings of security and well being which are essential to spontaneous smiling and laughter.

Children with peripheral deafness might cry often. Unlike laughing and smiling, crying is not deficient in extent. Perhaps, lacking verbal ability, these children find crying a means of readily expressing their wants. Also, parents find training and management more difficult, which adds to the child's frustration and displeasure. Diagnostically the most important aspects of the child's crying are the atypical tonal quality and the psychological integrity which it reveals. The child with deafness cries with vigor and feeling. It is a cry which expresses genuine emotional tones of anger, displeasure and desire; it is not a random whimper or whine. He sobs and sheds tears freely. His crying is persistent and demanding in nature, not unlike that of the normal child. It might be accompanied by gestures, vocalizing, stamping of the feet and genuine tantrums. These qualitative aspects of his crying reveal psychological integrity which frequently is lacking in other types of children with auditory disorders.

The characteristically atypical laughing, smiling and crying behavior in young children with deafness has other psychological and diagnostic implications. To illustrate, laughter is not only an expression of pleasure, acceptance and approval, it is an expression of understanding of a situation which is considered humorous. Such situations are abstract conceptually, often dependent on metaphor and analogy [14]. This type of behavior is highly symbolic and dependent on ability to fully appreciate variable symbolic meanings. The child with peripheral deafness who does not acquire language normally does not have this facility. His humor derives from situations which are concrete, visual and nonverbal. He laughs at "funny faces", peculiar movements or unusual sequences of pictures and drawings. All humor which is dependent on innuendo, inflection and rhyme, such as the pun, is meaningless to him. The child with deafness cannot be expected to find humor and laughter in situations which capitalize on verbalizations and other sounds. Furthermore, deafness results in more concrete behavior and humor is one of the most abstract forms of communication and expression.

The nature of laughter, smiling and crying is complex. However, it is significant behavior from the point of view of differential diagnosis of auditory disorders in infants and young children. Auditory behavior is related to laughing, smiling and crying because children with auditory disorders vary in their ability to laugh, smile and cry. They vary in this respect both in extent and in quality. Some emotionally disturbed children do not laugh, smile or cry. Likewise, the laughing, crying and smiling behavior of the aphasic child is characteristic. This is discussed in the following chapters. The diagnostician will find clinical observation of the child's laughing, smiling and crying behavior to be a significant source of diagnostic information. The crying, smiling and laughing behavior of the child with peripheral deafness is part of the behavioral syndrome of impaired acuity in infancy and childhood.

He is Unduly Sensitive to Movement and Other Visual Clues

Hearing and vision are the primary distance senses. Through these senses the normal child projects himself into space to determine the satisfactoriness or unsatisfactoriness of his environment. Gradually he learns to depend most extensively on his hearing for warning signals in regard to the threateningness or equilibrium of his environment [23]. The organism learns early and naturally that hearing explores the world in all directions simultaneously. The environment can be surveyed and scanned continuously through hearing, while vision is focused on those activities which are in the foreground of attention. While the psychology of hearing in early life remains to be studied extensively, the psychology of deafness assumes awareness of this highly significant function of the sense of hearing. Normally, hearing and vision function in a harmonious, reciprocal manner, but each has its major responsibility relative to the welfare of the individual. Hearing is the primary source of contact with the environment and, apparently, can be relied upon as the most generally effective warning sense. It generates security of relationship and well-being.

The child with impaired acuity has only one distance sense, which is vision. He must use his vision both for purposes of scanning and of contact with his environment. Vision is the only sense which he can use projectively and it seems less satisfactory than hearing for purposes of contact and exploration of the environment. This is critical inasmuch as the child with peripheral deafness cannot use hearing to supplement vision in the same manner that the normal child uses vision to supplement hearing. Vision must serve both foreground and background functions. It must scan the background environment and serve immediate foreground purposes. Furthermore, as suggested previously, vision is directional; it is limited to a more restricted field as compared to hearing. Vision cannot be projected into the dark, through walls or around corners, and it ceases to function during sleep. Regardless of these limitations of vision as an exploratory sense it is the sense on which the child with peripheral deafness must rely. He must use his vision for both exploratory purposes and immediate needs. Perhaps no other factor is of greater importance as a source of compensatory behavior in such children. This double function of vision and the child's resultant behavior is uniquely characteristic. For example, as a result of his unusual reliance on vision he becomes unduly sensitive to movement. Movements are his principal source of information and provide clues which are essential for his continuous evaluation of the situation in which he finds himself. He is constantly looking toward and following movements in his attempts to understand and to establish equilibrium with his environment. This means that his behavior is characterized by undue reliance on vision. He will attend to visual clues which the child with normal hearing can ignore. Moreover, the child with impaired acuity is not attentive to movement only, he is sensitive to light changes and shadows because all visual clues are a source of information concerning environment which he needs to maintain security.

Children with such deafness might seem unusually alert. Frequently they are described as being very intelligent because they notice many things that other children do not. This illustrates that the process of looking, of noticing, of continuous visual sensitivity is typical of this child. This process of continuous looking contributes to his motor behavior, which is also characteristic. If his position impedes visual contact he changes it so that he can again see and reestablish more adequate contact with the situation. Such movements are entailed in what parents frequently refer to as restlessness or nervousness. Moreover, seeing alone might not be sufficient; to satisfy his needs and curiosity more fully he needs to supplement his visual impressions with other sensory impressions. In order to do so he must go to the object or person and touch it because his second most useful exploratory sense is the tactual. Therefore, whenever possible he attempts to supplement visual impression with tactual impression, but the tactual sense cannot be used until the object has been located visually. This undue sensitivity visually and generalized behavioral orientation to vision is markedly suggestive to the astute observer. When the diagnostician observes a child who is unduly alert to movement and who, even while playing with an engaging toy, periodically looks up to survey the surroundings, he may consider the behavior as a part of the syndrome of peripheral deafness. It is apparent that such behavioral symptomatology must be corroborated by other findings.

He Attends to Facial Expression

In the pre-speech age normal children are especially responsive to vocal inflection and the facial expressions of the speaker. Vocal quality and facial expression are forms of nonverbal communication and are important conveyors of meaning to both children and adults, even after verbal facility has been established. To the child with peripheral deafness facial expression is a primary source of meanings. Inasmuch as he misses the vocal quality, the inflections, the ranges of intensity, and other tonal characteristics, he must rely on facial expressions for shades of meaning. This causes him to be unduly sensitive to the facial expressions of those around him, although he is unusually responsive to all types of nonverbal expression. He learns to interpret facial expressions as a primary source of security and acceptance and in this respect he seems even more responsive than the normal. Perhaps the normal child relies principally on his hearing for sensing the emotional tone of a given situation. The normal child might have learned that vocal inflection, intonation and intensity, communicate emotional connotations more efficiently than observations of facial expressions. Furthermore, the normal child can use vision to supplement hearing. The child with peripheral deafness compensates for his inability to hear the emotional content of speech by over-capitalizing the visual clues associated with it, especially the individual's facial expression. In early life this is an unconscious, automatic organismic compensation. As the child matures he consciously attends to facial expression and particularly to the speaker's lip movements.

Gradually the child with deafness acquires some ability to comprehend speech by reading the lip movements of the speaker. However, this is not possible until he has acquired a minimum of inner language. Just as the normal child cannot comprehend speech until he has heard it for some time, the child with such deafness cannot comprehend it until he has seen speech for some time. The hearing child must associate meanings with speech sounds and the child with deafness must associate meanings with lip movements. Appropriate and well timed training is necessary to assist the child with deafness to learn to speech read. Moreover, speech reading is not simply reading lip movements. It includes interpretation of many nonverbal clues, especially all facial expressions. Facial expressions become a substitute for inflection, intonation and general vocal quality. To the speech reader facial expression conveys emphasis and emotional tone which is an essential aspect of all communication. This means that the child with deafness becomes increasingly aware that facial expressions are an important source of information.

From the point of view of differential diagnosis, undue attention to facial expression is characteristic of children with peripheral deafness. It is not characteristic of children with other types of auditory disorders. While some aphasic children watch the face of the speaker it is not typical of them. Some emotionally disturbed children rarely look at the faces of those around them and they might even refuse, or ignore, all face to face contact. The child with deafness typically not only attempts to make facial contact, he responds to it. His behavior is influenced by what he perceives from glancing at, and watching, people's faces. This responsiveness is observable and assists in making a differential diagnosis. Such behavioral symptomatology is revealing in regard to the integrity of the entire organism. It is part of the syndrome of peripheral deafness in infants and young children. It provides the diagnostician with significant information.

He Is Unduly Sensitive to Tactile Sensation

The child with peripheral deafness uses his vision in a distinctive manner and this compensatory type of behavior is revealing in regard to the psychology of deafness and of sensory behavior in general. Schilder [24] emphasizes that there are no isolated senses; synesthesia is a basic aspect of perceptual behavior. Sensory impressions are not visual, auditory, or tactual, but are combinations of all three in most experience. Even when a stimulus is only visual, subjective auditory, tactual, and perhaps gustatory and olfactory experience is used in perceiving the visual sensation. That auditory deprivation resulting from deafness causes visual perception to be less effective has been demonstrated [19]. Therefore, increased reliance on vision as an all purpose distance sense by the child with peripheral deafness does not mean that his visual functioning is superior to the normal. However, it does signify that when a sensory avenue is deprived, the remaining sensory avenues serve the organism in a characteristically different manner. Due to his inability to use hearing, the child with peripheral deafness finds it necessary to be peculiarly dependent on his residual sensory capacities. This results not only in undue awareness visually but also in undue awareness of tactile sensation. Normally, hearing and vision function in a highly reciprocal manner. Auditory signals are received and immediately supplemented by visual impression, or, visual signals are received and immediately supplemented by auditory impressions. Lacking this possibility because of impaired auditory acuity, the organism uses vision and tactile sensation reciprocally. For example, the child is engaged in building with blocks. He must use his vision in this foreground activity and in so doing relies on tactile sensations to keep him in contact with his background environment, because when he feels footsteps he looks up to further identify and appraise the environmental circumstances. Such behavior is observable and diagnostically meaningful. Children with peripheral deafness attend to tactile sensations which are ignored by normal children and by children with other types of auditory disorders. It should not be inferred that the child with such deafness has greater capacity to use such sensations. It is the use of his other sensory avenues, his unusual dependence on them which causes his behavior to be qualitatively, rather than quantitatively, different as compared to the normal.

This type of compensatory behavior has significance in revealing organismic integrity. Some children with auditory disorders are not only unresponsive auditorially but they are unresponsive visually and tactually. Some diagnosticians overlook the importance of generalized reduction of sensory responsiveness and in such children make a diagnosis of peripheral deafness. Generalized unresponsiveness is not characteristic of children with such deafness. For example, they typically give undue responses to light tapping on the chair on which they are sitting, to light tapping on the floor, and to other mild tactile stimulations. Emotionally disturbed, aphasic and mentally deficient children often ignore vigorous tactile stimulation. The compensatory sensory responsiveness of the child with impaired acuity suggests normal integrative capacity. He maintains contact with his environment through his residual sensory avenues, and explores and integrates experientially to the extent that his sensory capacities permit. This is in contrast with children having marked emotional disturbances or central nervous system damage.

The compensatory sensory behavior of the child with peripheral deafness is characteristic and this behavioral symptomatology is an important aspect of the syndrome of such deafness in young children. The clinical observations of the diagnostician should include appraisal of the child's responsiveness tactually. Such observations of behavior add significantly to the interpretation of the child's inability to respond to sound normally and serve as an integral part of the process of differential diagnosis.

His Motor Behavior Is Characteristic

As indicated in the history of genetic development in Chapter V, motor development and loco-motor coordination are noteworthy aspects of behavior. Children with auditory disorders vary in their motor capacities and in the quality of their motor performances. Both developmental and qualitative factors of motor functioning are significant to the diagnostician. The child's motor functioning is illuminating whether he is engaging in spontaneous motor activity or whether he is being observed in a more standardized manner, such as during the administration of psycho-motor tests. Diagnosticians frequently do not include clinical observations of motor functioning because they are not familiar with its profound significance. As indicated in Chapter V, studies of maturational motor development by Gesell [8], Bayley [2] and Doll [6] have provided normative schedules which are useful in comparing a child with the normal. Furthermore, the data given in tables 10, 11, 12 and 13 indicate the importance of motor maturational factors in the differential diagnosis of auditory disorders. Children with peripheral deafness were not different from the normal in mean age of sitting or walking, whereas, the children with other types of auditory disorders differed significantly in both sitting and walking. Motor development is a significant indicator of organismic integrity. On the basis of clinical experience and research, marked delay in motor maturation should not be considered as typical of children with peripheral deafness. However, such delay might accompany other types of auditory disorders, especially as found in the aphasic and the mentally deficient. Emotionally disturbed children are not typically retarded in motor development. Aphasic children frequently are delayed in acquiring normal motor function.

In addition to these maturational factors of motor function, there are other characteristic patterns of motor behavior which warrant clinical appraisal. For example, many children with auditory disorders are hyperactive. Frequently, this hyperactivity is extreme and is one of the primary complaints of the parents. The quality of this motor activity is highly revealing because it varies for these various types of children. Some children engage in random, aimless, compulsive movement, their actions lack subjective direction, intent and purpose. They are easily dissuaded momentarily from one type of hyperactivity to another and they are lacking in persistence, even though they are attempting to adjust to their environment. This type of aimless hyperactivity typifies aphasic children, but it does not typify children with peripheral deafness. The motor deviation shown by children with emotional disorders also differs from those with impaired acuity. Their motor behavior is not random but it might be bizarre in rocking, turning, and in other ways. In general, each type of child with an auditory disorder presents a pattern of motor function which is consistent with his etiology and with his organismic adaptation. From this point of view the hyperactivity of the child with peripheral deafness is consistent and meaningful in terms of the limitations imposed by his inability to hear. As indicated previously, this child is primarily dependent on his vision and tactile sense for stimulation and impression. In order to use these two sensory avenues reciprocally he must be active because it is necessary for him to move frequently in order to maintain an optimum visual field. Moreover, he must go to objects before he can touch them, which necessitates a certain level of motor activity. Therefore, when the child with peripheral deafness is viewed as a unitary organism, and not only through his hearing impairment, his motor activity becomes meaningful. It is integrated behavior which is logical in terms of the organism's adaptation. His hyperactivity is not random, aimless and lacking in orientation or subjective direction. It is consistent, meaningful, intentional and persistent. This child wants to explore the situation so he moves to see. Then his curiosity requires further stimulation so he goes to touch and to feel. When he becomes familiar with the situation, such as in the home or in a nursery school, this behavior might be aggressive and relatively incessant. However, it is not behavior which is lacking in persistence and it is not random or dissuaded momentarily. This type of motor activity is observable by the diagnostician and it is decidedly characteristic of children with peripheral deafness.

There are other aspects of the motor behavior of children with impaired acuity. Because they are essentially nonverbal they must use motor activity as a means of communication. It is characteristic that the motor activity of normal children recedes as they acquire speech. Speech takes the place of gross and sustained motor activity because the child can satisfy many of its needs through speech. For example, he can ask "why" and "what" from a distance and does not find it necessary to first attain proximity and then to "act out" nonverbally. However, the child with peripheral deafness does acquire inner language, and he, like children with normal hearing, develops curiosity and has need for trial and error exploration. But he cannot use speech to take the place of walking, running and manipulation. He must continue to explore the world and to communicate through motor activity. In this respect his motor behavior is compensatory in nature because his lack of adequate social and emotional expression is expressed motorically. Moreover, like the normal child, as his ability to form identifications, and to communicate in other ways increases, he finds compensatory motor activity less necessary.

The child with peripheral deafness has another characteristic in regard to his motor functioning. He shuffles and drags his feet when he walks so that his gait is characterized by shuffling. This gait is characteristic long after school age and sometimes continues into adulthood. It might be caused by the inability to hear on the basis of inadequate auditory monitoring. The child does not hear the noise he makes by shuffling his feet and, thus, does not have the normal corrective stimulus to discontinue it. He does not hear that other people do not shuffle when they walk, that his way of walking differs from others. Apparently the normal child, through auditory monitoring, unconsciously learns to walk without shuffling his feet. It is interesting to note that children with peripheral deafness, whether or not they have concomitant vestibular dysfunction, usually have a shuffling gait.

Some children with deafness have severely diminished, or lack of, vestibular function. There is a direct relationship between vestibular functioning and loco-motor balance [18]. If the semicircular canals are non-functional balance will be disturbed. Poor balance sometimes can be observed in children with impaired acuity, but balance tests are useful in determining this type of motor disturbance. Schilder [24] suggests the psychological importance of vestibular functioning. The psychological significance of deprivation of vestibular functioning has not been ascertained. That it is a significant concomitant of peripheral deafness cannot be denied. Careful clinical attention should be given to this problem diagnostically because, perhaps, children with associated vestibular defects have complicating learning and adjustment difficulties. Several studies of motor capacity have been made of school age children and adults with peripheral deafness [15, 16, 18]. These studies are suggestive for making clinical observations in the young child with auditory disorders.

The child with peripheral deafness engages in motor activity which is characteristic developmentally and qualitatively. His motor function is clinically symptomatic in terms of auditory sensory deprivation. It can be contrasted with the motor function of other types of children with auditory disorders. Clinical observations of motor behavior constitute an important source of information in making a differential diagnosis of auditory disorders in infants and young children.

His Social Perception Is Characteristic

Social perception refers to the ability of the child to project himself into his environment and to relate to it. It emphasizes the ability to understand social situations, especially to comprehend what other people do and to behave appropriately. Social perception is characterized by the child's ability to include other people in his world [5]. Some aphasic children with auditory disorders have no shyness. They lack reserve and reticence and they are incapable of perceiving social circumstances or situations. However, these children attempt to relate to their environment socially, whereas, emotionally disturbed children with auditory disorders often ignore the social world. Their behavior is characteristically bizarre in that it does not include relationship with other people. Children with peripheral deafness have characteristic social perception in that their ability in this respect is superior to children having other types of auditory disorders. Therefore, clinical observations of the child's social perceptual functioning is helpful in making a differential diagnosis.

This concept of social perception includes other aspects of the child's behavior. Socialization is accomplished through the internalization of the social controls which the child encounters. In infancy his controls are external because the parents impose restrictions, restraints, expectations and demands. To illustrate, the parents restrict the child's touching certain objects, putting them in his mouth, and from wetting and soiling himself. Gradually these parental prohibitions and admonitions are internalized and the child begins to exercise control of himself. This process of internalizing the parents, and the social forces which they represent, is becoming increasingly pertinent to the differential diagnosis of language and auditory disorders in very early life. The emotionally disturbed child with language pathology is especially revealing in this respect and further discussion of this problem is given in Chapter VIII. The internalization of the social forces in his environment is accomplished by the normal child, to a certain extent, by one year of age but it begins to appear considerably earlier. Between one and two years of age the normal child can use symbols to represent external events and objects. Symbolic behavior, itself, is a manifestation of the internalized environment. When the child sees relationships mentally, when he "puts things together in his mind", when he integrates sensory experience meaningfully, he can be considered to be behaving socially; he has social perception, a concomitant of symbolic behavior. For example, even though he hears no conversation, the child who has been playing on the floor in the diagnostician's office, sees his mother pick up his cap and knows immediately that he is to leave. This type of social perception, this ability to interpret the behavior of others and to make highly appropriate adjustments characterizes the child with peripheral deafness. However, it is rare in other types of children with auditory disorders. Children with impaired acuity internalize their world symbolically, they do acquire an inner language and they do use it for social relationships. This is highly significant in differential diagnosis.

Although the child with peripheral deafness has social perception, this perception is essentially dependent on vision. He must see the social situation in order to adapt to it. Thus his social perception should be expected to differ from the normal even though it is qualitatively superior and different from the emotionally disturbed, the aphasic and the mentally deficient. Social awareness is peculiarly dependent on hearing. Not only for following conversation, the most significant aspect of social perceptions, but to hear all other types of sounds. All sound derives from the environment and is highly social. Sounds of traffic, telephones, dogs barking, trains, airplanes, automobiles, or of the wind, have social importance. They supplement the visual experience of normal children. Inasmuch as the child with peripheral deafness does not have such auditory experience, he behaves on the basis of his partial, incomplete social awareness which he acquires chiefly through vision. His social perception is effective, but it is inefficient as compared to the normal. His social and emotional contact with people is superficial, tenuous, and subject to unusual prerequisites. As a result he remains on the periphery of the social situation [11]. Perhaps, in a compensatory manner, he will withdraw from social participation and engage himself with objects. However, his preoccupation with objects is not compulsive in the manner that is so frequently seen in children with psychic deafness. The child with impaired acuity will forego his objects for social participation whenever these activities are sufficiently rewarding, enjoyable, and satisfying. He participates socially when the social situation is sufficiently visual in nature to be meaningful to him. For example, throwing a ball to him, especially if the examiner exaggerates the activity in a somewhat boisterous manner, often reveals that the child has good social perception when the situation lends itself to his social perceptual capacities.

The social perception of the child with peripheral deafness, irrespective of its limitations as compared with the normal, is a significant indicator of organismic integrity. His social perception is consistent with his sensory deprivation. He behaves integratively and responds to others accordingly. This behavioral symptomatology is observable and it can be compared with other children having auditory disorders. It is an important aspect of the syndrome of impaired auditory acuity.

His Emotional Expression and Development are Characteristic

An increasing awareness of the importance of early life on later emotional adjustment is apparent [3, 7]. There is increasing evidence that, from the point of view of language development, emotional factors during the first year of life are especially pertinent. This is discussed further in Chapter VIII. Clinical observations of emotional factors in children with auditory disorders are an essential aspect of making a differential diagnosis. Many such children present unusual behavior in terms of emotional adjustment. Childhood psychosis, neurosis and infantile behavior problems are encountered frequently. If these conditions are not recognized, and the children examined appropriately, errors in diagnosis will be common. All specialists should make careful observations of emotional factors and make the necessary adaptations in the use of auditory, or other types of tests with these children. Some specialists will find it necessary to refer these children to the clinical psychologist and child psychiatrist. However, the diagnostician having initial contact with the child must first recognize the emotional atypicality which is associated with psychic deafness and with other types of auditory disorders in young children. Trained and skilled observation usually reveals significant differences emotionally between the various types of children having auditory disorders.

The young child with peripheral deafness presents a characteristic pattern of emotional adjustment. That there is a relationship between peripheral deafness and emotional development has been suggested by a number of investigators [9, 20, 22, 26]. These studies have been limited to school age children; however, this research information is useful in clinically evaluating infants and young children with deafness. It is apparent that hearing plays a major role in the process of emotional development. It is a sensory avenue through which affectional relationships are stimulated and maintained. Furthermore, it is the sense through which verbal language is acquired. As indicated in Chapter II, the normal child comprehends verbal language even before he uses speech and as soon as he comprehends language, it serves to integrate his daily experiences. Thereby, the normal child not only hears and comprehends the speech of others, he acquires an efficient system whereby he can "talk to himself." Being able to use symbols effectively in an internal manner, also, aids him in integrating and structuring his experiences. Peripheral deafness precludes the integrating effect of hearing and verbal functioning. However, peripheral deafness does not preclude integration of experience in general. The child is delayed in integration, and the quality of his affectional experience is different, but he does develop emotionally. The aphasic child initially lacks capacity to integrate experientially. His emotional development is reciprocally highly disturbed. Children with marked emotional disorder, likewise, present problems of severe emotional disintegration or lack of normal development. The child with peripheral deafness is not bizarre in emotional development or expression. He might be demanding, fearful, aggressive or submissive, but he is in contact with his environment and, ordinarily, is making an adjustment to it. His emotional expression frequently is immature but not bizarre. Bizarreness usually suggests other problems than peripheral deafness. Even if severe emotional disturbance cannot be diagnostically differentiated from peripheral deafness in a particular child, it is an over-simplification to simply classify the child as having impaired acuity. Furthermore, some such children, after psychiatric treatment, have been found to have normal hearing.

The child with peripheral deafness usually is immature emotionally, but he has otherwise normal depth of emotional tone. He cries sobbingly, he becomes angry and has normally intense tantrums. He is aggressive, defending himself with perseverance. This is especially in contrast to aphasic children and to children with psychic deafness. Clinical observations of emotional factors frequently corroborate other findings. The psychology of deafness as it pertains to the emotional adjustment of very young children has not been established, but information is being accumulated rather rapidly. It is apparent that sensory deprivation such as peripheral deafness results in an altered emotional adjustment by virtue of the sensory deprivation. Such sensory deficiency has its own psychological implications which are different from those deriving from injury to the brain, or from other causes. The behavioral symptomatology varies accordingly.

SUMMARY

The diagnostician begins to observe the child's behavior with the first contact and he continues his observations throughout the history and during the examination. The peripherally deaf child, the aphasic, those with psychic deafness and the mentally deficient all have lack of speech in common; this usually is what prompts the parents to bring their child for diagnosis. But each of these auditory disorders will cause differences in behavior that can be observed and thus are helpful in making a differential diagnosis. Hearing has been called the social sense for it is used mainly to establish social relationships. The normal child is constantly reacting to the intonation of his parents' voices and he identifies himself with them largely through verbal communication. Hearing also affords the normal child his most basic contact with his environment in general. Vision functions only in front of the individual, in the light and while awake whereas hearing functions around corners, behind and in front, in the dark and during sleep. Thus the peripherally deaf child is deprived of one of his primary signaling or warning senses. Hearing and speech are related, therefore presence of speech, no matter how meager, means that the child can hear the spoken word or that deafness occurred after having acquired speech. The child with peripheral deafness does not vocalize for pleasure but he learns to use his voice to call attention to himself. Since he does not hear his own voice it has a characteristic non-melodious quality that can be identified as typical for the child having peripheral deafness. Moreover, this child uses gestures and understands the gestures of others. Since gestures are a form of symbolic behavior their presence means that the child can receive certain sensory impressions and utilize them integratively. This is the main incapacity of the aphasic. The peripherally deaf child uses his residual hearing to respond to loud sounds more consistently than children having other types of auditory disorders. He also uses his residual hearing projectively; he recognizes the relation between auditory sensation and his environment. He laughs less frequently than normal children and his laughter has a characteristic tonal quality. He is unduly sensitive to movement and other visual clues since he is deprived of contact with his environment through hearing. His continual use of vision is supplemented by tactual impressions so the child with peripheral deafness is unusually active, running about and touching things. He cannot hear the spoken voice but he learns the meanings of facial expressions and gradually learns to comprehend some speech by watching lip movements. This close attention to facial expression is not characteristic of children with other types of auditory disorders. Moreover, the child with peripheral deafness is unduly sensitive to tactile sensations; he requires help from other senses to keep him in contact with his environment so he is unduly responsive to footsteps, tapping on the chair on which he is sitting or to being touched. This is in contrast to the aphasic, those with psychic deafness and the mentally deficient all of whom often ignore this type of stimulation. The motor development of the peripherally deaf child is normal for his age and this is in contrast to the aphasic and the mentally deficient who are retarded motorically. A peculiarity of the deaf child's gait is that he shuffles and drags his feet while walking, probably because he does not hear it and therefore does not correct himself. In some children with peripheral deafness vestibular function is deficient and poor balance may be observed. The peripherally deaf child has social perception but it is largely limited to visually perceived situations; however, they are meaningful and well integrated. His emotional development is somewhat delayed and immature but he is not bizarre. A diagnosis of peripheral deafness should not be made on the basis of auditory tests alone. Corroborative evidence should be secured by carefully observing the child's pattern of behavior.

BIBLIOGRAPHY

1. Allport, G. and Vernon, P.: Studies in Expressive Movement. New York, Macmillan, 1933.
2. Bayley, Nancy: The Development of Motor Abilities During the First Three Years. Washington, Society for Research in Child Development, National Research Council, Mono. I, 1935.
3. Bowlby, John: Maternal Care and Mental Health. New York, World Health Organization, Columbia University Press, 1952.
4. Buhler, Charlotte: Testing Children's Development from Birth to School Age. New York, Farrar & Rinehart, 1935.
5. Cantril, Hadley: The "Why" of Man's Experience. New York, Macmillan, 1950.
6. Doll, Edgar A.: Measurement of Social Competence. Minneapolis, Educational Test Bureau, 1953.
7. Gerard, M. W.: Emotional disorders of childhood, in, Alexander, F. and Ross, H. (eds.): Dynamic Psychiatry. Chicago, University of Chicago Press, 1952.
8. Gesell, A. et al.: The First Five Years of Life. New York, Harpers, 1940.
9. —— and Amatruda, C.: Developmental Diagnosis, Ed. 2. New York, Paul B. Hoeber, 1947.
10. Goldstein, Kurt: Language and Language Disturbances. New York, Grune & Stratton, 1948.
11. Heider, F. and Heider, G.: Studies in the psychology of the deaf. Psychol. Monogr. No. I, 1940.
12. Hurlock, Elizabeth: Child Development. New York, McGraw-Hill, 1942.
13. Kanner, Leo: Child Psychiatry, Ed. 2. Springfield, Ill., C. C Thomas, 1948.
14. Langer, S. B.: Philosophy in a New Key. New York, Penguin Books, 1948.
15. Long, J. A.: Motor abilities of deaf children. New York, Teachers College Contributions to Education, Columbia University Press, No. 514, 1932.
16. Morsh, J. E.: Motor Performance of the Deaf. Comparative Psychol. Monog., No. 13, 1936.
17. Mowrer, O. H.: Learning Theory and Personality Dynamics. New York, The Ronald Press, 1950.

18. Myklebust, H. R.: Significance of etiology in motor performance of deaf children with special reference to meningitis. Am. J. Psychol. *59*: 249, 1946.
19. —— and Brutten, M.: A study of the visual perception of deaf children. Acta oto-laryng., Suppl. 105, 1953.
20. —— and Burchard, E. M. L.: A study of the effects of congenital and adventitious deafness on the intelligence, personality and social maturity of school children. J. Ed. Psychol. *36*: 321, 1945.
21. Piaget, Jean: Language and Thought of the Child. New York, Harcourt, Brace, 1926.
22. Pintner, R., Eisenson, J. and Stanton, M.: The Psychology of the Physically Handicapped. New York, F. S. Crofts, 1946.
23. Ramsdell, D. A.: The Psychology of the Hard of Hearing and the Deafened Adult, in Davis, H. (ed.): Hearing and Deafness, New York, Murray Hill Books, 1947, pp. 392–418.
24. Schilder, Paul: Mind: Perception and Thought in their Constructive Aspects. New York, Columbia University Press, 1942.
25. Spitz, R. and Wolf, K.: The smiling response: a contribution to the ontogenesis of social relations. Genet. Psychol. Mono., No. 34, 1946.
26. Springer, Norton: A comparative study of psychoneurotic responses of deaf and hearing children. J. Ed. Psychol. *29*: 459, 1938.
27. Vigotsky, L. S.: Thought and Speech. Psychiatry *2*: 29, 1939.
28. Yerkes, R. M.: Chimpanzees. New Haven, Yale University Press, 1943.

Chapter VII

Auditory Disorders Due to Aphasia

THE AREA OF DIFFERENTIAL DIAGNOSIS OF auditory disorders in young children includes consideration of the problem of aphasia. In early life aphasia is readily confused with other conditions which affect language growth and development. Furthermore, traditional orientation and diagnostic procedure might further such confusion because in the past auditory disturbances have been viewed mainly as deficiencies of acuity. It is becoming increasingly apparent that other types of auditory disorders might simulate deficiencies of acuity and one of these conditions is aphasia. Perhaps aphasia in early life is confused with deafness more frequently than any other condition. Children with deafness have been diagnosed as aphasic, and aphasic children have been diagnosed as deaf. Likewise, aphasic children have been diagnosed as mentally deficient, or as being emotionally disturbed. Erroneous diagnosis and classification of these children is unfortunate. Appropriate training programs for these groups of children are widely different [14]. From the point of view of auditory disorders the child with aphasia presents a substantially different syndrome than the child with peripheral deafness, psychic deafness, or mental deficiency. This chapter is a consideration of the behavioral syndrome associated with aphasia in young children. Auditory tests alone do not provide an adequate and valid basis for differentiating between aphasia and peripheral deafness. Therefore, it is necessary for the diagnostician to make clinical observations and to evaluate the total behavioral syndrome which the child presents. As indicated previously this is an essential step in making a differential diagnosis. However, before discussing the behavioral symptoms of aphasia it is necessary to consider its nature in young children.

143

TYPES OF APHASIA IN CHILDREN

The study of aphasia has been largely limited to adults [7, 8, 10, 16, 17, 23, 25]. Notable exceptions are the publications of Ewing [5] and Orton [18]. While the nature of aphasia in children is different from that which is sustained in adulthood, there is essentially no difference from the point of view of definition and classification. Aphasia is a language disorder which results from damage to the brain. Aphasia literally means lack of speech but this definition is inadequate because aphasia is not basically a speech disorder. It is a disorder in symbolic functioning. It is an inability to comprehend the spoken language of others, an inability to speak, or an inability to use language internally for purposes of thinking to oneself. It must be emphasized that none of these incapacities of the aphasic can be attributed to peripheral defects or to mental deficiency. For example, the inability to comprehend is not due to peripheral deafness, the inability to speak is not due to impairment of the speech mechanism, and the language deficiency itself is not due to mental deficiency. Other clarifications must be made. Some authorities have considered that an essential aspect of aphasia was to have had normal language function and then to have lost it, due to damage to the brain through injury or disease. This position interprets aphasia as a loss of language once acquired; it has added to the confusion of diagnosis of aphasia in young children. Aphasia in children usually is congenital because the condition which results in the aphasia is present at the time of birth. However, the condition might have been sustained prenatally, at the time of birth, or it might have been caused by damage during the pre-speech age. Therefore, although central nervous system damage occurred previously, the aphasia is not apparent until the resultant language disorder can be determined. This is typical of aphasia in children. Rather than sustaining the language disorder after normal language has been acquired, the aphasia is present congenitally, or from very early in life. The child does not lose his language, he does not initially acquire normal symbolic behavior. The concept of aphasia used here includes symbolic disorders of comprehension, expression and of inner language, irrespective of the age of onset. Moreover, it includes various degrees of language disorder. The term aphasia literally means complete inability to use language symbolically. Aphasia of this severity is rare. The term dysphasia means partial incapacity to use language symbolically. Comparable to the term deafness in the preceding chapter, the term aphasia will be used to include all degrees of symbolic disorder.

Aphasia is a disorder in the use of the symbols which constitute language. To illustrate, language is a system of symbols which can be used in place of, or to represent, objects, ideas and feelings. The process of acquiring this system of symbols and its relationship to auditory disorders was discussed in Chapter II. Furthermore, the three major functional classifications of language, inner, receptive and expressive, were shown diagrammatically in figure 2. This functional classification is useful in categorizing different types of aphasic disorders. For example, the language which is used to communicate verbally is referred to as speech and this is expressive language. Thereby, if damage to the brain causes an incapacity to relate the heard symbol (spoken word) to the central motor speech mechanism, expressive aphasia is present [25]. Frequently, such children can comprehend well auditorially but they cannot speak, or can speak only intermittently and inadequately. Their expressive deficiency is not due to defects of articulation because the peripheral speech mechanism might be normally intact. If damage to the brain causes an incapacity to comprehend speech, receptive aphasia is present, because although speech is heard it cannot be interpreted. Such children cannot normally associate meanings with words. Words continue to be empty and meaningless, just as they are initially for the infant before he learns that they have meaning. If damage to the brain causes inability to develop inner language, central, or global, aphasia is present. Such children cannot use symbols for any purpose, including thought. They lack ability to internalize their world symbolically. This is the most severe form of aphasia. It seems to be rare in occurrence but it must be considered in the differential diagnosis of auditory disorders in young children.

It seems pertinent to emphasize further that an aphasia derives from damage to the brain and that it is a symbolic disorder. Lack of speech, or inability to comprehend spoken language are symptomatic of aphasia. However, these incapacities, likewise, are symptomatic of peripheral deafness. Moreover, lack of speech and inability to comprehend auditorially might be due to emotional disturbance rather than to aphasia or deafness. A diagnosis of aphasia is made only when the disorder is due to a central nervous system lesion and only when this lesion has disturbed symbolic behavior. Many children sustain brain lesions without concomitantly sustaining aphasia. For example, some children, as a result of brain damage, have conditions such as dysarthria and central deafness. These conditions should be differentiated from aphasia and they are discussed below. The critical facet of aphasia, remedially and diagnostically, is the disturbance of symbolic behavior. This disturbance affects behavior in a characteristic manner and has far reaching consequences. Symbolic behavior is essentially a human achievement [3, 11, 26]. As suggested in Chapter II, it is the capacity to use words in place of the actual objects, ideas or feelings. These words (symbols) can be used to refer to the past, present or future. This makes abstraction and abstract behavior possible. Disorders of symbolic functioning disturb a basic facet of human behavior.

Several classifications of aphasic disorders have been used by authorities in connection with their work with adults. Comparable classifications have not been developed for aphasic children. Additional clinical experience and research is necessary before types and appropriate classifications can be more satisfactorily evolved. However, for purposes of differential diagnosis of auditory disorders it is possible to classify broadly the types of aphasia that are clinically apparent in young children. The classifications used by Wiesenberg and McBride [25] in their work with aphasic adults is highly useful for this purpose. They used four classifications—predominantly expressive, predominantly receptive, expressive-receptive and amnesic. While all of these classifications are useful in work with aphasic children, the designation of amnesic aphasia can be used only after language functioning has been appreciably established. With this type of aphasia the individual knows what he wishes to say but he cannot remember the words, although he recognizes the correct word when it is given to him. In congenital aphasia this condition can be diagnosed only after the child has acquired sufficient language so the amnesic component becomes apparent. Expressive and receptive aphasic disorders can be diagnosed earlier because of the nature of the symbolic disorders which these conditions include.

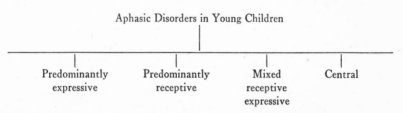

Fig. 4. — Classification of aphasic disorders in young children.

However, specific classification of any type of aphasia usually cannot be accomplished before two years of age.

Another classification is useful in work with young children. This is the designation of central aphasia. Goldstein [7] has emphasized the importance of this classification for adults. Wepman [23], for a similar purpose, used the designation of global aphasia. While its occurrence is relatively rare there are some children who have this severe aphasic disorder to the extent that symbolic functioning is lacking. There is no expressive, receptive, or inner language function as far as can be ascertained. Such children are classified as having central aphasia. The classifications which have been found to be most useful for young children are shown diagrammatically in figure 4. For purposes of reference to the literature expressive aphasia is fundamentally synonymous with motor aphasia and receptive with sensory aphasia.

Predominantly Expressive Aphasia

Children having predominantly expressive aphasia are not frequently presumed to have an auditory disorder. These children respond well to their auditory world. They comprehend language and are in good auditory contact with their environment in other respects. However, because of their inability to speak they are occasionally presumed to have auditory disorders, especially when superimposed involvements, such as emotional problems, are present. In this connection it is important to emphasize that the behavioral symptomatology of the predominantly expressive child differs significantly from the child with receptive, mixed or central aphasia. The child with predominantly expressive aphasia, in general, is considerably less disturbed behaviorally. This is in agreement with the observations given by Orton [18]. Expressive aphasia is symptomatically peculiarly limited to the lack of speech. Unlike other aphasic children, the expressive aphasic child is not markedly disturbed psychologically. In this respect he is not characteristic of brain injured children in general. He is quiet, amenable, and has a good relationship with his environment. He might be exceedingly mute, rarely vocalizing to the extent of using jargon, imitative speech, or echolalia. Frequently he lacks normal facial animation and he might be lethargic and somewhat phlegmatic emotionally. Motor functioning, likewise, usually is superior to children having other types of aphasia. This substantial organismic intactness observed in children with predominantly expressive aphasia is in agreement with the findings of Wepman [23] in the retraining of adults. He has reported that the expressive group attained the highest level of educational achievement. However, the difficulty of developing ability to speak in children with expressive aphasia should not be minimized. Clinical experience indicates that it is a slow, arduous task. Clinical experience, also, indicates that predominantly expressive aphasic children are highly homogeneous as a group, especially as compared to predominantly receptive and mixed aphasics. It should not be inferred that there are no variations in the extent, or degree, of expressive aphasia encountered in children. Some are lacking in ability to speak while others have minimal disability which is not readily determinable. Intermittent ability to use words, phrases, or sentences is common and frequently symptomatic.

Predominantly expressive aphasia apparently is not common in children. Usually more extensive involvements are present. This group will not be considered further inasmuch as these children present a minimal problem in the differential diagnosis of auditory disorders. Moreover, this group does not manifest the behavioral symptomatology which is discussed in this chapter. As indicated below, this symptomatology pertains to the predominantly receptive, mixed-expressive-receptive, and central aphasic conditions, not to the predominantly expressive. In this connection, it seems that the neurological damage sustained by the expressive aphasic child is markedly specific in its effect. The damage sustained by the other groups is characteristically more generalized, affecting the entire organism, not specifically nor as markedly only the language function. There is substantial agreement in neurology that predominantly expressive aphasia results from lesions in Broca's Area, the third left frontal convolution (area 44) [6].

Predominantly Receptive Aphasia

Predominantly receptive aphasia refers to the incapacity to understand the speech of others. Other terms which have been used to designate this condition are sensory aphasia, word deafness, auditory aphasia and Wernicke's aphasia. From the point of view of language pathology the term receptive aphasia is desirable because it emphasizes the nature of the defect, which is inability to receive and to interpret language symbolically. The child with receptive aphasia can hear the speech of others but he cannot comprehend it. The consequences of this incapacity are numerous. Frequently, these children ignore, not only speech, but sounds in general and thereby are presumed to be peripherally deaf. They are typically erratic in auditory behavior. They commonly comprehend a word intermittently and unexpectedly. It is of considerable significance diag-

nostically that there is a direct reciprocal relationship between receptive and expressive language function. Comprehension is possible
without expression. However, except in echolalia, expression is not
possible without comprehension. Therefore, the receptive aphasic
has a reciprocal expressive limitation. Because he cannot understand
what he hears, he has no language for expression. This does not
mean that he is mute because, unlike the expressive, he might use
jargon freely. The general behavior of the receptive aphasic is
characteristically disturbed. On the basis of his incapacity auditorially, and his corresponding lack of speech, he is frequently presumed to have peripheral deafness. Because of this common confusion and the necessity for differential diagnosis a comparative
analysis is made of the behavioral symptomatology of children with
receptive aphasia and children having other types of auditory disorders. There is general agreement in neurology that receptive
aphasia results from lesions in the second and third temporal gyri
(area 41) [6]. Varying degrees of involvement are observed clinically.

Mixed Receptive-Expressive Aphasia

A number of authorities have observed that the most common
type of aphasia seen clinically in adults is the mixed receptive-expressive. Presently, clinical experience suggests that this is true, also, of
children. However, inasmuch as most aphasia in young children is
congenital it is often difficult to differentiate between predominantly
receptive and mixed receptive-expressive conditions. As additional
clinical experience and research are accomplished more specific
statements relative to incidence will be possible. It is apparent, however, that the most satisfactory classification currently for many
children having a receptive component is receptive-expressive rather
than predominantly receptive. This means that more children are
classified as mixed receptive-expressive than in any other category.
The mixed receptive-expressive classification assumes that the child
has sustained brain lesions which have caused both receptive and
expressive aphasias to be present. He cannot understand or produce

speech normally because of defects of symbolization in both respects. The expressive limitation is not due exclusively to the reciprocal effect of receptive aphasic incapacity; rather, a superimposed deficiency of an expressive type is present. Varying degrees of each type of aphasia can be observed in some children. The corresponding relationship between receptive and expressive components should be described when possible because of its importance in remedial training. The behavioral symptomatology of children with mixed receptive-expressive aphasia cannot be differentiated from those with predominantly receptive aphasia. The behavioral symptomatology as discussed in this chapter includes both of these groups and the group with central aphasia.

Central Aphasia

Goldstein [7] has described central aphasia in some detail. This discussion, while it pertains to adults, is provocative in its implications for central aphasia in children. As suggested previously, central aphasia is a severe language disorder. It is characterized by marked deficiencies in both receptive and expressive capacities. Clinically the child seems to be devoid of capacity to behave symbolically. As Goldstein suggests, this severe disorder seems not to derive only from the combined effects of incapacities of reception and expression but from additional involvement; central aphasia is characterized by its disturbance of inner language functioning. To illustrate comparatively, expressive aphasia is an impairment of language used to speak to others, receptive aphasia is an impairment of the capacity to comprehend the spoken language of others, and central aphasia is an impairment of the capacity to use language to communicate with oneself. Goldstein states that this involves a brain lesion which is different from, but usually simultaneous with, those lesions which cause receptive and expressive aphasias. This position, apparently, is in agreement with Vigotsky's [22] statement that inner language is subject to its own laws, which differentiate it from both expressive and receptive language. From the point of view of differential diagnosis, children with central aphasia present marked disturbances of all language functioning and of general behavior. These children have extreme deviations of behavioral symptomatology as discussed in this chapter. On the basis of clinical experience, and as compared to work with adults, central aphasia appears to be more common in children. Perhaps the brain lesions sustained prenatally, or in early infancy, are more often generalized. Children with central aphasia usually can be differentiated from the mentally deficient, the emotionally disturbed and those with peripheral deafness, and clinical observation of behavioral symptomatology is an important step in making such diagnoses. The nature of the language and auditory disorders in these various types of children is significantly different, with concomitant differences in organismic behavioral adjustments and compensations.

OTHER AUDITORY DISORDERS CAUSED BY BRAIN LESIONS

Aphasia is not the only condition resulting from brain lesions that causes disturbances of auditory functioning. Children with other types of central nervous system involvements are seen by the diagnostician of auditory disorders in infants and young children. These conditions include central deafness, auditory agnosia, and disturbances of auditory perceptual functioning. These conditions should be differentiated from peripheral deafness and from other types of disorders but knowledge of these conditions is highly inadequate and definitive clinical experience is meager. However, a brief discussion of these conditions is included as an attempt to emphasize their importance and to clarify their relationship to auditory disorders in young children.

Central Deafness

Central deafness is an inability to hear normally because of lesions in the auditory pathways in the brain. Central deafness is differentiated from receptive aphasia, by definition, on the basis of the site of the lesion. Receptive aphasia results when the primary auditory area in the temporal lobe has been damaged. Central deafness is present when lesions occur at points in the auditory pathways from the cochlear nucleus in the medulla to the temporal lobe. Central deafness is a deficiency in transmitting auditory impulses to the higher brain centers while receptive aphasia is a deficiency in the interpretation of these impulses after they have been delivered. This distinction is useful for clinical and research purposes although it is not possible at this time to describe definitely the syndrome of central deafness. Several authorities have outlined present neurological knowledge of the central auditory pathways [6, 20, 24]. Each ear has auditory nerve fibers leading to both hemispheres of the brain. Therefore, complete destruction of the nerve pathways from one ear would not result in central deafness because the intact pathways from the other ear would transmit auditory impulses to both brain hemispheres. However, the possibility that destruction of the pathways from one ear would influence auditory functioning cannot be denied. The auditory nerve fibers reach the brain stem from the inner ear and end in the cochlear nucleus in the medulla. Here nerve projections join cranial nerve nuclei which provide for reflexive responses to auditory sensations. Other nerve radiations run directly upward through tracts on each side called the lateral lemniscus. There are various interruptions along this pathway but some of the fibers extend upward to the medial geniculate body or to the inferior colliculus. From here the final nerve fibers relay the impulse to the temporal lobe and the specific area in the temporal lobe is referred to as area 41.

Audiometric patterns have not been determined for central deafness. Likewise clinical experience has not revealed a behavioral syndrome because definitive diagnoses of central deafness have not been possible in young children. Inasmuch as central deafness results from injury to the brain it seems probable that these children would be comparable behaviorally to others with brain damage, such as those with receptive aphasia. However, central deafness might result primarily from damage to lower brain areas, such as the medulla or mid-brain and such brain lesions might not be as detrimental to general behavior. Moreover, there are a number of young children who have auditory disorders who are not typical of the known types of disabilities. Perhaps some of these children with advancement of knowledge will be found to have central deafness. For example, some children are seen who have good reflexive responsiveness, even at moderate intensities, but who cannot profit from auditory stimuli in other respects. Because they have symbolic behavior and are in normal contact with their environment in other respects, they cannot be considered aphasic, emotionally disturbed or mentally deficient. Perhaps such children have brain lesions which prevent auditory sensations from reaching the higher brain areas, but these sensations do reach the cranial nerve nuclei and thereby serve the organism for reflexive purposes only. Continued clinical and research evidence from these children can be expected to clarify this problem. All diagnosticians encounter children who cannot be adequately diagnosed and classified. Whenever possible these children should be examined periodically in order to ascertain the nature of their auditory disorder. Central deafness in young children currently cannot be differentially diagnosed, but this should not be reason to ignore it as a diagnostic possibility.

Auditory Agnosia

Another auditory disorder resulting from brain lesions is auditory agnosia. This condition has a substantially longer history of clinical attention than central deafness. Authorities who have discussed the clinical and neurological aspects of auditory agnosia include Head [10], Gardner [6], Wepman [23] and Nielsen [16]. These discussions relate to adults, thus, to the individual who had normal language function prior to sustaining the agnosia. As far as can be determined there is no discussion in the literature concerning auditory agnosia in young children. Clinical experience suggests that this condition occurs in children and, thereby, it is necessary to consider it in making a differential diagnosis. Agnosia literally means lack of knowledge. In clinical diagnosis it refers to a generalized inability to understand the sensations from a given sense modality. Receptive aphasia is the incapacity to comprehend spoken language but ability to interpret other types of auditory stimuli is intact. Auditory agnosia is the incapacity to understand the meaning of environmental sounds in general. For example, such sounds as the ringing of a telephone, an auto horn, or the common sounds associated with the preparation of food, are not interpreted. The auditory world is meaningless. Nielsen states that auditory agnosia can occur without receptive aphasia being present, but, however, that this is rare clinically. Whether auditory agnosia can occur in children without simultaneous receptive aphasia is not known, but clinical experience suggests that it does not. When auditory agnosia can be differentially diagnosed in young children it is a severe condition which includes incapacity to interpret any auditory sensation, verbal or nonverbal. This indicates that receptive aphasia frequently occurs without auditory agnosia but that auditory agnosia does not occur without simultaneous receptive aphasia. Children with auditory agnosia present a behavioral syndrome which is similar to those having central aphasia. From the point of view of auditory capacities the central aphasic is capable of comprehending nonverbal environmental sounds. However, both auditory agnosia and central aphasia are marked disturbances with behavioral manifestations revealing organismic deficiency and deprivation.

Other agnosias commonly referred to in the literature on adults are tactual and visual agnosia. These conditions are the equivalent of auditory agnosia for these respective sense modalities. Occasionally in severe brain pathology, such as might follow encephalitis in children, it appears that agnosias of more than one sense modality occur concomitantly. Such conditions are not necessarily synonymous with mental deficiency because even low grade mental deficiency does not typically imply presence of agnosias. The central lesion which causes auditory agnosia presumably is extensive damage to the auditory cortex, including the general receptive areas for hearing. Gardner [6] suggests that it especially includes association fibers adjacent to the primary receptive areas.

The differential diagnosis of auditory agnosia in children perhaps can be accomplished only when the condition is severe. This condition seems to be rare but it warrants attention on the part of the diagnostician. It is easily confused with other types of auditory disorders. Perhaps the primary differentiating characteristic is the child's ability to note the presence and absence of sound without making any meaningful interpretation of it. Procedures for such auditory evaluation are given in Chapter XI. The history and the behavioral symptomatology provide essential corroborative evidence and the behavioral symptoms discussed in this chapter are pertinent.

Alexia and Agraphia

Some authorities include alexia and agraphia under the aphasias. Alexia is a language disorder in which the individual, although he has normal vision, cannot read; he is incapable of interpreting written words. This condition is analogous to receptive aphasia. In young children it is desirable that the terms aphasia and alexia be differentiated. While alexia might be present it is not possible to so determine until the child is approximately six years of age. However, both are symbolic disorders and might be considered together for purposes of schooling [14]. Diagnostically, aphasia can be determined much earlier.

Agraphia is an inability to use written language although motor functioning is normal. This, too, is a symbolic, or language disorder. Again, this condition should be differentiated from aphasia in children. Like alexia, it cannot be diagnosed until the age at which the child normally learns to write. Ability to copy words does not necessarily preclude the presence of agraphia because it is spontaneous writing which is usually impaired. Alexia, agraphia and aphasia are disorders of different aspects of language functioning and all are due to lesions of the brain. These symbolic disorders apparently are more common in children than has been generally assumed. From the point of view of auditory disorders in young children it is the aphasias which must be differentially determined. The problems of alexia and agraphia are not discussed further although they are significant factors in language pathology.

Disturbances of Auditory Perception

Strauss and Lehtinen [21] have demonstrated the importance of perceptual disturbances consequent to injuries to the brain. Visual, tactual and auditory perceptual functions might be affected. Diagnosis of auditory disorders in young children includes continuous appraisal of visual and auditory perceptual behavior. Auditory perceptual disorders are directly related to the problem of differential diagnosis and visual perceptual capacities are remarkably useful as corroborative evidence. Perceptual disturbances are manifested in behavior and thus are directly related to behavioral symptomatology as discussed below. Clinical evidence suggests that all children with receptive aphasia are not disturbed in auditory perception. Likewise, all children with auditory perceptual disorders are not aphasic. This means that a certain number of young children have disturbances of auditory perception without symbolic language disorders. Such children are encountered by the diagnostician of auditory disorders. The differentiating factor is whether a deficiency of symbolic functioning is present. The child with an auditory perceptual disturbance, but without aphasia, can comprehend the meaning of words when the total auditory world has been appropriately simplified and structured. Because the differential diagnosis between receptive aphasia and auditory perceptual disturbances is complex in young children the distinction is sometimes impractical clinically. Moreover, the behavioral symptomatology is highly similar.

The differential relationship between auditory perceptual disturbances and behavior is discussed under behavioral symptomatology of aphasia. However, a brief discussion is given here of the nature of auditory perceptual functioning. Various workers have shown that while each sensory avenue functions with considerable autonomy, there is a high degree of intersensory behavior [9]. In vision and hearing, especially, there is a reciprocal supplementation perceptually. This relationship has been emphasized in the discussion of the behavioral symptomatology of children with peripheral deafness

(Chapter VI). Study of the organismic behavior of peripherally deaf children is rewarding from the point of view of the psychology of perceptual functioning [15]. Likewise, the study of brain injured children has been fruitful because such studies have revealed that auditory behavior has been over-simplified. Most studies involving audition, including studies using typical auditory tests, have assumed normal auditory perceptual functioning. Therefore, if auditory perception was disturbed the deficiency would have been erroneously attributed to peripheral deafness. An auditory perceptual disturbance precludes normal listening behavior; the child can hear but he cannot structure the auditory world and select those sounds which are immediately pertinent to adjustment.   To illustrate, it is apparent that the environment is comprised of multiple auditory stimuli at all times. It is a primary function of auditory perception to hold a conglomeration of auditory stimuli in the background of attention while selecting other specific stimuli for purposes of immediate attention and behavior. There are many sounds present but only certain ones are pertinent to a given situation.   When auditory perception is disturbed this normal selective process is deficient or impossible; all sounds are of equal importance and make continuous demand responsively on the organism. Therefore, the child, while attempting to attend to all sounds, is incapable of listening to a given sound. Instead of responding to his name he might be responding to a minor noise from the street which is even unrecognized by the parent or examiner. Such a lack of response to a given sound occurs relatively irrespective of the intensity of that sound. Calling of his name might be very loud but the child will respond to an incidental environmental sound of moderate or even mild intensity. This is high-lighted by the insistence of parents that their child will respond to sounds of which they have no prior awareness but he will not respond when called. Because the child's ability to respond auditorially is grossly disturbed he is frequently erroneously presumed to be peripherally deaf. Furthermore, inasmuch as the child cannot respond selectively to the common tests of hearing he might be considered as having impaired acuity, also, by some diagnosticians. Moreover, some of these perceptually disturbed children, to prevent severe distintegration psychologically, learn to ignore the auditory world to the extent that they appear to have severe impairment of auditory acuity. Inability to listen, to give sustained selected responses auditorially, is a characteristic of disturbed auditory perception. Such disturbances frequently are associated with analogous disorders in the area of vision. However, auditory perceptual disorders are not necessarily associated with visual perceptual disturbances, either can occur as distinct from the other. Perceptual disorders are markedly disturbing psychologically and the behavioral symptomatology is characteristic. Many young children having auditory disorders are disturbed in auditory perception. Certain tests of auditory perceptual capacity are discussed in Chapter XI.

Dysarthria

Dysarthria is a condition in which the individual is deficient in normal use of the speech muscles because of injury to the brain. It is a motor deficiency rather than a symbolic deficiency but this distinction has not always been made and there is confusion in the literature accordingly. Dysarthria means partial lack of motor control of the speech mechanism and anarthria means total loss of control. It must be emphasized that this condition does not include malformations or other peripheral defects but results from central nervous system damage. Dysarthria is commonly associated with aphasia in children and when it is present the diagnostician should include a statement concerning it. The primary difficulty diagnostically is to differentiate dysarthria from expressive aphasic components. For example, it is difficult to differentiate between dysarthria and possible expressive aphasic components in children with receptive aphasia. The history and tests of muscular oral functioning are useful in this diagnostic differentiation. In expressive aphasia the condition is symbolic, and therefore the speech muscular system is intact for purposes of chewing and eating. History information is pertinent specifically in this connection. Dysarthria is seen frequently in children with cerebral palsies. It warrants attention diagnostically in connection with auditory disorders because it is a complicating factor and because special remedial procedures are indicated when it is present.

ETIOLOGY AS A DIFFERENTIATING FACTOR IN BRAIN INJURY

As clinical experience and research are increasingly achieved the relationships between types of brain damage and behavior disturbances will be further clarified. Strauss and Lehtinen [21] have compared brain injured children behaviorally with other types of disturbances, but comparison of children having different types and degrees of brain injury remains to be accomplished. However, it is interesting to note that on the basis of clinical experience, etiology of brain injury and behavioral sequelae might be significantly related. Aphasia in children commonly is caused by anoxia, injury during birth and by diseases such as rubella during pregnancy. To these must be added agenetic causes because it is not always possible to find evidence of exogenous factors in children with aphasia. The history might be devoid of such evidence and, furthermore, more than one child in a given family might be aphasic. This suggests the possibility of endogenous factors in some cases. Agenetic aphasia in children has been described by Orton [18]. He described it as a failure of development of certain brain tissues and nerve associations. Agenetic aphasia perhaps occurs with or without endogenous factors being present. Clinical experience suggests that predominantly expressive aphasia might often be due to agenetic development.

As indicated above, the predominantly expressive child differs behaviorally from the predominantly receptive child. This difference might reflect different etiologies with concomitant different brain pathology. Other comparisons can be made clinically. When there is strong presumption of anoxia the child usually presents a problem of generalized effect and deficiencies are noted in motor, perceptual and symbolic behavior. However, when there is a strong presumption of forceps injury the impairment seems to be more specific, perceptual disturbances are minimal and the deficiency might be limited to motor or symbolic functioning. When the brain lesion is due to encephalitis the behavioral syndrome usually differs significantly from the sequelae of anoxia and of forceps type injuries. The behavior of post-encephalitic children has been studied extensively [1, 2, 13]. They are aggressive, impulsive, unstable emotionally and difficult to discipline. Frequently, they are not deficient in inner language and they might perform well on certain tests of intelligence. They might not speak or respond to sound. Peripheral deafness must be suspected, but due to the generalized nature of their auditory disturbance a diagnosis of auditory agnosia often is indicated. If the encephalitic involvement was severe, tactual and visual agnosia also might be present. The presumption is that encephalitis frequently is markedly damaging to lower brain areas, leaving relatively intact the areas which serve cognitive intelligence. Therefore, such children might not present the typical incapacity perceptually and intellectually which so often accompanies other types of brain injury. If the higher brain areas have been affected correspondingly then mental deficiency usually is present, but aphasic components still are not obvious. Research on etiology and its implications can be expected to be rewarding both in terms of diagnosis and therapeutic measures.

The etiology of the auditory disorder is related to the behavior of the organism in other ways. If the auditory disorder is due to peripheral deafness the organism makes different adjustments than when the disorder is due to brain damage, emotional disturbance or mental deficiency. Moreover, each of these groups differs from the other. This is apparent, also, from the data on genetic development as shown in tables 10 through 15. This is the basic assumption of the behavioral symptomatological approach to diagnosis. When such a basic disorder as language deprivation occurs, the organism is forced to make adjustments, and characteristic adjustments are necessitated on the basis of the causative agent. A central nervous system damage is substantially more organismically disturbing than peripheral deafness, therefore, the behavioral symptoms of receptive aphasia differ from those deriving from peripheral deafness both qualitatively and quantitatively. The behavioral symptoms described below apply primarily to receptive aphasia; however, these behavioral sequelae, also, are useful in the diagnosis of auditory agnosia and central aphasia, but they should not be considered as directly related to predominantly expressive aphasia.

BEHAVIORAL SYMPTOMS OF APHASIA IN YOUNG CHILDREN

He Does Not Acquire Speech

The child with receptive aphasia from infancy does not acquire speech naturally. His inability to acquire speech is a primary concern of his parents and it is one of the reasons these children might be presumed to have peripheral deafness. It is significant diagnostically that speech attempts are characteristic of the young receptive aphasic child. These speech attempts are most often in the form of jargon. The vocalizations are not direct attempts to imitate the speech used by others. Even urging the child to imitate results in failure. The child's jargon is spontaneous but characterized by meaninglessness. Therefore, he does not look at an object and make deliberate speech attempts in connection with this object. His jargon is random, occurring as a generalized indication of tension and confusion on the part of the child. However, a word such as "mom" might be used, but such words are used indiscriminately and might refer to food, pets or furniture. Furthermore, when the condition is moderate certain words are used correctly but inconsistently. For example, in a given situation words such as spoon, chair, candy, and bye-bye, might be used, but a moment later the child finds it impossible to use the word again. This is exasperating to the parents, teachers and diagnosticians. Frequently, they erroneously interpret this inconsistency as stubbornness and refusal. This inconsistency is due characteristically to the fluctuating state of the organism in regard to integration and mobilization responsively. Experience in training such children reveals that patience, not urging, often will bring about repeated successful use of language. Occasional meaningful use of words expressively, without ability to do so volitionally, is highly symptomatic of receptive aphasia. It is indicative, further, that gradual improvement can be expected.

Diagnosticians have not capitalized the importance of this type of speech behavior. Parental reports of such speech and clinical observations have been ignored because the child did not respond adequately to tests of auditory acuity. Even in very young children such speech attempts are characteristic of receptive aphasia. Jargon, vocalizing, and use of words, are not characteristic of children with peripheral deafness, emotional disturbance or mental deficiency.

His Vocalizations Do Not Have a Characteristic Tonal Quality

The monitory function of hearing in relation to the tonal quality of the vocalizations produced has been discussed in Chapter VI. This monitory function is not characteristically disturbed in children with receptive aphasia. Although he cannot comprehend speech, he can hear it. He naturally uses the inflection, intonation and pitch patterns with which he is surrounded. Obviously this might not be true of children with more generalized disorders such as auditory agnosia and central aphasia. The receptive aphasic can be expected to manifest vocal tonal quality which does not deviate significantly from the normal.

He Uses Improvised Sounds in a Characteristic Manner but Does Not Use Vocalizations Projectively

Although the child with receptive aphasia might vocalize randomly, and although the vocalizations are normal in tonal quality, his vocal behavior deviates substantially in important aspects. His vocalizations lack directed intent and purpose because they are lacking in normal psychological content. The child with peripheral deafness learns early that vocal projections cause others to respond with attention. The aphasic child typically is highly deficient in this manner. He does not use his vocal capacities to influence others. Such behavior, apparently, involves perceptual and symbolic integration to an extent which is impossible for him. This inability to use his voice projectively, for control of his environment, presumably is reciprocally related to his inability to attend meaningfully to the vocalizations of others; he does not find the vocal utterances of others meaningful, therefore, he does not use vocal utterances meaningfully. This reciprocal relationship is inherent in a symbolic disorder such as receptive aphasia. Furthermore, in this connection, it is suggested that receptive aphasic children apparently do not babble normally. More evidence is necessary but the inability to relate with others auditorially seems to include the incapacity to babble at the expected age, if at all. Moreover, the inability to use vocalizations normally usually includes the play situation. The child does not use typical vocalizations while playing with a train or a toy gun. Such improvisation involves abstractions, percepts and symbolic functioning, which is precluded by the nature of his defect. He not only does not vocalize in his play, the play itself is typically deficient. This is discussed below in connection with social perception.

The diagnostician will find that clinical observations of vocalizations are useful in making a differential diagnosis. A child is not necessarily peripherally deaf because he does not relate to the vocalizations of others. Such relating, or responding, requires a certain capacity to associate meanings with the vocalizations and to integrate these meanings organismically. The receptive aphasic is especially deficient in such capacities. His vocal behavior is observable and can be compared differentially with children having other types of auditory disorders.

He Does Not Use Gesture

The nature and importance of gesture in language behavior has been discussed. Goldstein [7] has discussed disturbances of ability to gesture in aphasic adults. He states that when abstract ability is reduced, the use of gestures increases. This illustrates the observation that gestures are more concrete than verbal language. In children, however, gesture is related to symbolic functioning in general and to inner language in particular. Because the child with peripheral deafness can integrate experientially, he develops inner language, and uses gestures to express himself. Likewise, the predominantly expressive aphasic child might use gestures effectively. The receptive aphasic child deviates singularly in this connection. His receptive capacities are meager so his inner language is reciprocally reduced and he cannot use gestures effectively. His use of gestures varies from complete inability to frequent but inconsistent use. Typically the receptive aphasic is grossly deficient in gesture. His deficiency is not one of refusal but a manifest inability to use gesture as a means of relating to his environment. His inadequate use of gesture frequently includes the inability to understand the gestures of others. Gesticulation is symbolic in nature and requires social perceptual orientation and ability to relate to others in a meaningful way. The receptive aphasic child is particularly disintegrated experientially. He cannot grasp the significance of the gesture because the total situation is lacking in psychological structure and normal content. Therefore, attempts to gesticulate the concept that you want him to play ball with you might be meaningless. His inability to comprehend the gestures of others might be a reciprocal effect of his inability to use inner language and thereby, to relate normally to others. Inner language develops through reception of language.

Clinical observations of the child's use of gesture are revealing diagnostically. The use of gestures has far reaching significance and as a symptom it should be evaluated in terms of a given syndrome. Deficiency of gesture is characteristic of children with receptive aphasia.

He Does Not Respond to Sound Consistently and Does Not Use His Hearing Projectively

Inconsistent responses auditorially have been widely interpreted as manifestations of fluctuations of hearing acuity. Clinical experience with young aphasic children has demonstrated the importance of central nervous system lesions in this respect. Brain injury causes the organism to behave differently in general and thresholds of responsiveness vary greatly, not primarily because of shifts in acuity, but because of the organism's inability to relate and integrate experientially. Therefore, receptive aphasic children are highly variable to all stimuli, including sound. Typically, they respond inconsistently to intensity and to variations in pitch or frequency. For example, they might respond to a mild intensity of a given sound but not respond when this sound is used at higher intensities. Moreover, they might respond to a given intensity once, but not respond to this same intensity even if it is given a great many times thereafter. Their auditory behavior is erratic and is usually described in this manner by the parents.

The aphasic child's inconsistency of response auditorially is explained by the nature of his defect. His responsiveness is a reflection of his incapacity to integrate organismically. In audition this can be described as his ability to listen. Hearing and listening are significantly different. A child might hear but be unable to integrate what he hears. To use hearing consistently assumes ability to integrate and to shift attention selectively in a sustained manner. Such behavior is notably absent or deficient in children with receptive aphasia. This is discussed further in connection with auditory tests in Chapter XI.

The aphasic child does not use his hearing projectively. As indicated previously he does not use his vocalizations projectively. In the same manner, and perhaps for the same reasons, he does not relate his hearing meaningfully to his environment. For example, he might not respond to being called, or to other common sounds, although it is apparent clinically that he responds erratically to sounds of less intensity. He does not use his hearing to systematically scan, and to keep in touch with his environment. Such use of hearing is dependent on integration, normal perception and listening. The aphasic child's auditory functioning is disintegrated and aimless, so it cannot be used volitionally. His entire organism is a victim of the environment; he cannot separate himself from the environment and select stimuli which are meaningful and appropriate to the situation. He responds indiscriminately, with resultant confusion and inconsistency. These disintegrated responses auditorially frequently are interpreted as deficiencies of acuity, especially when inappropriate use of auditory tests suggest such deafness. Clinical observations are an important source of information in this connection. Such observations might be more revealing and more valid than formal tests of acuity. The aphasic child's disintegrated auditory behavior is highly observable to the experienced diagnostician. This behavior is an important aspect of the syndrome of receptive aphasia and it is helpful in making a differential diagnosis of auditory disorders.

His Laughing, Smiling and Crying Are Characteristic

The psychological significance of laughter, smiling and crying has been referred to in Chapter VI in connection with peripheral deafness. These behavioral manifestations are characteristically atypical, also, in children with receptive aphasia because the emotions themselves are notably deficient in depth and quality. When the child laughs or smiles this behavior is lacking in intensity of feeling and reflects insecurity and poor organismic integrity. Likewise, his crying is deficient in depth of emotional content because his cry typically is a whine. Crying rarely is associated with persistence of emotion such as typifies a tantrum. Therefore, laughing, smiling and crying in these children are manifestations of the generalized lack of psychological integrity which accompanies brain injury. Such basic damage to the organism is reflected in generalized emotional inadequacy.

The child with receptive aphasia does not laugh or smile freely. Some such children rarely laugh normally. At times, however, they laugh compulsively, in a defensive manner. Such laughter reflects over-fatigue, over-stimulation, and inability to cope with the situation at hand. It is important to recognize this laughter as a symptom of disintegration in order to assist the child in overcoming the situation more successfully. The aphasic child's laughter does not deviate in tonal quality and thereby, does not suggest inability to hear himself or others laugh. However, his inability to relate adequately to the social situation in order to appreciate humor is obvious. He does not respond even in the concrete manner of the young child with peripheral deafness. It is difficult for him to show amusement because he does not comprehend amusing situations. As indicated previously, humor implies abstraction and imaginative ability. Such behavior is possible for the young aphasic child only after training, greater maturation and development. In early life he manifests in a multiple manner that brain injury which precludes the acquisition of language is a profound deterrent to normal behavior.

The laughing, smiling and crying behavior of the receptive aphasic is characteristic and differentiable by clinical observation from other children with auditory disorders. His behavior in this respect is consistent with the syndrome of brain injury and receptive aphasia. These behavioral symptoms warrant the attention of the diagnostician and emphasize the problem of the aphasic child.

He Is Not Unduly Sensitive to Movement or Other Visual Clues

The child with deafness compensates for his sensory deprivation by using his vision in a unique manner. The child with receptive aphasia cannot compensate for his auditory disorder by unusual application of his other senses. Such application of his other sensory impressions are fruitless because his deficiency is in the central nervous system. His is not a sensory defect, it is an incapacity to use such sensations. This incapacity in the receptive aphasic is rarely limited to the auditory area. Usually there are disturbances of visual or of tactual perception. His general inability to relate to his environment perceptually and symbolically precludes use of his other senses in a compensatory manner. This is not without exception. Through assistance, especially, some aphasic children do use their vision and tactile avenues for exploratory and compensating purposes. However, such use is intermittent, usually erratic and in general quite different from the sustained visual compensation of the child with peripheral deafness.

Receptive aphasic children are highly distractible visually but this is not comparable to the use of vision in a compensatory manner. Rather, these are symptoms of the generalized organismic psychological disintegration which derives from injury to the brain in early life. The diagnostician can observe this inability to use vision in a compensatory manner.

He Does Not Attend to Facial Expression

In contrast to children with peripheral deafness, most receptive aphasic children do not attend unduly to the faces of persons around him. However, some aphasics do make attempts to read the speaker's lips and to interpret facial expressions in other respects, but such use of visual clues is not characteristic. Ordinarily the receptive aphasic is incapable of the sustained attention and social perceptual functioning which are entailed in such compensatory behavior. He is not oblivious to people in his environment and he does attempt to relate to them. Furthermore, he does not avoid face-to-face contact but he cannot use facial expressions significantly as clues for his actions. As a result he does not relate well with others. When a given situation is structured and concretized for him, he does find it possible to integrate experientially and to profit from more subtle social interaction. This is one of the ways in which his behavior differs from the mentally deficient.

The lack of ability to use facial expression, as compared to children with peripheral deafness, is characteristic of the child with receptive aphasia. This inability is related basically to the nature of his disorder. Even direct urging of the attention to the face is unsuccessful. The underlying organismic confusion and disintegration must be alleviated before such functioning is possible. This inability to profit from the use of facial expressions in a compensatory manner is noteworthy and observable clinically, and can be evaluated as a behavioral symptom of receptive aphasia.

He Is Not Unduly Sensitive to Tactile Sensation

The receptive aphasic child is not unduly sensitive to tactile sensation. This, again, is in contrast to children with peripheral deafness. The aphasic child's inability to systematically select and organize experientially greatly impedes his use of all sensory impressions. In this respect there is a generalized reduction of sensory thresholds. He does not respond normally to sound but clinical observation frequently reveals that he does not respond more successfully to tactile sensation. Such comparison of the use of other sensory capacities is highly rewarding in differential diagnosis. The child with peripheral deafness shows compensatory use of other sensory avenues. The aphasic shows a generalized reduction of response to all stimuli; his threshold of responsiveness has been impaired, whereas, generally, his thresholds of sensory acuity are normal. A common diagnostic error is to confuse the nature of the aphasic's central disorder with peripheral deficiencies. Therefore, he is diagnosed as having peripheral deafness without due awareness that his capacity to respond auditorially is determined by the damage to the brain and his auditory capacities are not more deficient than his capacities to respond in other ways.

The aphasic child does not use tactile sensations to keep in contact with his environment. Furthermore, he does not differentiate between background, and the immediate or foreground. He does not use one sense modality to maintain contact with the background while another sense modality is used for foreground activity. Likewise, he is impaired in his capacity to use synesthesia. He is highly dependent on one sensory avenue at a time. Instead of finding supplementary sensory impression beneficial he seems to find it disturbing and confusing. This is logical clinically because the brain damage results in a basic impairment in ability to integrate experientially. Therefore, if sensory impressions are leading in from two or more sensory avenues simultaneously it overloads the organism more than if the sensations derive from one sensory channel at a time. This might explain the receptive aphasic's ability to respond more successfully auditorially when he can be impeded from engaging himself visually, or in other ways. These children are remarkable in their capacity to ignore other sensory stimulation while they are engaged in some activity, irrespective of how aimless the activity might be, and such atypical behavior sensorially is characteristic. It is diagnostically revealing and directly related to making a differential diagnosis of auditory disorder.

His Motor Behavior Is Characteristic

The clinical significance of motor behavior has been suggested previously. One of the most observable aspects of the behavioral syndrome in aphasia is the characteristic motor disturbance. The child with receptive aphasia rarely manifests motor function which is within the limits of normal. Furthermore, his motor development is retarded maturationally. (See tables 10, 11, 12 and 13.) Frequently, it is qualitatively, more than quantitatively, different. His motor coordination is inferior in a generalized manner. Obvious motor impairment such as spastic paralysis is not characteristic; rather, his motor inferiority is an undue awkwardness and clumsiness. He is not especially disturbed in balance but walking, throwing and kicking are poorly executed. Grasping and manual dexterity, also, are inferior. These typical motor problems are apparent by clinical observation but they can be further revealed by psycho-motor tests which are discussed in Chapter XI.

There is another feature of the receptive aphasic's motor functioning which warrants attention diagnostically. His motor behavior is psychologically characteristic. The psychological content of his motor activity is deficient. In contrast to the child with deafness, his motor activity lacks normal subjective direction, purpose and intent. His activity is random in nature and it is easily impeded; persistence of motor activity is deficient. Success of the manipulation, throwing, or running seems inconsequential and there is a generalized incapacity to cope with the environment motorically. Motor activity is present much of the time and compulsive hyperactivity is common, but the motor activity is not deliberate, volitional, intentional and in pursuit of a goal. It is characterized by superficiality; it reveals attempts to manipulate and to relate to the environment, but it manifests only spasmodic or accidental successes. This generalized inadequacy of the motor functioning is highly characteristic.

The central nervous system involvement of the receptive aphasic ordinarily includes some impairment of motor capacity. This impairment is further characterized by the inferior psychological integrity.

This motor behavior is a significant aspect of the syndrome of receptive aphasia. It reveals contrasting behavioral symptomatology between children with peripheral deafness and children with aphasia. Furthermore, it is differentiable from children whose auditory disorders are due to emotional disturbance or mental deficiency.

His Social Perception Is Characteristic

The social perception of children with receptive aphasia is characteristic. The nature of social perception has been indicated in Chapter VI. It includes the ability to psychologically organize and to relate to a given situation. Appropriate adjustments to the persons present is a substantial factor in social perception. For example, when a young child encounters strangers it is normal and appropriate to behave with shyness and reticence and children with peripheral deafness do behave in this manner. The child with receptive aphasia, on the contrary, often makes little distinction between friends and strangers. He is characteristically lacking in shyness and social decorum and might approach the diagnostician immediately by being momentarily attracted to his tie, pencil or other details, without reacting appropriately to the social situation as a whole. Other aphasic children react in a different way, but in a manner which reveals incapacity to cope with the social situation perceptually and conceptually. In general, ability to engage in typical play activities is grossly inadequate.

There are various factors involved in the aphasic child's deficiency in social perception. A basic factor seems to be his inability to normally identify with his parents. Such inability might derive from his symbolic disorder and resultant incapacity to internalize his environment. Social perception is to a considerable extent the internalization of environmental social forces. Furthermore, it entails ability to perceive and to react to many cues and subtleties simultaneously. The receptive aphasic's language and integrative deficiencies make such behavior difficult and sometimes impossible. It is simultaneity of sensory and perceptual functioning which is characteristically lacking in the brain injured child with receptive aphasia and social perception is dependent on such simultaneity. The normal child uses background sounds, all stimuli from the visual field and language reception and expression simultaneously to direct his behavior in a given social situation. The receptive aphasic cannot use language even in isolation from other stimuli, he is deficient in his capacity to integrate other sensory impressions and perceptual synesthesia and simultaneity are grossly disturbed. His social perception reflects this generalized disturbance. Clinical observation of his social perceptual functioning is corroborative of other findings. His behavior auditorially requires validation by this type of evidence in order to differentiate his problem from other types of auditory disorders.

His Emotional Expression Is Characteristic

Damage to the central nervous system is directly related to disturbances psychologically. The emotional development of the young aphasic child might be reciprocally retarded with his language. Such psychological processes as identification, projection, internalization, perception and conception are notably disturbed in these children. The importance of normal symbolic development to emotional factors has not been generally recognized. However, the receptive aphasic child is not only retarded in emotional development, and, thereby, simply emotionally immature. He lacks certain basic means of developing and of expressing his emotions. He is severely deficient in language and cannot compensate for this deficiency. He does not comprehend words and cannot use word substitutes. This greatly impedes his emotional development and his emotional relationships with other persons.

From the point of view of clinical observations this is revealed by a superficiality of emotional tone. The receptive aphasic child lacks depth of feeling, strength and persistence of his emotions. He is not bizarre emotionally because his emotions usually are appropriate but they lack heartiness and integrity. His emotions reflect the organismic confusion, insecurity and weakness which derive from damage to the central nervous system. He expresses feelings appropriately through crying, laughing and anger, but his emotional outbursts are weak and lacking in intensity. In this respect he differs significantly from children with peripheral deafness and from children having auditory disorders due to emotional disturbance.

Goldstein [7] and Strauss and Lehtinen [21] have emphasized a special aspect of the emotional disturbance of persons having injury to the brain. This characteristic emotional reaction was referred to by Goldstein as catastrophic behavior. This is a sudden emotional reaction characterized by psychological disintegration and accompanied by such emotional manifestations as uncontrollable weeping, screaming or laughing. Both Goldstein and Strauss mention the intensity of these emotional outbursts. While catastrophic behavior is common in young aphasic children, it is rarely of severe intensity, or aggressive in nature. Rather, it reflects considerable disintegration and incapacity to cope with the circumstances even with anger or aggression. The catastrophic behavior itself, apparently, is an organismic protective reaction. By this reaction the child can reject oncoming stimuli rather completely and, thereby, again establish relative equilibrium with his environment. This behavior occurs mainly when the child has been subjected to tasks and situations which require greater integrative capacities than he possesses. Catastrophic behavior is not characteristic of other types of children having auditory disorders. It is clinically recognizable and symptomatic.

He Has Disturbances in Visual and Auditory Perception

The importance of auditory perceptual disturbances in the differential diagnosis of auditory disorders in young children has been discussed previously. These deficiencies are common in children with receptive aphasia. This is significant diagnostically inasmuch as this deficiency is not characteristic of children with peripheral or psychic deafness. Some mentally deficient children are disturbed in auditory perception. Disturbances of visual perception, likewise, are characteristic of receptive aphasic children. They can interpret visual stimuli only when they are sufficiently outlined, simplified and segregated from a conglomerate visual field. Perceptual disorders are not synonymous with symbolic incapacities. The aphasic child is limited in his ability to select stimuli which are appropriate to his needs and he frequently mis-perceives objects or sounds. For example, he might engage in examining a spot on a ball instead of perceiving it as an object to play with. Likewise, he might engage himself in looking at a button on the diagnostician's coat rather than perceive that he is to respond to sounds being produced.

The receptive aphasic's characteristic perceptual disturbances result in fleeting fluctuations of attention, marked hyperactivity, confusion and bewilderment. Unless this behavioral symptomatology is recognized and the child managed accordingly, his responses to auditory stimuli are generally meaningless. This is discussed further in connection with auditory test results in Chapter XI. The child's inappropriate behavior, reflecting his inability to function normally in regard to visual and auditory perception usually is observable clinically and warrants careful differential evaluation diagnostically.

He Is Echolalic

Some children with receptive aphasia are echolalic. Echolalia is the automatic and immediate imitation of the speech of others without ability to comprehend it. Other descriptive terms which have been used for this phenomenon are "parrot speech" and "echo speech." Echolalia is not voluntary imitation; rather, when echolalia is present the child usually finds volitional imitation impossible. To illustrate, if the examiner says "Throw the ball," the child immediately says "Throw the ball," without knowing the meaning of the words. Then if the examiner urges the child to "say ball," the child repeats "say ball," without ability to grasp the meaning of the instruction and to volitionally imitate the word "ball". There is substantial variation in the extent of echolalia present. In some children it is marked but in others it is so mild that careful observation is required to detect it. As a behavioral symptom it is a significant indicator of auditory disorder. Children with peripheral deafness are not echolalic; however, occasionally it is confused with symptoms of deafness.

As a symptom of language pathology due to lesions in the brain, echolalia is a provocative phenomenon. In instances of extreme echolalia, the entire language process is intact with the exception of comprehension. The child receives and expresses verbal language but cannot associate meanings with the symbols. Another factor must be emphasized. The imitation lacks intention and volition; therefore, the child is a victim of circumstances, repeating the heard speech in an automaton manner. The problem is complex because similar echolalic behavior is associated with severe emotional deviations such as infantile autism. This is discussed in Chapter VIII. The neurological involvements resulting in echolalia have not been well defined. Goldstein's [7] discussion of echolalia in brain injured adults is pertinent in this connection. From the point of view of auditory functioning and the central nervous system, echolalia reveals that auditory impulses might be delivered to the brain and that these impulses can be related to the central speech mechanism without being interpreted. The suggestion is that brain areas which receive sounds and transmit them into verbal speech have not been damaged, but areas which make it possible to relate auditory symbols to experience are defective.

Because echolalia is not well understood and because it is readily confused with other symptoms, it has not been used extensively as a symptom of auditory disorder, but it is observable and relevant to differential diagnosis.

He Is Perseverative, Distractible and Disinhibited

The atypical behavioral syndrome which accompanies brain injury in adults has been emphasized by Goldstein [7], Wiesenburg and McBride [25], and Wepman [23]. Strauss and Lehtinen [21] and Doll [4] have stressed this syndrome in children. From the point of view of psychological manifestations of brain injury in children, perhaps the most significant clinical symptoms are perseveration, distractibility and disinhibition. The young receptive aphasic child's behavior is highly characterized by this syndrome. Perseveration means performing an activity over and over again without intent and purpose and the activity is performed without regard to needs or circumstances. Distractibility is the incapacity to maintain sustained attention to an activity and it is characterized by fleeting attention to minor details without attention to major aspects. This distractibility is manifested toward objects, such as toys, and in social situations. Disinhibition is incapacity to normally restrain distractions from within. This is revealed by the child's inability to restrain himself from erratically pursuing his impulses to look out the window, go to another child, vocalize, run to the door, and many others, in spite of the situation or circumstances. Although perseveration, distractibility and disinhibition are common in all young children, it must be emphasized that this syndrome in the receptive aphasic child usually far exceeds expectations for the normal. Moreover, this behavior is highly significant in terms of the differential diagnosis of auditory disorders in early childhood. This is discussed, also, in terms of the clinical examination in Chapter XI. From the point of view of behavioral symptomatology this syndrome does not occur in children with peripheral deafness. Likewise, it differs in extent and in quality from children with psychic deafness and mental deficiency. Psychological disintegration such as is manifested by this syndrome is directly related to receptive aphasia. The assimilative, organizing and integrating capacity of the organism has been disturbed. The organism cannot forego the environment, nor can it assimilate and internalize it. The organism is psychologically suspended and thus in a compulsive manner continues attempts to establish equilibrium. Inasmuch as these attempts are basically unsatisfactory the syndrome of perseveration, distractibility and disinhibition occurs, apparently on a preservation of the organism basis. The organism prevents more disastrous disintegration, or annihilation by the development of these symptoms. To illustrate, if the child continues an activity unduly, such as is seen in perseveration, he finds it unnecessary to expose himself to a new activity which might be more difficult to relate organismically. Likewise, distractibility prevents more serious disintegration resulting from inability to structure and to select appropriate stimuli, because distractibility is continuous erratic scanning without ability to relate meaningfully. Disinhibition is continued attempts at integration. Sensations from within cannot be adequately integrated experientially. Therefore, they continue to come into the foreground of attention in order to give the organism repeated opportunity to make attempts at assimilation. Piaget [19] has discussed similar concepts in relation to the development of intelligence in normal children. May [12] has indicated the relationship of such behavioral manifestations to anxiety because similar psycho-dynamics occur without central nervous system impairment. However, this behavior in receptive aphasic children is remarkably symptomatic. Like other behavioral manifestations it must be related to the total syndrome as it is revealed by all of the steps in the differential diagnosis. Clinical observation of the behavioral symptomatology of these children is especially necessary because they are often incapable of the level of cooperation which is necessary for more formal evaluation procedures.

SUMMARY

Aphasia is a language disorder which results from damage to the brain. It is a disorder in symbolic behavior with inability to comprehend speech (receptive aphasia), inability to use speech (expressive aphasia) or inability to use language for any purpose (central aphasia). Children with expressive aphasia have a good relationship with their environment and typically respond normally to sound. Receptive aphasia, the inability to interpret the verbal language symbols, is more common than pure expressive aphasia and it is frequently mis-diagnosed as peripheral deafness. Being unable to comprehend the significance of speech sounds these children often ignore speech and other types of sound, hence are presumed to be deaf. Mixed receptive and expressive aphasia is common and the behavioral disturbance which results is not distinguishable from the receptive. The young child with predominantly receptive aphasia does not acquire speech. He attempts to use sound by engaging in meaningless jargon but he cannot use a particular sound as a symbol for a particular object. If the aphasia is moderate he may use names for objects correctly at times but a moment later he cannot repeat the name of the object. This inconsistency is characteristic and usually indicates a favorable prognosis. The jargon of the receptive aphasic while meaningless has good tonal quality in contrast to the vocalizations of the peripherally deaf child. However, he does not use his voice to call others and he does not vocalize for pleasure during play. He does not gesture since gesture is a form of symbolic behavior and he does not comprehend gesture normally. His response to sound characteristically is erratic and inconsistent; he may respond to a sound of mild intensity once but not when it is repeated even though it is made much louder. His auditory function, like his other sensory functioning, is disintegrated and results in inconsistency and confusion behaviorally. His laughing and crying are deficient in intensity of feeling, manifesting emotional inadequacy. Most often his laughter reflects over-fatigue, over-stimulation and inability to cope with the situation at hand. He is not unduly sensitive to movement or other visual clues, is not attentive to facial expression and is not unduly sensitive to tactile sensations; usually he is equally insensitive to all sensory stimulation. The motor development of the receptive aphasic child usually is retarded and his motor coordination is inferior, showing clumsiness in walking, throwing and kicking. Moreover, his motor activity lacks direction, purpose and intent; it is random, easily impeded and distracted. He is deficient in social perception making little distinction between friends and strangers; shyness may be lacking. His emotional development is not only retarded but lacks depth of feeling and intensity. A special aspect of his emotional reaction, known as catastrophic behavior, consists of uncontrollable weeping, screaming or laughing and occurs mainly when the child is confronted with tasks and situations requiring greater integrative capacities than he possesses. Disturbances of visual perception often accompany disturbances of auditory perception and are manifested through fluctuation of visual attention, confusion and apparent bewilderment. Some receptive aphasic children are echolalic; the child repeats phrases in a parrot-like manner without comprehending their meaning. The aphasic child shows perseveration, distractibility and disinhibition. Perseveration means performing the same activity over and over again without intent and purpose and without regard for environmental needs. Distractibility is the incapacity to maintain sustained attention to one activity with fleeting attention to irrelevant and minor details. Disinhibition is the inability to restrain himself normally; he erratically pursues impulses to look out the window, run to the door or go to another child without regard to the situation or circumstances. Perseveration, distractability and disinhibition are common to a certain degree in all young children but are greatly exaggerated in most receptive aphasic children. These three symptoms show failure in structuring and resultant psychological disintegration when the child is confronted with multiple sensory stimuli. This behavioral symptomatology of the receptive aphasic child is markedly different from the peripherally deaf child.

BIBLIOGRAPHY

1. Bender, L.: The Goodenough Test in chronic encephalitis in children. J. Nerv. & Ment. Dis. *91*: 277, 1940.
2. Bond, E. D. and Appel, K. E.: The Treatment of Behavior Disorders Following Encephalitis. New York, Commonwealth Fund, 1931.
3. Cassirer, Ernst: An Essay on Man. New Haven, Yale University Press, 1951.
4. Doll, E. A.: Neurophrenia. Am. J. Psychiat. *108*: 50, 1951.
5. Ewing, A.: Aphasia in Children. New York, Oxford University Press, 1930.
6. Gardner, Ernest: Fundamentals of Neurology. Philadelphia, Saunders, 1948.
7. Goldstein, Kurt: Language and Language Disturbances. New York, Grune & Stratton, 1948.
8. Granich, Louis: Aphasia. New York, Grune & Stratton, 1947.
9. Harris, J. D.: Some Relations between Vision and Audition. Springfield, Ill., C. C Thomas, 1950.
10. Head, Henry: Aphasia and Kindred Disorders of Speech. London, Cambridge University Press, 1926, vols. 1 and 2.
11. Langer, S.: Philosophy in a New Key. New York, Penguin Books, 1942.
12. May, Rollo: The Meaning of Anxiety. New York, The Ronald Press, 1950.
13. Myklebust, H. R.: Significance of etiology in motor performance of deaf children with special reference to meningitis. Am. J. Psychol. *59*: 249, 1946.
14. ———: Aphasia in children. J. Exceptional Child. *19*: 9, 1952.

15. —— and Brutten, M.: A study of the visual perception of deaf children. Acta oto-laryngol., Suppl. 105, 1953.

16. Nielsen, J. N.: Agnosia, Apraxia, Aphasia, Ed. 2. New York, Paul B. Hoeber, 1946.

17. Ombredane, André: L'Aphasie. Paris, Presses Universitaires de France, 1951.

18. Orton, S. T.: Reading, Writing and Speech Problems in Children. New York, W. W. Norton, 1937.

19. Piaget, Jean: The Origins of Intelligence in Children. New York, International Universities Press, 1952.

20. Spiegel, E. A. and Sommer, I.: Neurology of the Eye, Ear, Nose and Throat. New York, Grune & Stratton, 1944.

21. Strauss, A. and Lehtinen, L.: Psychopathology and Education of the Brain-Injured Child. New York, Grune & Stratton, 1947.

22. Vigotsky, L. S.: Thought and speech. Psychiatry 2: 29, 1939.

23. Wepman, J.: Recovery from Aphasia. New York, The Ronald Press, 1951.

24. Wever, E. G.: Theory of Hearing. New York, Wiley, 1949.

25. Wiesenburg, T. and McBride, K.: Aphasia. New York, The Commonwealth Fund, Division of Publications, 1935.

26. Yerkes, R. M.: Chimpanzees. New Haven, Yale University Press, 1943.

Chapter VIII

Auditory Disorders Due to Psychic Deafness

SOME YOUNG CHILDREN DO NOT USE THEIR auditory capacities because they are emotionally disturbed. Such children have psychic deafness. There are various types and degrees of this involvement. Some children are grossly disturbed emotionally with extensive incapacity to function auditorially. Others have minor disturbances with auditory incapacities limited to specific situations. Before discussing the common types of emotional disturbances which are related to psychic deafness in children, it is necessary to consider the relationship between auditory behavior and emotional development in normal children.

In Chapter II it was suggested that both sensory and psychological avenues must be functioning adequately in order for the child to develop language normally (see fig. 1). In children with psychic deafness it is the psychological avenues which are impaired. The psychological significance of hearing in young children has not been generally recognized. With the increasing awareness of the significance of very early life to later emotional development the importance of hearing is becoming clarified. Furthermore, it is increasingly apparent that auditory functioning, especially in young children, cannot be disassociated from the child's general responsiveness because emotional disturbance will be reflected in organismic changes, including shifts in sensory behavior. As stated previously, hearing is a primary sense for purposes of maintaining contact with the environment. Ramsdell [19] first emphasized this aspect of the psychology of hearing in connection with deafened veterans. Hearing is the distance sense which serves the organism in a continuous scanning manner. It provides the organism with mandatory environmental contact under normal circumstances. This is significant in connection with emotional disturbances because emotional disturbances derive from conflict between the organism's inner requirements and external demands of the environment. When this conflict reaches certain proportions the organism compromises by relinquishing at least part of its contact with the environment and a highly significant manner in which this can be achieved is to relinquish use of hearing. This type of compromise has many advantages from the point of view of resolving, although unsatisfactorily, the conflict which exists. For example, it is not as necessary to relinquish vision because simply closing the eyes will serve to sever visual contact with the environment. Whereas, the ears cannot be closed except through relinquishing their use. Furthermore, if hearing is relinquished, closing the eyes can be used in addition at times of extreme psychological distress.

The function of hearing as a primary source of sensory contact environmentally is not the only way in which it forbodes emotional problems. It is the sense through which verbal language is acquired. Speech is the fundamental means of establishing contact with people, and people are the major part of the environment, especially for infants and young children. Perhaps one of the most apparent oversimplifications in the past has been the tacit assumption that the child would use his hearing and acquire language irrespective of the psychological climate. Clinical experience with children having psychic deafness denies this assumption. Moreover, research is being accomplished which relates directly to this problem. Such work includes studies by Spitz [21], Bowlby [3], Mowrer [16] and Gesell [8]. These studies are in agreement in suggesting that psychological factors, especially between six and twenty-four months of age, are markedly significant in the development of speech. The psychology of language development and the psychology of hearing, while not synonymous, are related. When language development is impeded by psychological factors, hearing is one of the avenues through which this impairment is sustained. Mowrer stresses that unless speech sounds are reacted to as "good" sounds, the child will be impeded in his acquisition of speech. This highlights the nonverbal psychological aspects of the speech sounds themselves. Any sound might be frightening and otherwise threatening to an infant. In order for speech sounds to be pleasant and generally satisfying experientially they must be associated with individuals who are affectionate, warm, accepting and sympathetic. For example, Spitz has shown that normally, between three and six months of age, the infant smiles, babbles and gurgles at any human face because the face has become associated with comfort and well-being. After six months of age the child differentiates between faces. This is one of the child's earliest perceptions. If the child does not associate sound with the comfort and well-being which normally derives from the parents he might be impeded in the use of his auditory capacities and in the acquisition of speech. Use of his hearing is reciprocally related to general psychological well-being. This is further emphasized by Mowrer's finding that talking birds do not learn to talk until they have become pets. Similarly the child must find his environment friendly, accepting and lacking in threateningness if he is to relate favorably to speech sounds. Such relating in a psychological sense implies identification. For the child to use his hearing and to develop verbal language he must feel that he is integrally related to his parents and that speech sounds have autistic value accordingly. Perhaps, in other words, if infants are not made to feel that they are "pets", they cannot develop normally in regard to language. It is necessary to recognize in this connection that threateningness psychologically derives freely through speech. Before the infant can comprehend verbal symbols, speech is used to scold, reprimand and inhibit. This is seen in connection with eating and sleeping, when a mother says, "You cannot have any more milk because you spilled," or, "Now you go to sleep, you bad girl." Such use of language with infants, perhaps, is not unusually damaging except when it reflects and is associated with genuine feelings of rejection on the part of the mother. The child reacts primarily to the psychological dynamics and associates the spoken language with these dynamics.

As the child increasingly learns to use verbal language, especially between twelve and twenty-four months of age, other threats might occur. This is the age at which a great deal of restraining is done through language and toilet training is stressed, with concomitant use of language to influence the child. Moreover, this is the period during which many "No, No" commands are used. In some respects it might be described as a period of scolding and nagging for many children. It is a critical age, also, from the point of view of language development. Normally, the child is acquiring a verbal vocabulary rapidly because this process of symbolic development, the internalization of the environment, is paramount between one and two years of age. Clinical experience indicates that many children develop psychological difficulties in connection with hearing and speech during this time. On the basis of clinical experience, the peak of these difficulties occurs between the ages of eighteen and twenty-four months. This is discussed further below in connection with childhood schizophrenia.

Scolding and nagging the child obviously does not cause the child to relate hearing and speech to pleasant and satisfying contacts with other persons. In certain instances, there are even more overt threats. Some children are told to be quiet and not speak again for a period of time. Others are told that if they say a certain word, or phrase, they will be "slapped" or punished in other ways. This is an obvious example of how the acceptance of hearing and speech results in emotional conflict. Moreover, a young child cannot differentiate between words that are acceptable and words that are not, so in order not to be rejected for the use of specific verbalizations he must generalize and relinquish use of words completely. An effective way to do this is to relinquish use of his hearing. Sometimes he might relinquish hearing of speech only and retain use of his hearing for nonverbal sounds. More frequently he again generalizes and relinquishes his hearing for all sounds at least to some extent. This concept of the threateningness of speech emphasizes that verbalization can be a weapon which is used against the child. The child learns to fear this weapon because it becomes a primary source of anxiety. Moreover, according to dynamic psychiatry, anxiety derives not only from the threatening situation itself, such as fear of speech because it is a weapon which is used against them, but even greater fear might be aroused by the desire to fight back [6]. In this instance, the child might fear the use of hearing and speech as a weapon with which to fight back and, thereby, cause his rejection to be intensified.

The study of psychogenic deafness in adults and in adolescents is related to psychic deafness in children. Etiology, means of detection and therapy might differ, but study of adults assists in clarifying the problem in children. All psychogenic deafness is essentially defensive in nature. The organism's endurance, tolerance and survival are challenged. Defensive measures are used in a compensatory manner in an attempt to assure self-preservation. Such behavior is not volitional, it is unconscious and organismically motivated. Pearson [17] gives two cases, both adolescents, of partial deafness due to psychological conflict. In one case the child's mother scolded a great deal and made contradictory statements. The child felt rejected and in order to avoid intense anxiety, she learned not to hear what her mother said. This reaction became generalized so she had difficulty in hearing what anyone said. In the other case there was much argument and disagreement between the parents. When arguments ensued the parents made statements which they did not wish to have repeated. When the child referred to these statements they denied them and said she was lying. The child reacted by attempting to convince herself that she had not heard the comments and this necessitated actually not hearing. These illustrations are meaningful in terms of the psychology of hearing and speech development in infants and young children. It is becoming increasingly clear that in order for the child to use his hearing normally, the sounds he hears cannot be unduly threatening. Frequently parents are greatly concerned that the child not see what is "bad", but comparatively little attention has been given to what the child hears. Sounds should be "good", but foster acceptance of reality through relief and satisfaction. Undue use of speech in discipline, punishment and restraint can be expected to be influential in the use of hearing and in the development of speech. The psychodynamics of auditory behavior in early life is directly related to the problem of differential diagnosis of auditory disorders.

TYPES OF EMOTIONAL DISTURBANCE

There are types of peripheral deafness and types of aphasia. There are, also, types of emotional disturbance. A child with psychic deafness, even in very early life, is not simply atypical psychologically. Rather, his emotional disturbance will be characterized by certain patterns of behavior and these patterns comprise his symptoms. As in other areas of diagnosis and therapy, the symptoms are used as a basis of diagnosis and classification. To illustrate, some children with psychic deafness are extreme deviates, bizarre, withdrawn and out of contact with their environment, while others are aggressive and dominant. Children presenting these dissimilar patterns of behavior, in general, have different emotional problems quantitatively and qualitatively. However, some types of emotional disturbances are associated with psychic deafness more frequently than others. Only the most common are included for discussion. It is apparent that this consideration of emotional disturbances in children is limited to the language and auditory aspects. The discussion, furthermore, is in terms of the problem of differential diagnosis.

Childhood Schizophrenia

Schizophrenia has long been known as a mental illness occurring primarily in youth or early adulthood. Despert [5], Bender [1], Lourie [14], and Pearson [18] have emphasized the nature and etiology of schizophrenia in young children. In this connection Pearson [17] makes the observation that all psychotic behavior in children usually is designated as schizophrenia, although the psycho-dynamic processes might be different from those associated with schizophrenia in adulthood. He makes another observation which is especially pertinent to auditory disorders in emotionally disturbed children. He observes that schizophrenic children almost invariably have a history of extreme fear of sounds during infancy. This is in agreement with clinical experience with such children when psychic deafness is present. Perhaps the greatest number of children having auditory disorders which derive from severe emotional disturbances in early life are those who are designated as schizophrenic. These children have not been duly considered by the diagnostician of auditory disorders. Because of the child's inability to respond appropriately to formal appraisals of auditory acuity he has been most often diagnosed as having peripheral deafness. It is apparent from experience with many such children that they are not peripherally deaf. Furthermore, even when the presence of peripheral deafness cannot be definitively eliminated diagnostically, to designate these children as simply peripherally deaf is a marked over-simplification. A diagnosis of severe emotional disorder with possible peripheral deafness is exceedingly more accurate and beneficial to the child. Such diagnoses should be made only by the specialists with appropriate background and experience. However, all specialists encountering children with auditory disorders should be competent to suspect an emotional disturbance and to make referrals correspondingly. This is one of the most apparent needs in this area of differential diagnosis and one of the ways in which such children can be tentatively identified for further evaluation is through recognition of their behavioral symptomatology. The diagnostician can make clinical observations of their behavior and compare the syndrome clinically with the syndromes of other children presenting problems of auditory disorders.

Study of schizophrenic children who have been presumed to have peripheral deafness is revealing relative to the psychology of auditory behavior in early life. The importance of hearing as a means of maintaining contact with the environment has been stressed. This is an important concept from the point of view of schizophrenia in early life. Hearing is a primary source of environmental demand and in a predominant way reality is auditory in nature. Perhaps this explains the characteristic history as reported by Pearson, that marked fear of sound has occurred in these children during infancy. Reality might have been too demanding and threatening, with a primary anxiety symptom of fear of sound. Some of these children might later show the symptom of lack of adequate response auditorially. This is in agreement with the histories of schizophrenic children who are presumed to have deafness. Usually the history is one of their having used hearing and of having developed some use of verbal language, but then gradually becoming abstracted and withdrawn with simultaneous decreasing use of speech and hearing. The history might be complicated by such factors as hospitalization of the child. However, usually the most significant aspect from the point of view of emotional disorder is that the home is psychologically demanding and generally inadequate. The schizophrenia becomes apparent between the ages of eighteen and twenty-four months in most instances. It is during this period that, because of the child's lack of continued development of speech and poor auditory behavior, he is presumed by the parents to be developing a peripheral deafness.

One of the fundamental characteristics of schizophrenia behaviorally is extreme withdrawal from reality. The child is bizarrely out of contact with his environment. This detachment includes lack of contact with the environment auditorially. However, in this connection it is interesting to consider the problem of auditory hallucinations. This is symptomatic of some schizophrenic adolescents and adults in which they have subjective auditory experiences. The individual "hears voices" talking to him and he behaves as though these voices are real, although they are actually non-existent. This is a challenging phenomenon from the point of view of the psychology of auditory behavior. The question which must be considered is why hallucinations are usually auditory; why does the schizophrenic have a subjective auditory experience more commonly than he has other subjective sensory experiences, such as visual hallucinations. It seems that relinquishing auditory contact environmentally is a more effective withdrawal from reality than a comparable suspension of the use of vision. Also, through auditory hallucinations the individual can "hear without hearing"; he can have the experience of hearing without accepting the demands of the environment. Thereby, hearing can serve only the distorted purposes of his seriously disintegrated personality. The auditory nature of the schizophrenic's inner world remains to be explored experientially. Whether the very young schizophrenic child has auditory hallucinations is not known. His verbalizations usually are so limited that clinical evidence is meager. However, his nonverbal behavior is determined essentially by subjective motivations, without regard for external stimulation and circumstances, and conceivably could include subjective auditory experience. In any event, the relinquishing of hearing makes it unnecessary to maintain contact with the environment in general because the "all-purpose" scanning sense is suspended while more restricted environmental contact is maintained visually. After hearing is relinquished it can be reinstated subjectively through hallucination for purposes of phantasy and unrealistic behavior in general.

The behavioral symptomatology as discussed in this chapter includes the young child who is schizophrenic and who is presumed to have an auditory impairment. Many schizophrenic children do not relinquish speech development and use of their hearing, so the behavioral syndrome is discussed only in relation to those who do have these symptoms. Children with other types of emotional disturbances, also, are included in the syndrome. An attempt has been made to indicate the characteristic behavioral differences between these primary types of emotionally disturbed children who present problems of psychic deafness.

Early Infantile Autism

Another emotional disorder which is associated with psychic deafness is infantile autism. This condition usually is considered as a form of psychosis in young children and, therefore, as a type of schizophrenia in childhood. It was first described by Kanner in 1943 [11]. The syndrome has been rather extensively discussed since that time. Recent discussions include those of Mahler [15] and Kanner [12]. The infantile autistic child is commonly presumed by his parents to have peripheral deafness and because of his inability to respond adequately to formal tests of hearing some diagnosticians, too, have erroneously concluded that the problem was simply impaired acuity. Some autistic children have been considered deaf and managed accordingly for a period of several years. Such erroneous diagnosis and consequent inappropriate management is unfortunate for the welfare of the child. The confusion of infantile autism with peripheral deafness occurs because many autistic children do not use speech and do not attend to their auditory world. Furthermore, in some instances these children are confused with the aphasic and the mentally deficient.

Infantile autism is a condition which derives from very early life. Typically, these children do not have a period of relative normal development emotionally and then regress. This is a significant difference in their history as contrasted with the more typical schizophrenic child. The autistic's involvement is more pronounced from the preverbal age. Because the history does not reveal a period of relative normalcy some specialists have concluded that the condition must be a cerebral dysgenesis; however, in general, autistic children differ significantly in behavioral symptomatology from those with known brain lesions. Moreover, gradually authorities are agreeing that the usual organic syndrome is absent. Infantile autism usually can be explained on a psychological and psychiatric basis. For example, Kanner [10] has observed that the parents often are engaged in professional pursuits. There is an unusually high incidence of scientists, physicians, teachers, artists and other professional groups represented among the parents of these children and, in general, the parents lack warmheartedness. Apparently, they are more concerned about the intellectual and the abstract than they are about their children. This is in agreement with clinical experience generally. However, as Mahler [15] has stated, not all of the parents of autistic children lack this capacity to love their child. The etiology then is obscure, but emotional starvation cannot be revealed in all cases.

Children with infantile autism must be included in the problem of diagnosis of auditory disorders in young children. Many such children do not use verbal language and are markedly disturbed in auditory behavior. They must be differentiated from children having other types of language and auditory disorders. Not all autistic children have symptoms which cause parents, and others, to suspect deafness or aphasia. The behavioral symptomatology as discussed in this chapter pertains only to those having such symptoms.

Other Emotional Disturbances

Childhood schizophrenia and early infantile autism are the most common types of emotional disturbances associated with auditory disorders in young children. Other types of emotional disturbances are encountered, however, and these usually are referred to as the neuroses, or as primary behavior disorders. These conditions include mainly obsessional and anxiety neurosis. Obsessional neurosis is characterized by rigid adherence to certain orderly routines. Frequently these routines are related to obsessive need for cleanliness. For example, if the child accidentally spills food on himself he insists on having a clean bib, a clean shirt, or he might insist on being bathed. This behavior apparently derives from conflict regarding toilet training and other societal demands in early life. The obsessive need for cleanliness often masks a fundamental rebellion against demands to be clean. This emotional conflict can include the suspension of normal auditory contact with the environment because if the child does not hear the demands, adjustment to them is precluded. However, the psychic deafness associated with this emotional disturbance, usually, is not as complete as that found in schizophrenia and autism. This is true, in general, of all of the neuroses. However, obsessional behavior should not be minimized because it is far reaching in its effects in later life if it is not corrected. It might be associated with concomitant peripheral deafness and it is apparent that undue emphasis on remedial training procedures by parents and teachers causes some young children to react with such obsessional behavior. The differential diagnosis includes determining whether partial peripheral deafness is present.

Anxiety states are seen in children presenting problems of psychic deafness. These conditions vary from extreme incapacitating dread to more mild specific fears. Many diagnosticians do not distinguish between anxiety states and normal apprehension, shyness and ret-

icence. The histories of children with severe anxiousness might include illness and hospitalization. Bowlby [4] has shown the relationship between anxiety and hospitalization in young children. He
found that the child's reaction might be one of intense clinging to
the mother thereafter, or one of rejecting the mother. Both of these
reactions are seen in children with auditory disturbances. The histories, also, might include surgery experience. Jessner, et al. [9] have
studied the emotional implications of tonsillectomy. These studies
are provocative and challenging. Children might develop anxiety in
relation to any surgery but when auditory disorders are present there
is a manifest relationship to tonsillectomy. For example, the child
might have been told that the surgery is to help him hear. Such suggestion is relevant to anxiety as it pertains to auditory function.
Marked anxiety is not necessarily related to hospital or illness experiences. It can derive directly from inadequate affectional contact with
the parents. As indicated previously, relinquishing the use of hearing
is an effective way for the organism to prevent anxiety producing
stimuli from becoming overwhelming. Anxiety states, therefore,
must be considered in the differential diagnosis of auditory disorders.
Such emotional involvement usually does not cause the severity of
incapacity that is seen in children with psychosis. The auditory disturbance might be intermittent and situational. Clinical experience
with children presenting problems which are primarily auditory in
nature indicates that profound psychic deafness occurs most frequently in children with psychosis. Marked psychic deafness is rarely
seen in children with the neurotic type of emotional disturbance.
This does not minimize the importance of determining the presence
of partial deafness due to emotional factors.

Inhibition of hearing only for certain situations is not common in
children below four or five years of age. It occurs more frequently
in children above six years of age. The very young child seems not
to differentiate between situations in regard to suspension of the use
of his hearing. His immaturity genetically, perhaps, makes such differentiation impossible. He does not differentiate between parents
and other speakers; rather, he relinquishes use of hearing in general,

usually including sounds other than speech. Such children characteristically are grossly disturbed psychologically; minor emotional deviations presumably do not include such drastic withdrawal of sensory functioning. Perhaps this explains the higher incidence of
psychotic children with presumed deafness.

When psychological disturbances occur in early life, and when
language and auditory behavior are disturbed reciprocally, the behavior of the child is symptomatic. This behavioral symptomatology
is characteristic because when the organism is disintegrated on a
psychological basis the resultant behavior differs from disintegration
due to central nervous system damage, sensory deprivation, or mental
subnormality. The psychologically disturbed organism behaves primarily on the basis of subjective stimulation, sensory stimulation, and
thereby, the environment no longer is a predominant determinant of
behavior. This is fundamental in the nature of the behavioral symptomatology of the emotionally disturbed child with psychic deafness.
Children with peripheral deafness, aphasia or mental deficiency do
not relinquish contact with the environment; their behavior is characterized by the manner in which they attempt to relate to their
environment. The behavioral symptomatology of the emotionally
disturbed child is characterized by the manner in which he disasso-
ciates himself from the environment and behaves as if the only significant stimulation is that which he senses internally. He essentially
denies the external world.

This discussion of the behavior symptoms of children with psychic
deafness includes the schizophrenic and autistic primarily because
these types comprise most of the cases. However, these behavioral
symptoms apply, though less directly, to children with anxiety states
and obsessive and compulsive conditions. An attempt has been made
throughout the discussion of this behavioral symptomatology to
describe the differences between these types of emotionally disturbed children. Furthermore, the data given in tables 10, 11, 12, 13,
14 and 15 should be considered in relation to this symptomatology.
In general, these data support the differences betwen the groups as
revealed by clinical observation and in this manner these data are

helpful in clarifying the diagnostic categories for the various types of auditory disorders.

BEHAVIORAL SYMPTOMS OF PSYCHIC DEAFNESS IN YOUNG CHILDREN

He Does Not Acquire Speech

Like other young children having auditory disorders the emotionally disturbed child usually does not use verbal language and characteristically the autistic child has never spoken. However, Kanner has observed that some autistic children speak rarely and others speak freely. Even those who speak rarely might be erroneously presumed to have deafness. The schizophrenic child who is presumed to have such deafness typically has shown no marked deviations during his first year of life. Therefore, he has a history of normal language development until between one and two years of age. At this time speech might have ceased, or have been used infrequently. Complete muteness is not uncommon, but muteness is rare in peripherally deaf, aphasic and mentally deficient children. Marked mutism, therefore, should be evaluated clinically as a possible manifestation of emotional involvements. The child with psychic deafness is, perhaps, the most speechless of children with auditory disorders. Because of his concomitant marked lack of response to sound he has been diagnosed as having profound peripheral deafness. Extensive contact and therapy with these children has revealed normal speech and hearing in some instances.

Use of speech is closely related to contact with the environment, especially with people. Severe emotional disorder is characterized by an inability to develop and maintain contact with other persons and the lack of use of speech is one way in which the child manifests his rejection of people and of the world. He frequently rejects speech more completely than hearing. Appropriate examining procedures usually elicit auditory responses but speech most frequently cannot be elicited except under prolonged psychotherapy. Such children make no attempt to speak and urging is fruitless. This in itself is diagnostically revealing because it is readily possible to persuade children with peripheral deafness to attempt speech by imitating the visual movements of the speaker's lips and tongue. Such imitation cannot be elicited from the child with psychic deafness. In general, lack of speech must be evaluated and related to the total syndrome, particularly to other language behavior.

His Vocalizations Do Not Have a Characteristic Tonal Quality

Many of the emotionally disturbed children are mute, making it impossible to evaluate the tonal quality of their vocalizations. However, when vocalizations are produced, usually the acoustic quality is normal. The vocalizations, typically, do not signify an inability to monitor auditorially. This has been emphasized, also, in connection with psychic deafness in adults. Nevertheless, some severely disturbed schizophrenic children might vocalize in a bizzare, atypical manner. For example, they might scream, make guttural or unusual nasal sounds. In addition to usually having a normal acoustic quality vocally, the child with psychic deafness does not use jargon. Furthermore, his vocalizations relate essentially to his inner world rather than to his environment, or to reality in general. This is primarily what is meant by the bizarreness of his vocal behavior. He may be sitting quietly, then begin to smile and suddenly blurt out a vocalization without regard to those around him. Such vocal activity does not characterize other types of children with auditory disorders.

He Does Not Improvise Sound for Pleasure and Does Not Use Vocalizations Projectively

Like the child with peripheral deafness, the child with psychic deafness does not vocalize, or use other sounds to entertain himself. He does not engage in vocalizations for pleasure, nor does he use his voice to call the attention of others. In this behavior he is especially in contrast to the child having peripheral deafness. The aphasic might use jargon, the child with peripheral deafness uses his voice projectively, the emotionally disturbed child usually does neither. Autistic children relate well to objects, such as blocks, but they do not vocalize while engaging in activity with such objects. The schizophrenic child is more vocal but his vocalizations derive from internal phantasy, his vocalizations do not relate to objects, or to people. His vocal behavior characterizes his detachment from his environment. Furthermore, when autistic or schizophrenic children do use words they are not for purposes of communication. Rather, their verbalization serves their own subjective worlds and is not for purposes of relationship with others. In general, however, verbalization even for subjective purposes is rare in these children.

Significantly, the emotionally disturbed child does not use his voice to call his parents, or to directly influence his environment in other ways. Such behavior assumes psychological functioning which is precluded by marked emotional disorder. The aphasic child, likewise, does not use his voice projectively, but his behavioral symptomatology manifests real need to come to terms with his environment. The emotionally disturbed child's behavior is characterized by his rejection of the environment and his ability to behave as though the external world is nonexistent. Therefore, the lack of use of his voice to control the environment is qualitatively different and is one of the symptoms which manifests a general withdrawal and detachment from reality.

Children with less severe emotional disorders such as anxiety states, do vocalize during play activity and some do use their voices projectively. Such vocal behavior might be erratic and intermittent, and it might include the use of words. When this occurs the tonal quality, the psychological content and the symbolic functioning are differentiating in terms of the nature of the auditory disorder.

He Does Not Use Gesture

The importance of gesture in differential diagnosis has been indicated previously. The lack of gesture in emotionally disturbed children is highly symptomatic because their lack of gesture is in marked contrast to children with peripheral deafness. For example, the autistic child does not point to an object with a pleading expression, indicating that he wishes the adult to get it for him. Rather, without preference he takes an adult, parent or stranger, by the hand then attempts to place this hand on the object without looking into the face of the adult while indicating his wishes in this manner. However, this behavior reveals intact symbolic functioning, inner language is highly developed. His lack of gesture is not due to an inability to function symbolically. The autistic's rejection of reality is specifically in the area of human relationships. He maintains contact with inanimate aspects of his environment, and significantly, he incorporates people into his world as though they, too, are inanimate. This means that he manifests a high degree of inner language and symbolic behavior but he does not need a means of communication because his world consists only of inanimate objects and it is not necessary to hear speech, to speak, or to gesture in such a world. Neither is it necessary to relate to people by looking at their faces and interpreting facial expressions. This type of behavior when associated with lack of gesture is markedly characteristic of autistic children with psychic deafness. It is highly differentiating and such children should be examined and managed accordingly in all ways.

Likewise, the schizophrenic child does not use gesture but he differs in some respects from the autistic child. The schizophrenic child typically has not only rejected the people in his world, he has rejected his entire environment. While he might engage in stereotyped manipulation of an object, the object is not used meaningfully. His rejection of his environment makes relation to objects and to people unnecessary. Such complete withdrawal obviously makes gesture, and other use of language for communication purposes reciprocally impossible. Such children might use language internally, however. This is revealed by the changes of facial expression, their motor behavior, and even by their vocalizations. For example, the child might be sitting placidly, relatively oblivious to his surroundings, and then without any notice of his environment, he might suddenly laugh, scream or run to the window. Such behavior usually reveals psychological functioning of a complex nature, often entailing a high degree of symbolic integrity. It suggests, not the lack of ability to function symbolically, but rather a distortion of the use of symbolization. The child internalized the world symbolically but, apparently, simultaneously rejected the world. It is as though the incorporation of the world symbolically made existence of the concrete world untenable. Therefore, use of symbols is for subjective purposes only. Words and certain gesticulations might be used, not for communication, but only for phantasy. Facial grimacing, or pushing objects off from the table, have no direct relationship to those present but simply are manifestations of inner phantasy and mental activity.

Lack of gesture is a significant symptom diagnostically. Children with peripheral deafness gesticulate freely. Aphasic and emotionally disturbed children are especially deficient in the use of gestures. However, clinical observation reveals significant differences between the aphasic and the emotionally disturbed in this deficiency. The aphasic are deficient in symbolic behavior in general, whereas the emotionally disturbed manifest intact symbolic capacities.

He Does Not Respond to Sound and He Does Not Use His Hearing Projectively

The auditory responses of emotionally disturbed children are characteristic. Parents do not describe them as being inconsistent in the same manner as the responses of aphasic children. Rather, the emotionally disturbed child's inadequate auditory behavior is described as being willful in nature. The parents state that he seems to hear but refuses to give attention to them. These parental reports are consistent with clinical observation because schizophrenic children, especially, manifest willful attitudes in their rejection of the auditory world. This quality of the schizophrenic's behavior has been described by psychiatrists [22]. Loud intensities do not alter the child's responsiveness. Characteristically schizophrenic and autistic children do not respond directly to an auditory stimulus irrespective of the level of intensity. This usually includes sounds even at the pain level of intensity. This is important in auditory testing and is discussed further in Chapter XI. From the point of view of clinical observations, no direct responses to sound, irrespective of intensity, should be evaluated in terms of possible emotional involvement.

Such children, in clinical parlance, might be "too deaf to be deaf," because such auditory inhibition can occur only on the basis of concomitant shifts in general responsiveness, such as associated reduction in the threshold for pain.

Close prolonged contact with schizophrenic and autistic children reveals that although they do not respond directly even to intense sounds, they do use their hearing in a superficial manner. For example, the child might smile in a manner manifesting willful rejection when his name is spoken softly. Likewise, if his vocalizations are imitated softly, he might cease vocalizing abruptly. Other observations can be made, especially of autistic children and children with anxiety states. If the examiner, or parents, make incidental comments relative to concrete situations in the child's life, such as "Where is sister," or "Mommy go bye-bye," these children frequently manifest changes in motor activity or give other indications that the statements were heard. Clinical observations, therefore, should be directed primarily to detecting indirect responses to sound rather than to obvious and overt reactions. Many parents, after having been informed that their child seems to hear, can detect subtle but definite indications of good auditory acuity from the child's daily routine. Emotionally disturbed children do not respond directly to their auditory world but their auditory behavior is qualitatively characteristic. Clinical observations also might reveal normal ability to comprehend if indirect reactions are noted.

Normal projective use of hearing likewise is grossly deficient. For example, although superficial use of hearing can be observed, or manifested by special procedures, these children lack the ability to respond normally to information which derives from their auditory environment. They will not react by crying, or running away, even from sounds which are normally considered threatening or dangerous. They will ignore such sounds in the same willful manner as they reject speech sounds. It is apparent, however, that they use sounds somewhat more effectively for background than for foreground purposes. Thus, although projective use of hearing is markedly disturbed, frequently they do manifest indirect responses to peripheral, or background sounds, while simultaneously rejecting immediate, or foreground sounds. This should not be interpreted as indicating an auditory perceptual disorder. The indirect responses of the emotionally disturbed child do not manifest an inability to structure the auditory world, because structuring the sound field for them has no effect on their behavior, whereas, the child who has an auditory perceptual disturbance responds immediately to such structuring.

Uncritical use of auditory tests with emotionally disturbed children might erroneously suggest peripheral deafness. Clinical observation of their auditory responses reveals a characteristic pattern as compared to other children with auditory disorders. Such observations are essential for interpretation of test results and for differential diagnosis.

His Laughing, Smiling and Crying Are Characteristic

The laughing, smiling and crying of children with psychic deafness is characteristically atypical as compared to other children with auditory disorders. One of the most obvious ways in which this behavior deviates is in quantity. Autistic children, in general, can be described as lacking laughter, smiling and crying. They do not even laugh and smile bizarrely. Furthermore, on rare occasions when they do cry they typically do not shed tears. Thus, when impeded vigorously a simulated, superficial type of crying might be elicited, but tears and sobbing are notably lacking. Schizophrenic children do laugh and smile, but in a bizarre manner. They engage in laughing and smiling for phantasy purposes only. They do not laugh with others as a reaction to a humorous situation. They laugh only in a preoccupied, detached manner and as a result of subjective sensations. Likewise, they might begin to cry without obvious reason or provocation. Such crying might be accompanied by tears but in general it is not intense. Schizophrenic children, too, might be grossly deficient in laughing, smiling and crying behavior. Some parents report that such behavior has never been observed. When laughter and crying are observed the tonal quality does not suggest incapacity to monitor auditorially.

Clinical observation of laughing, smiling and crying is significant in other respects. Such observation reveals the nature of the emotional disorder and its far reaching consequences. Normal laughter and smiling are direct manifestations of emotional responsiveness to other persons. Such behavior reflects psychological integrity and well-being. Crying is a normal reaction in children when they feel threatened, distressed, or when they are in pain. This is significant clinically because many autistic and some schizophrenic children do not cry even when injured. For example, an autistic child injured his thumb in a door to the extent that bleeding was profuse. He showed no reaction of pain, he did not cry, nor did he seek assurance from his mother. This reduction of sensitivity to pain is directly corroborative of their lack of response to sounds, even at the threshold of discomfort. It highlights the importance of considering the unitary responsiveness of the organism when making a diagnosis. When a child is insensitive to auditory stimulation and is simultaneously insensitive in other respects, a diagnosis of peripheral deafness should be questioned.

Children with less severe emotional disturbances might laugh and cry with intensity and appropriateness, especially when their anxiety has been relieved. Such children, likewise, might respond auditorially to the extent that their fears and apprehensions can be overcome. Observation of laughing, smiling and crying behavior is useful, however, in all children presenting problems of auditory disorder. Such information makes definitive differential diagnosis more possible.

He Is Not Unduly Sensitive to Movement or to Other Visual Clues

Children whose auditory disorders are due to psychological disturbances do not manifest organismic adjustment to compensate for their suspension of hearing. For example, they do not use vision differently because their behavior deprives them of normal auditory function; compensatory behavior is lacking. Clinical observations accordingly are diagnostically helpful. When a child has an auditory disorder but other sensory avenues are not used to compensate organismically the presence of peripheral deafness might be questioned. Characteristically, children with psychic hearing disorders are not atypical only in the area of auditory behavior. Their emotional disturbance is more generalized in its effect. Ordinarily they are disturbed in the use of other sensory functioning simultaneously. For example, the schizophrenic and autistic children show little awareness, or recognition, of parents as compared to strangers. They see their parents daily but make no distinction between them and individuals whom they are encountering for the first time. Likewise, as indicated above, they might give no reaction to pain. Despite these generalized effects of severe emotional disorders, some diagnosticians conclude that the child is peripherally deaf on the basis of his reactions to auditory tests alone. From the point of view of differential diagnosis consideration of the child's marked inability to respond in general provides a basis for the interpretation of all test results. Furthermore, the behavioral syndrome of emotionally disturbed children is contrasted with the behavioral syndrome associated with peripheral deafness, and with the syndromes of children who are aphasic or mentally deficient. Aphasic children cannot integrate sensory experience normally and thus do not compensate effectively through compensatory use of other sensory channels. However, aphasic children do not reject sensory impressions. They react to them erratically and at the level of their integrative capacity. The emotionally disturbed child rejects sensation at the point of its entering the organism [17]. Therefore, his behavior is as though the sensations do not exist and this makes compensatory behavior unnecessary. The organism which is deprived of auditory experience because of peripheral deafness makes shifts on the basis of that deprivation, which implies reactional patterns deriving from a realistic need to overcome that which has been deprived. The aphasic child's behavior manifests an incapacity to cope with the sensations after they have been delivered to the brain. Each of these children's behavioral symptomatology is consistent with the nature of his deficiency organismically. This emphasizes the need to make clinical observations regarding compensatory use of sensory avenues. Emotionally disturbed children typically do not compensate by shifts in their use of vision.

He Does Not Attend to Facial Expression

Children with peripheral deafness use visual clues, including facial expressions, as a source of contact with their surroundings. Aphasic children attempt to use such clues for action but are generally unsuccessful in such attempts. Emotionally disturbed children are remarkable in the way in which they ignore face to face contact. One of the most observable behavioral symptoms of autistic children is their rigid refusal to attend to the faces of others. Mothers have reported that their autistic child has never looked into their faces. This child might approach an adult, take his hand, lead him to the door and place his hand on the door knob, indicating that he wishes him to open the door. During such activity, even under stress and duress, the child will not look at the face of the adult. Perhaps no other child refuses facial contact to the extent which is typical of autistic children. Their rejection of the world of people is manifested particularly in rejection of people's faces. They will accept people as objects but not as animate beings and this is achieved largely by lack of recognition of their faces.

Schizophrenic children, too, are characteristic in the manner in which they reject people's faces, but these children achieve such rejection in a less direct manner. While the autistic refuses to look at the face, the schizophrenic will look at the face without recognition or awareness. It is as though he looks through the face. When he looks at an individual's face he remains preoccupied, lacks eye contact and gives the impression of willful ignoring of intimate relationship. This behavior is consistent with his attitudes and lack of normal emotional expression in other respects.

Children with anxiety states, or less extensive emotional disorder, do not reject facial contact in this manner. They do manifest fear of face to face contact but they will relate more satisfactorily and they will use facial expression as a guide to action. There is a marked difference between the types of children presenting problems of auditory disorder in regard to their responsiveness to people's faces. This is a significant behavioral symptom and should be evaluated differentially.

He Is Not Unduly Sensitive to Tactile Sensation

Emotionally disturbed children do not use other sensory avenues to compensate for their lack of use of hearing. Their behavior organismically is as though hearing is nonexistent and, therefore, compensatory behavior is unnecessary. This behavior is in marked contrast to children with peripheral deafness. Autistic and schizophrenic children are unresponsive to environmental stimulation in general. They might not respond overtly even to vigorous tactile sensation. It is essential diagnostically to relate their unresponsiveness auditorially to their lack of response through other channels. An auditory disorder which is accompanied by lack of response to the environment in general has specific implications for emotional involvement. It is in this respect that the lack of tactile response in the emotionally disturbed child is symptomatic because he rejects contact with reality in general, not only by rejecting auditory sensations. The psychology of tactile sensitivity in early life has not been investigated. Schilder [20] suggests its importance as the avenue through which feelings of warmth and well-being derive in infancy. It is apparent that coddling, caressing and fondling are all tactile means of conveying affection to the child and that these means, though qualitatively different, are used by adults. Emotionally disturbed children in their rejection of normal affectional relationship and contacts, also might reject tactile sensations because of the psychological aspects. Generalizations are difficult, however, because while autistic children reject tactile sensations in general, some schizophrenic children seek coddling and caressing unduly. To illustrate, a four year old schizophrenic child might seek coddling in a manner as though he were six months of age. This emphasizes

Bleuler's [2] concept that the schizophrenic does not reject that aspect of reality which conforms to his affective purposes. From the point of view of differential diagnosis, however, emotionally disturbed children do not use tactile sensations normally or in a compensatory way. Therefore, they differ especially from children with peripheral deafness. Aphasic children do not use tactile sensation normally; rather, they manifest that such sensations are disturbing; while they cannot integrate the sensations they do not behave as though the sensations are nonexistent. Tactile responsiveness is readily observable clinically and it is an important indicator of organismic integrity.

His Motor Behavior Is Characteristic

The motor functioning of children with marked emotional disturbances is characteristic. In general, autistic children have good motor abilities. They not only perform well motorically, but as Kanner [10] suggests, they appear healthy and robust. The history usually reveals that they walked at twelve months of age or earlier. They have no difficulty in performing motor tasks involved in eating, drinking and buttoning, except as they might reject the entire activity in preference to having someone perform it for them. When they make no attempt to perform the act, they do not lack ability to do so. In contrast, many aphasics attempt such motor tasks but cannot execute the coordination entailed. Likewise, the histories of autistic children do not suggest problems of cerebral dominance, handedness and ambidexterity. This, too, is in agreement with clinical observations. There is an absence of awkwardness and clumsiness, they are motorically intact and well developed physically.

Schizophrenic children present a similar but not identical motor pattern. In some respects their motor capacities are within normal limits of expectation. They might grasp a spoon well, hold a glass normally, and manifest good motor control in walking. However, they are characteristically depressed and unresponsive motorically. They do not run or throw with vigor. This depression of motor activity has been described by Bender [1].

The motor behavior of both schizophrenic and autistic children includes ritualistic and stereotyped activities. They might rock themselves while in a standing position, remain in a fixed position for an unusual period of time, and twirl themselves, or twirl objects, in an incessant manner. These stereotyped activities are performed usually without regard to their surroundings. These activities usually manifest a good quality of motor performance. Parents describe them as being able to climb upon anything in the home and that such climbing is done without apparent fear. It is interesting to note from tables 10, 11, 12 and 13, however, that the emotionally disturbed child is delayed as compared to the normal, in sitting and beginning walking. Inasmuch as these children do not manifest motor problems clinically there is a suggestion that severe emotional disturbances in early life may impede the acquisition, or use of certain motor capacities. Moreover, parents report, and it is apparent from clinical observation, that some schizophrenic children will walk only when they are permitted some type of superficial support. For example, one such child would walk only when permitted to hold on to the finger of an adult, but it was obvious that the holding on to the finger was not for support or balance. This child occasionally took a few steps inadvertently, then as though realizing that she had revealed herself, she would immediately sit down. The neurologist described her as being capable of walking but that she did not want to. This type of deviation motorically is not typical of the other types of children with auditory disorders.

His Social Perception is Characteristic

Autistic and schizophrenic children are seriously impaired in social perception. As indicated previously social perception is characterized by the ability to behave appropriately according to the wishes and feelings of the individuals present in a given situation. It implies ability to accept and to adjust to societal requirements in general. Autistic and schizophrenic children behave essentially according to their own subjective needs and feelings. In most respects they have no regard for the wishes and needs of others. If the parent prepares to leave the room, they do not conclude that it is time to return home, because usually they ignore the fact that the parent is leaving. They behave substantially as though people are not present, which means that they do not use social perception. The autistic child does include people in his world but he includes them as inanimate objects and relates to them on this basis. He uses people to open doors, and to accomplish other ends, in the same manner as he uses a chair or a hammer.

Play activities provide a means of observing the child's ability to socialize. Children with peripheral deafness engage in socialized play readily when the activities are essentially visual in nature. Aphasic children attempt to play but they lack imagination and ability to grasp the many subtleties involved, so they become lost in a detail instead of grasping the significance of the total situation. However, they do make attempts and they do not reject the persons involved. Autistic children engage in play of a highly specific type but it is not socialized play. They are greatly attracted to blocks [13]. They prefer blocks which are neutral, without pictures or letters on them. They build intricate designs and patterns with these blocks. Parents report that they will engage in such activities for several hours without interruption. Furthermore, they have unusual memory for the patterns which they construct. If the parent, or diagnostician, removes a block it disturbs the child and he will put forth vigorous effort to replace it. He does not look at the person who took the block while he is attempting to replace it. His building with blocks is stereotyped, perseverative and repetitious. Nevertheless, his rejection of the world, apparently, is less complete than the schizophrenic's. The autistic child has contact with reality through his identification with inanimate objects because his rejection is specific to animate objects. He generalizes from people to other living things, because he rejects pets as well as people.

Schizophrenic children do not engage in play activities. They might perform the routine of throwing a ball but they will not relate emotionally to the activity. They will engage in the activity but it is performed as though they are not doing it. There is no enjoy-

ment, no recognition of other persons, and no manifestation of emotion. If left to himself such a child moves about or remains inactive
on the basis of his subjective world, as there is no object or goal
directed behavior. Therefore, he is devoid of social perceptual functioning.

Children with anxiety states usually do manifest social perceptual
awareness. They might react intensely to their mother's rising from
her chair even though there is no direct indication that she is preparing to leave the room. In extreme anxiety conditions these children, too, might reject their environment to the extent of not manifesting social perceptual awareness. Fraiberg [7] has described the
symptoms and treatment of such a child.

Clinical observation reveals that the social perception of emotionally disturbed children is characteristic. Most testing procedures
assume normal social perceptual functioning. Thus when social perception is disturbed the use of clinical and testing procedures must
be adapted correspondingly.

His Emotional Expression Is Characteristic

The history and behavior relative to emotional expression is characteristic in autistic and schizophrenic children. Parents report that
autistic children have never demonstrated normal emotional reactions to coddling and affection. As Kanner has indicated, in some
instances this seems to be reciprocally related to the parents' inability
to feel love for their child. However, Mahler [15] has oberved that
autistic children might occur in families where the parents are not
incapable of affectional feelings and attitudes. Schizophrenic children usually have not manifested a rejection of normal emotional
expression during the first year of life. However, their histories do
suggest some undue fretting behavior, poor eating habits and considerable demand for attention prior to the onset of their severe
withdrawal psychologically. For both schizophrenic and autistic
children, at the time that they present problems in auditory functioning, the primary behavioral symptom is lack of normal expression of emotion. They do not laugh or show other signs of normal

joviality, they show no emotion for their parents, they rarely show normal anger and aggression, they have mask-like expressions and they show little fluctuation of moods and attitudes. In general, their disorder is characterized by an inability to express feeling and emotion. Knowledge of the etiology of these early life disorders is inadequate, but the behavior of these children suggests that the organism is compensating for traumatic psychological experiences. For example, the autistic's behavior indicates that the organism rejects people because it senses psychological deprivation and annihilation. To prevent further disintegration organismically the child rejects the world of people and identifies with the world of inanimate objects. Moreover, the world of inanimate objects does not include communication but to acquire verbal language necessitates identification with the world of people. Perhaps this explains the common symptom of lack of speech and inadequate auditory behavior in autistic children.

Schizophrenic children, likewise, behave as though emotions are threatening and, therefore, must be denied and rejected. Identification is not made with the world of people nor with the world of inanimate objects. Internal needs subdue and overcome sensory functioning, so the external world is denied except in instances when external circumstances are incorporated for subjective purposes.

Children with anxiety states usually do express emotions. They might manifest marked fear of leaving the mother, insisting that she be in the same room with them, even while in the home. They are severely apprehensive regarding other children or adults. They cry and reveal intense fright and apprehension. With prolonged assurance they might relate with others to the extent of smiling and cooperating for brief periods. Many such children, however, are too severely disturbed to be able to respond to direct psychological assurances.

Clinical observation of emotional expression is informative in regard to the differential diagnosis of auditory disorders. These various types of children differ widely in their characteristic emotional expression. Observation of this aspect of the child's behavior is basic to management of him while proceeding with the other steps in making a differential diagnosis.

His Auditory and Visual Perceptual Behavior Is Characteristic

Another behavioral difference between children with psychic deafness and children having other types of auditory disorders is their characteristic functioning perceptually. Sensory experience precedes perception. If sensory experience is rejected, perceptual functioning, likewise, will be absent. It is the absence of normal perceptual functioning which is manifested in schizophrenic children. Their perceptions derive from their subjective worlds only. Therefore, they are bizarre, showing no perceptual response to sensory impressions. The child with peripheral deafness structures the world psychologically and behaves on a foreground–background basis. The aphasic child is perceptually disturbed and confuses foreground and background. The schizophrenic child structures the world but only in terms of his grossly distorted emotional needs. Sensory experience is not used, or it is used only incidentally. There is no foreground and background interaction and structuring. His world is essentially foreground and this foregroundedness is determined only by subjective, affectional needs. His perceptual behavior, thereby, is characteristic. He perceives only on the basis of internal sensations, rejecting his sensory impressions. However, he does not manifest perceptual disintegration such as characterizes the aphasic.

The autistic child does not reject sensation as completely as the schizophrenic child. He engages himself in foreground activities such as building with blocks. His activities reveal intactness of perception within the limits in which he permits it to function. He is not disturbed in his ability to integrate the sensory experience which he accepts. In general these children are unusually competent in visual perceptual functioning as it pertains to inanimate objects and this characterizes their perceptual behavior. They structure their world psychologically but they do not include people in their world. They, too, are directed essentially by subjective sensation and affect, rather than by sensory stimulation. Those with psychic deafness especially reject auditory sensations, perhaps, because it is the avenue through which speech is perceived and speech is identified with people.

Children with anxiety states do not reject the world of sensory experience as extensively or in the same manner. Their perceptual behavior is more normal accordingly. Their difficulty derives primarily from fear of sensory experience rather than rejection of it. Therefore, although they cannot accept sensory stimulation normally, their behavior is characterized by attempts to escape from such stimulation rather than behaving as though it did not exist. These children structure the world psychologically in a normal manner, but they are threatened by their environment and manifest marked fear and anxiety relative to all stimulation. They are not perceptually disturbed. They integrate sensory experience but are fearful of this experience.

The perceptual functioning of emotionally disturbed children, therefore, is characteristic and it is apparent in their behavior. The organism behaves perceptually according to its acceptance, rejection, integration or deprivation of sensory experience. If it rejects sensory experience it behaves as though sensations derive only from within. If it cannot integrate sensory experience, because of damage to the central nervous system, it behaves in a confused, disturbed manner but makes continuous attempts to relate organismically. If it is deprived of sensory experience, such as in peripheral deafness, the organism uses vision and tactile sensation to compensate for the deprivation. These characteristic patterns of behavior perceptually provide significant information for the diagnostician.

Echolalia

Emotionally disturbed children with psychic auditory involvements usually do not use speech echolalically and, often, these children are mute and nonverbal. However, it is noteworthy diagnostically that some autistic children do engage in an echolalic type of speech. Such echolalia usually is superior qualitatively to the echolalic production of the receptive aphasic. Clinically, it seems that autistic children who engage in echolalia have not rejected people as completely as those who do not. By reacting echolalically the child can maintain a minimum of contact with people and with the auditory world. The echolalic reaction precludes the necessity of adjusting to what others say, but it affords a verbal contact with them. Schizophrenic children typically do not use echolalia. They might use words but they are not imitations of those heard. The language used spontaneously by autistic and schizophrenic children is characteristic [13]. It is symbolic, but the symbolic content has been distorted according to their subjective needs. Their word associations and meanings, therefore, are not those commonly used by others. This characteristic of their language functioning has been recognized and described by various authorities.

From the point of view of auditory disorders, echolalia is a manifestation of integrity of the auditory mechanism. It should be considered as symptomatic of conditions other than peripheral deafness.

SUMMARY

Hearing is a primary sense for purposes of maintaining contact with the environment. When conflict arises between the child's inner needs and his environment he protects himself by relinquishing part of his contact with the environment; he "closes his ears." Speech sounds to be pleasant and satisfying must be associated with individuals who are affectionate, warm, accepting and sympathetic. It has been shown that talking birds do not learn to talk until they become pets. Similarly, if infants are not made to feel that they are loved, they may not develop speech normally. The critical age for speech development is between twelve and twenty-four months. This also is the age for much restraining through language, such as use of "no, no," urging of toilet habits and other demands by the parents. This seems to be the age at which most emotional delay and imposition of speech development occurs in early life. Important restraints and influences at this time include telling the child to be quiet and not to speak again for a period of time and that he is not to say a certain word or phrase or he will be punished. Since the young child cannot differentiate between words that are accept-able and those that are not, he must generalize and relinquish all words. An effective way for him to do this is to relinquish all hear-ing. This means that speech which is threatening causes fear of speech because it is a source of anxiety. It is becoming clear that in order for the child to use his hearing normally, sounds and especially speech sounds, cannot be unduly threatening. One type of emotional disturbance which causes psychic deafness is childhood schizophre-nia which frequently has been found to show a history of extreme fear of sounds during infancy. Furthermore, usually children with this type of emotional problem give a history of having used hear-ing and of having developed some verbal language but then gradu-ally becoming withdrawn with decreasing use of speech and hear-ing; this occurs mainly between eighteen and twenty-four months of age. Some children with psychic deafness give up contact with their environment and their detachment includes relinquishing con-tact through hearing. Another emotional disturbance which causes psychic deafness is infantile autism which has been considered a form of childhood schizophrenia. Unlike the more typical schizophrenic child, the infantile autistic child does not give a history of a period of relatively normal emotional development followed by a regres-sion. Rather, his behavioral deviation dates from early infancy. Generally it can be explained on a psychological and psychiatric basis; the parents often are highly intellectual, professional people who are lacking in warmheartedness, causing the child to be emo-tionally starved. The child reacts to this lack of love and affection with a disturbance of his feelings toward people, sometimes includ-ing the relinquishing of his use of hearing. Less common and milder emotional disturbances of hearing include certain of the neuroses. For example, obsessional neurosis often manifested by abnormal and compulsive need for cleanliness may be associated with psychic deafness. Likewise severe anxiety states may interfere with the child's normal use of hearing. Such interference usually is not as complete as that found in the psychoses. Inhibition of hearing only for certain situations occurs more often in children above six years of age because younger children do not differentiate between sounds and situations and, therefore, more often inhibit hearing for all sounds. The behavior of the child with psychic deafness is characteristic. Like the peripherally deaf and the aphasic he does not use speech; he might, however, show complete muteness in contrast to the peripherally deaf and the aphasic. He is the most speechless of all children with auditory disorders; when vocalizations do occur they are normal in tonal quality. He does not improvise sound for pleasure and in this regard is like the child with peripheral deafness, but he does not use his voice to call attention to himself. Moreover, he does not gesture which also is in striking contrast to the peripherally deaf child. Nor does he look at the faces of people to note their expressions or communicate with them by gesture. This is not because the child with psychic deafness cannot use symbolic behavior but that he shuts himself off from his environment. Actually these children have an inner world with a high degree of symbolic behavior but these symbols do not relate to the environment normally. The child with psychic deafness does not respond to sound of loud intensity, often not even to loud sounds low in pitch, which produce a simultaneous tactile sensation, but they do respond to faint sounds in an indirect manner. Thus soft imitation of his vocalizations may cause him to cease vocalizing abruptly. He may smile when his name is spoken softly, but without responding in other ways, manifesting a willful rejection of sound. The parents often observe other subtle indications of good auditory acuity. Autistic and schizophrenic children lack laughter, smiling and crying; when they do cry they do not shed tears or sob. Characteristically they do not cry when injured; reaction to all sensory stimulation is markedly impaired. Likewise, the child with psychic deafness is not unduly sensitive to movement or to other visual clues. He rejects all sensory stimuli at the point of their entrance to the organism and behaves accordingly; this is in contrast to the aphasic child who is confused and erratic by sensory stimulation because of inability to integrate his experience. The child with psychic deafness ignores facial expression and may refuse all face to face contact, indicating his rejection of the world of people. He is unresponsive to tactile sensation in marked contrast to the peripherally deaf child. His motor functioning is good and this is in contrast to the delayed motor development of the aphasic and the mentally deficient. His motor-behavior, however, often is ritualized and stereotyped in the form of rocking, remaining in a fixed position, twirling and many other forms. His social perception is unusually deficient; he behaves as though people are not present or are exceedingly unimportant to him. The autistic child with psychic deafness characteristically plays compulsively with blocks; the schizophrenic does not play but usually remains lost in phantasy. Some autistic children engage in echolalia thus maintaining a minimum of verbal contact with people but this is not characteristic of the more typically schizophrenic child. The psychic deafness of the emotionally disturbed child is a manifestation of their generalized relinquishment of the environment.

BIBLIOGRAPHY

1. Bender, L.: Childhood schizophrenia. Am. J. Orthopsychiat. *17*: 40, 1947.
2. Bleuler, Eugen: The basic symptoms of schizophrenia, in, Rapport, D. (ed.): Organization and Pathology of Thought. New York, Columbia University Press, 1951, pp. 581–641.
3. Bowlby, J.: Maternal Care and Mental Health. New York, World Health Organization. Columbia University Press, 1952.
4. ——, Robertson, J. and Rosenbluth, D.: A two-year-old goes to hospital, in: Psychoanalytic Study of the Child. New York, International Universities Press, 1952, vol. 7, p. 82.
5. Despert, L.: Psychotherapy in childhood schizophrenia. Am. J. Psychiat. *104*: 36, 1947.
6. Fenichel, Otto: The Psychoanalytic Theory of Neurosis. New York, W. W. Norton, 1945.
7. Fraiberg, Selma: A critical neurosis in a two-and-a-half-year-old girl, in: Psychoanalytic Study of the Child. New York, International Universities Press, 1952, vol. 7, p. 173.
8. Gesell, A. et al.: The First Five Years of Life. New York, Harpers, 1940.
9. Jessner, Lucie, Blom, E. and Waldfogel, S.: Emotional implications of tonsillectomy and adenoidectomy on children, in: Psychoanalytic Study of the Child. New York, International Universities Press, 1952, vol. 7, p. 126.

10. Kanner, Leo: Child Psychiatry. Springfield, Ill., C. C Thomas, 1948.

11. ——: Autistic disturbances of affective content. Nervous Child *2*: 217, 1943.

12. ——: A discussion of early infantile autism. Digest Neurol. & Psychiat. *29*: 158, 1951.

13. ——: Early infantile autism. J. Pediat. *25*: 211, 1944.

14. Lourie, R. S. et al.: Studies on the prognosis in schizophrenic-like psychoses in children. Am. J. Psychiat. *22*: 542, 1943.

15. Mahler, M. S.: On child psychosis in schizophrenia; autistic and symbiotic infantile psychosis, in: Psychoanalytic Study of the Child, New York, International Universities Press, 1952, vol. 7, p. 286.

16. Mowrer, O. H.: Learning Theory and Personality Dynamics. New York, The Ronald Press, 1950.

17. Pearson, G. H. J.: A survey of learning difficulties in children, in: Psychoanalytic Study of the Child. New York, International Universities Press, 1952, vol. 7, p. 366.

18. ——: Emotional Disorders of Children. New York, W. W. Norton, 1949.

19. Ramsdell, D. A.: The psychology of the hard of hearing and the deafened adult, in, Davis, H. (ed.): Hearing and Deafness. New York, Murray Hill Books, 1947, pp. 392–418.

20. Schilder, Paul: Mind: Perception and Thought in their Constructive Aspects. New York, Columbia University Press, 1942.

21. Spitz, R. A. and Wolf, K. M.: Anaclitic depression, in: Psychoanalytic Study of the Child. New York, International Universities Press, 1946, vol. 2, p. 313.

22. Sullivan, Henry: The Interpersonal Theory of Psychiatry. New York, W. W. Norton, 1953.

Chapter IX

Auditory Disorders Due to Mental Deficiency

SOME CHILDREN PRESENT PROBLEMS AUDI-torially because of mental deficiency. This is revealed by the data given in table 1 because eleven per cent of the children in the sample were found to be mentally deficient. Auditory disorders associated with mental deficiency differ from peripheral deafness, and from those associated with aphasia and emotional disorders. The mental defective's inadequate auditory behavior is a manifestation of his generalized retardation. He cannot respond to sound normally because of his limited mental ability. In general, his auditory behavior is equivalent to his mental level. However, it is necessary to consider his auditory functioning diagnostically because the mentally deficient child might be presumed to have peripheral deafness. Another reason for including these children in relation to auditory disorders is the frequent confusion of mental deficiency with aphasia and emotional disturbance. Marked deviations of language development in early life, with corresponding auditory involvements, must be differentiated from generalized mental subnormality. Like most other children seen by the diagnostician of auditory disorders, the mentally deficient child is presumed to have deafness because he does not acquire speech at the usual age. Moreover, because he cannot respond appropriately to formal tests of auditory capacity, he might be erroneously diagnosed as having peripheral deafness. The problem of differential diagnosis of auditory disorders in connection with mental deficiency again emphasizes the importance of evaluating the child's responsiveness unitarily and organismically. The intellectual retardation is the basic problem. Consideration of language and auditory aspects must be in terms of this problem. Perhaps the most common error diagnostically is to proceed with appraisal of auditory capacity without regard for the child's mental level. It is assumed that the child is capable of behaving in a normal manner relative to the use of his hearing despite his mental retardation. Another error in this connection is to proceed with appraisal of language and auditory functioning without realization that the child is mentally deficient. All specialists should consider the possibility of mental deficiency. Through the history and clinical observations the diagnostician might tentatively conclude that the problem is subnormality. A complete psychological examination should then follow as a part of the total diagnosis of auditory capacity.

AUDITORY DISORDER AND THE DEGREES OF MENTAL DEFICIENCY

One of the ways in which mental deficiency can be considered is through the extent of the defect. This seems to be the most useful for the diagnostician of auditory disorders. Clinically there is a relationship between the extent of the mental inferiority and the presumption of auditory disorder. Not many idiots are presumed to have auditory impairment. The idiot's marked mental deficiency is apparent and recognized as the cause of his lack of language development. Likewise, children with minor mental retardation usually are not presumed to have auditory disorders. Such children are not sufficiently retarded in language acquisition for the presumption of deafness to be common. It is those children whose mental deficiency is not immediately apparent, but who do not acquire speech by two years of age, who are commonly presumed to have deafness. To illustrate, if a child has an intelligence quotient of 75 his intellectual growth is proceeding at three-fourths of the average rate. He will not use his first words when he is twelve months of age because his mental age at this time is only nine months. He will not have a mental age of twelve months until he is sixteen months of age. However, this degree of retardation will not preclude his using speech with some facility before he is two years of age, the critical age at which parents and specialists become concerned about deafness. When the intellectual level is below an intelligence quotient of 50 the child does not acquire speech until he is above two years of age. It is these children who might be presumed to have deafness and the diagnostician of auditory disorders in young children must make a differential diagnosis accordingly.

Idiot Level of Mental Deficiency

The category of idiocy is used for the greatest degree of mental defect. This classification includes those whose rate of mental growth is less than one-fifth of the average (I.Q. 20 and below) [4]. This means that if the child's mental level falls at the upper limit of idiocy, five years will be required for him to attain a mental age of one year. At ten years of age his mental age will not exceed two years and at fifteen years, or at adulthood, his mental age will not exceed three years. Children with this degree of mental deficiency usually do not acquire speech. They require complete custodial care. Many do not learn to walk and all are incapable of dressing and feeding themselves without direct assistance [5, 13]. Responses to sound can be observed in these children. Their responses are similar to those described by Piaget [15] in normal children below one year of age. They learn to respond to sounds in their environment, such as vocalizations and feeding sounds, but they are incapable of responding to formal tests of auditory capacity. An essential of appraising the auditory integrity of these children, as it is with all children, is that the methods of appraisal be suitable to the genetic and mental level. Methods which are applicable are discussed in Chapter XI. Idiocy is always associated with marked retardation in all respects. The child's capacity to respond auditorially is commensurate with his general incapability. In general idiocy is caused by exogenous factors [4].

Imbecile Level of Mental Deficiency

The imbecile level of mental deficiency ranges from the rate of one-fifth (I.Q. 20) to one-half (I.Q. 50) of normal progress in mental growth. Many of these children are presumed to have auditory disorders. As indicated by table 1, eleven per cent of the sample analyzed were found to be mentally deficient. Most of these children were developing mentally at the rate of one-third of normal to one-half of normal. If the child is developing at the rate of one-third of normal he will be approximately three years of age when he begins to use words. If he is developing mentally at the rate of one-half of normal he will be approximately two years of age before beginning to speak. This characteristic delay in speech development seems to explain the higher incidence of imbeciles who are presumed to have deafness. Imbeciles do acquire speech but as Doll [5] has emphasized, they have limited capacity to express ideas. Imbeciles usually do not learn to read. They do learn to feed themselves and to perform other simple functions with supervision and direction. Their capacity to respond auditorially is equivalent to their mental level. To illustrate, an imbecile, typically, is between two and three years of age when he is presumed to have an auditory defect. His mental age at this time ranges from approximately eight months to one and one-half years. His capacity to use his hearing and to profit from auditory experience will be equivalent to this mental age level. This might be overlooked diagnostically. Children have been diagnosed as having impaired acuity when their deficiency was an inability to profit normally from auditory experience. These children must be differentially distinguished from those presenting other types of auditory disorders. Imbecility, like idiocy, is due essentially to exogenous causes, with a mixture of familial factors [4].

The Moron Level of Mental Deficiency

Moronity represents the highest level of mental deficiency. This category includes those whose mental growth is not less than one-half (I.Q. 50) or more than seven-tenths (I.Q. 70) of normal. Children falling at the lower half of this range (I.Q. 50 to 60) are sometimes presumed to have auditory impairments. Such children will be approximately eighteen months to two years of age when they begin to use words expressively. This is sufficient delay for concern to arise regarding auditory capacity. Children falling at the moron level mentally do acquire speech and limited capacity to read and write. Their academic achievement rarely exceeds the fourth grade level. Morons frequently make an adequate adjustment to society, assuming appropriate training and some supervision. Moronity is primarily endogenous in origin [4]. Their capacity to respond auditorially is commensurate with their mental level. However, their mental retardation precludes capacity to profit normally from auditory experience, but their incapacity auditorially is less than that of the idiot or the imbecile.

It is apparent that language acquisition is related to intelligence. Karlin and Strazzula [11] have shown the difference between idiots, imbeciles and morons relative to the age of acquiring words as compared to the age of sitting and walking. They found that speech was more retarded than motor development. This is pertinent in connection with presumed auditory impairment. The mentally deficient child must experience the hearing of speech for a longer period of time before words become verbal symbols. It is apparent, also, that the greater the mental defect, the less words become verbal symbols, irrespective of the length of time they are heard.

Sensory capacities of the mentally deficient have not been studied extensively. However, authorities are agreed that their generalized incapacities are not attributable to sensory impairments. Landis and Bolles [14] state that gross sensory impairments do not seem to exist but that grave sensory defect might be presumed because of the lack of alertness. They observe that some low-grade mentally deficient children do not respond to odors or tastes which are highly unpleasant to the normal. This is explained on the basis of deficiency of perception. The higher brain centers are deficient. Therefore the meaningfulness of sensation, the ability to make associations and to differentiate between them qualitatively, is grossly reduced. This illustrates the clinical experience with audition. The mentally deficient child lacks capacity to respond normally to auditory stimuli but he responds to concrete sounds, comparable to the very young normal child. Auditory stimuli which entail abstractedness and experiential associations beyond his level of capacity are ignored, therefore, such stimuli are unsuitable for evaluating his auditory capacities [2].

The differential diagnosis of auditory disorders in young children includes ascertaining whether the child's lack of language is due to mental deficiency rather than impaired hearing. Clinical observations and behavioral symptomatology are essential for this purpose. However, other diagnostic possibilities must be considered. For example, Hardy [9] has emphasized that children might be diagnosed as mentally deficient when their basic impairment is peripheral deafness. Furthermore, a problem in this area is the confusion between aphasia and mental deficiency [16]. Children with congenital aphasia are sometimes diagnosed as mentally deficient without regard to the language involvements. A diagnosis of aphasia might be made even in some cases of mental deficiency if a significant discrepancy exists between mental age and language functioning. This is an essential whenever a diagnosis of aphasia is made because a significant discrepancy between symbolic functioning and capacity to function in other respects is assumed. Karlin and Strazzula [11] have indicated the importance of such language disabilities in the mentally deficient. Many aphasic children have mental levels within the normal range despite their deficiency in the area of symbolic behavior. Another consideration diagnostically is the differentiation between children with psychic deafness and the mentally deficient. Many emotionally disturbed children present a problem of generalized reduced ability to profit from sensory stimuli. Such children have been referred to as the pseudo-feebleminded. From the point of view of auditory disorders this problem is to differentiate between children whose auditory disorder is due to emotional disturbance and children who do not respond auditorially because of marked deficiency in mental development. Such differentiations usually can be achieved when the child is evaluated as a unitary functioning organism, and not only in terms of his auditory responses.

BEHAVIORAL SYMPTOMS OF MENTAL DEFICIENCY IN YOUNG CHILDREN

The behavioral symptomatology of the mentally deficient can be contrasted with the other types of children presenting problems of language development and auditory disorders. When sensory deprivation such as peripheral deafness is present, the organism's adjustment consists essentially of compensatory use of other sensory avenues and the behavior is characterized by this adjustment. When the organism is deprived of normal integrative functioning, but general capacity is within the normal range, such as in aphasia, tension and disequilibrium results. Then behavior is characterized by a need to relate more effectively to the environment without ability to do so and the organism remains in an unusually distraught and dissatisfied state. When sensory functioning is inadequate because of marked emotional disturbance the organism characteristically is directed by subjective sensation without due regard for external stimulation or circumstance. The behavior of children with mental deficiency, likewise, is characteristic. Even though the exogenous and endogenous mentally deficient can be contrasted in behavior, these children in general manifest their inadequacy in a uniform manner. The mentally deficient child comes to terms with his environment in a realistic way at the level of his intellectual ability to do so. His behavior is characterized by generalized inability to perform at his age level but with ability to perform when the task is appropriate to his mental age. The behavior of the mentally deficient child is compared briefly with other children presenting problems of differential diagnosis relative to auditory disorders.

He Acquires Speech but at a Later Age Than the Normal

Most mentally deficient children do acquire speech; the idiot is the principal exception. However, speech is acquired at a later age because more time is required for the child to reach the necessary mental level. It is noteworthy diagnostically that the mentally deficient child is not only retarded in language acquisition. He is retarded in most other aspects of his genetic development (see tables 10, 11, 12, 13, 14 and 15). This is one of his predominant character-istics. Generalized retardation is predominant and this is in contrast to the child with peripheral deafness, psychic deafness and usually, also, to the child with aphasia. When delayed language development is associated with generalized retardation of a marked degree, a clinical presumption of mental deficiency is warranted. Such a pre-sumption should be followed by appropriate adjustment of examina-tion procedures auditorially and by appropriate referral. The men-tally deficient child's generalized retardation includes his ability to respond   auditorially. Inability to profit normally from auditory experience, and, thereby, to acquire speech, should not be confused with peripheral deafness. Clinical observation and appropriate tests of auditory capacity makes this distinction possible in most instances.

His Vocalizations Are Not Characteristic in Tonal Quality

The vocalizations of mentally deficient children do not deviate significantly in tonal quality because the monitoring function of audition is not appreciably disturbed. The vocalizations of the men-tally deficient do vary, however, on the basis of the degree of the mental defect. Kennedy [12] found that mutism was characteristic of idiots and approximately twenty per cent of imbeciles were mute, with no mutism in the moron group. Gesell [8] observed that the vocalizations of the low grade mentally deficient are sparse and poorly controlled in articulation. Relative to auditory disorders, the mental deficient's vocalizations are not symptomatic of peripheral deafness. The tonal quality is not unusual but the quality in other respects is suggestive. Vocalizations are used as a social response even in early life by the imbecile and moron but such use of vocal-ization is delayed according to the mental levels. This characteristic use of vocalization, sometimes as a substitute for speech, is highly differentiating. It can be compared with other children presenting problems of auditory behavior and with the normal. For example, a two year old child making one-half of normal progress in mental growth might vocalize in a manner comparable to a normal child of twelve months. This comparison emphasizes the ways in which the mental deficient's vocalizations differ from those of children with deafness, aphasia or emotional disturbance. Clinical observations are useful and warranted accordingly.

He Improvises Sound for Pleasure and Uses His Voice Projectively

The idiot does not vocalize for pleasure. His vocalizations are essentially involuntary, with varied ability to use his voice to signal the need for attention. Children with less severe mental deficiency do vocalize for pleasure. They coo and gurgle with enjoyment. This activity might continue beyond the age at which it is expected. Some mentally deficient children are still cooing and babbling at twelve to eighteen months of age but such vocalizing, also, is begun at a later age. A history of phlegmatic behavior, genetic retardation, late onset of babbling and vocal play, with persistence of babbling after twelve months of age is symptomatic of mental retardation.

Gradually the mentally deficient child acquires ability to use his voice projectively and vocalizes in a manner which the parents recognize to mean that he is calling for attention. This use of his voice usually does not occur until he is above two years of age. Normal children acquire this utilitarian use of their voice earlier. In general the mental deficient's vocal behavior is consistent with his organismic hypoplasia. He uses hearing and vocalization for pleasurable and utilitarian purposes in a reciprocal manner, but only at the level of his genetic maturation. Such use of hearing and vocalization is characteristic and it can be compared clinically with other children having auditory disorders.

He Uses Gesture

The mental deficient's use of gesture is in proportion to his degree of mental development. Unlike the child with peripheral deafness he does not use gesture in a compensatory manner. If he lacks speech he also lacks gesture. If he has ability to speak and to behave symbolically even to a slight degree, his ability to gesticulate is proportionate. His use of gesture and nonverbal body language differs widely from the autistic and schizophrenic. His gesture lacks ideation and complexity just as he is limited in ideation and abstraction in other respects. He manifests integrative capacity of a limited type and uses gesture appropriately to the extent of these capacities. The mental defective is not characterized by his inability to use language, including gesture, like the aphasic child. Rather, he is characterized by his ability to use language at the level of his mental ability. However, the exogenous mental defective might have a specific language disability in addition to generalized mental inferiority. In such instances the areas of the brain which make language behavior possible have been damaged to a greater extent than other areas. Thus, although intellectual capacity has been substantially impaired, language function has been impaired to a significantly greater extent. Such children will not use gesture to the level of their mental capacity and they will be comparable to aphasic children in this respect.

The use of gesture by the mentally deficient child will be reduced as compared to the child with peripheral deafness and as compared to the normal. This sparse use of gesture is attributable to his reduced capacity to express ideas in general. He can function symbolically only at the level of his mental ability. Although gesture is a more concrete means of expression than speech, the mentally deficient child does not use gesture extensively.

He Responds to Sound and Uses His Hearing Projectively

The primary difficulty in evaluating the auditory behavior of mentally deficient children is to determine their general level of responsiveness. Some of the exogenous children are inconsistent in their auditory responses for the same reason that the aphasic are inconsistent. However, in general the mentally deficient child responds consistently to those sounds which are suitable to his genetic immaturity. Parents might report that the child's responses are inconsistent but usually clinical observation reveals that the inconsistency can be explained on the basis of the varying difficulty of the auditory responses which have been demanded. For example, the child might respond to feeding sounds, vocalizations and to sounds of simple toys, but not respond to music or even to conversation. Such inconsistency can be attributed to the degree of abstractness of the auditory situation. As Landis and Bolles [14] observed for the olfactory and gustatory senses, mentally deficient children are incapable of responding differentially in regard to many auditory stimuli. They ignore sounds which have abstract relationships or connotations. Such auditory reactions assume perceptual and conceptual functioning which is precluded by virtue of their mental deficiency. Clinical observation suggests that these children most often respond consistently to sound if the auditory situations are equivalent in terms of difficulty, or the degree of abstractness.

Mentally deficient children do use their hearing projectively. They learn to explore their environment auditorially, and to maintain contact with it, to the level of their ability to profit from such auditory experience. Their behavior in this respect is characteristic. Much of their auditory world is ignored because they cannot comprehend it, the organism can make no use of it, so the organism behaves as though the stimulation is not present. However, observation reveals that the mentally deficient child responds to environmental sounds which have become useful to him. If he is evaluated verbally, such as by numbers or through formal auditory tests, he might be considered peripherally deaf. If he is evaluated according to sounds which he has found useful organismically he might be found to have intact auditory capacities. Clinical observations should be made accordingly because his auditory responses in general are consistent and he uses his auditory capacities to the extent permitted by his limited mental capacities.

His Laughing, Smiling and Crying Are Characteristic

The low grade mentally deficient child is lacking in laughter. Smiling is present but all social responsiveness is grossly inadequate. Children who are less severely retarded and who are presumed to have auditory impairment do laugh and smile. Their laughter is not atypical in tonal quality and is in contrast to children with peripheral deafness. They smile in response to other persons. Such behavior is elicited especially when the social situation does not require normal alertness and curiosity. These children are markedly reduced in their ability to perceive humor. Crying is frequent and might be used in attempts to indicate that the demands of the situation are too great. In this respect it is defensive. The crying is not atypical in tonal quality. Many mental deficients reveal that organismic functioning is poor by the way in which they laugh, smile and cry. This is especially apparent in the exogenous group. The most notable aspects of this behavior diagnostically are that laughing, crying and smiling are present and have a normal acoustic quality. However, usually other qualitative differences can be observed.

He Is Not Unduly Sensitive to Other Sensory Stimulation

The mentally deficient child does not compensate by peculiar use of other sensory avenues. His unresponsiveness auditorially is characteristic of his incapacity to respond normally to sensory stimulation in general. Diagnosticians might overlook this significant aspect of the child's limitations. A diagnosis of peripheral deafness is made without awareness of the child's generalized inability to respond sensorially. The child lacks normal curiosity and capacity to profit from sensory stimulation, therefore, compensatory use of other sensory avenues is impossible. Furthermore, inasmuch as the auditory avenue is being used to the extent of the organism's capacity, compensatory use of other avenues is unnecessary. Sensory deprivation is not present. The sensory avenues are providing stimulation and the organism is using these impressions without awareness of limitation. The mentally deficient's behavior organismically is characterized by the use of sensory stimulation in a realistic manner according to his limited capacities to do so. Clinical observations of his generalized unresponsiveness to sensory stimulation are diagnostically useful accordingly. His capacity to respond visually and to tactile sensation is commensurate with his responsiveness auditorially. All responsiveness sensorially is commensurate with the degree of his mental retardation.

He Attends to Facial Expression

The mentally deficient child is responsive to facial expression. This is especially apparent in those who are presumed to have hearing impairment. This group has mental capacity which is adequate for purposes of responding to facial expressions. This does not imply that these children are capable of subtleties of social perception. However, they are responsive to expressions of warmth, friendliness, smiling and other manifestations of acceptance. Like the normal young child, they use facial expression to determine the threateningness or security of the immediate situation. Mentally deficient children do not reject people's faces, nor do they behave as though they are unaware of them. It is, also, differentially significant that they do not attend unduly to facial expression, in the manner of the child with peripheral deafness. It can be stated that, as in most other respects, the mentally deficient's attention to facial expression is not compensatory but it is realistic to the extent of his capacity to profit from such attention. Clinical observations in this connection are useful in making a differential diagnosis.

His Motor Behavior Is Characteristic

As indicated previously, there is a relationship between intellectual development and genetic maturation in general. Some diagnosticians, however, proceed as though no such relationship exists because they do not recognize that the child develops as a unitary organism. Maturational age, not chronological age, is the determining factor and motor behavior is no exception. The child's motor development can be compared with the normal through norms provided by Bayley [1], Doll [6], and Gesell [7]. Furthermore, various authorities have studied the motor functioning of mentally deficient children. Heath [10] contrasted the motor capacities of the exogenous and the endogenous and found the endogenous to be superior. Karlin and Strazzula [11] showed the relationship between ages of sitting alone and walking for idiots, imbeciles, and morons. The findings for the mentally deficient, as shown in tables 10, 11, 12 and 13, are in close agreement with those presented by these workers. They found a mean for sitting of 11.2 for the imbeciles and 10.6 for the morons. The mean age for sitting for the sample presumed to have auditory disorders was 10.33 (table 10). Likewise, Karlin and Strazzula reported a mean age for walking of 23.5 for the imbeciles and of 14.4 for the morons. The mean age for walking for the group who were seen for differential diagnosis was 21.15 (table 12). These findings are in close agreement and corroborate the observation that mentally deficient children who are presumed to have impaired auditory acuity usually fall in the intelligence range of imbecile or low grade moron.

Tables 11 and 13, also, are suggestive concerning the importance of motor maturational factors in the differential diagnosis of auditory disorders. These data reveal that the mentally deficient were more delayed in both sitting and walking than any of the other groups. These data are in disagreement especially with those who make no distinction between the aphasic, the severely emotionally disturbed and the mentally deficient. From the point of view of auditory disorders, moreover, it is apparent that the peripheral auditory mechanism is useful only to the extent that the central nervous system functions normally in general.

The primary characteristic of the mentally deficient child is generalized retardation. He is not only retarded in sitting and walking, he is retarded in feeding, dressing, grasping, throwing, and in many other aspects of his motor development. Clinical observations can be made because usually his motor deficiencies are observable. However, a careful genetic history is essential. Furthermore, the diagnostician should be thoroughly familiar with the norms for normal children so that he can make immediate comparative observations of the child with auditory disorder. It is important to note that the child with peripheral deafness was not found to deviate significantly from the normal in either sitting or walking (tables 10 and 12).

His Social Perception Is Limited

The mentally deficient child's social perception is appropriate to his mental age. He is aware of persons around him and adapts to their presence at his level of capacity. He is not unduly alert visually to those in his environment like the child with peripheral deafness. Moreover, he does not reject or lack awareness of other persons. He is slow in his reactions and incapable of comprehending many social situations and circumstances which are automatically perceived by the normal child of his age. For example, he might show no awareness when his mother gets his coat and prepares to leave. Likewise, he might show little response to games, such as roll the ball or patacake [8]. His response is characterized by lack of comprehension, not by shyness, reticence or rejection. His play, furthermore, lacks imagination, ideation, and it is limited and repetitive. His social perceptual behavior is characteristic and suggestive in its appropriateness, but with marked immaturity. It is comparable to a child approximately one-half of his age, or less. Clinical observations of his social perception are revealing diagnostically.

His Emotional Expression Is Characteristic

When normal genetic maturation is impeded, emotional development and expression are arrested accordingly. Blatz, et al. [3] have shown genetic stages of observable expressions of emotion in normal children under two years of age. Crying and screaming occur before four months of age. Refusing, resisting, throwing and calling by vocal projection occur between four and eight months of age. Clinging, throwing self back and stiffening occur between eight and twelve months of age. Running away occurs between twelve and sixteen months, hiding the face and saying "no" are observed between sixteen and twenty months, and slumping, crying and asking in a demanding manner, are observed between twenty and twenty-four months. Many clinical observations can be added to this genetic evaluation of emotional expression. Mentally deficient children do show emotional expression. In this respect they are more natural than autistic or schizophrenic children. They show joviality and resentment which is appropriate to the circumstances but their responses are immature as compared to the normal. For example, at two years of age the mentally deficient child might respond emotionally in a manner which characterizes the average child of one year of age but his emotional expression, or behavior, is not bizarre. It is in marked contrast to the autistic and schizophrenic child in this respect. Likewise, his emotional expressions are more limited and retarded than those associated with peripheral deafness. Shyness, reticence, apprehension, clinging, resistance and running away are less apparent as compared to children with peripheral deafness. As compared to aphasic children, the mentally deficient's emotional expression is more appropriate to his mental age. Moreover, while some exogenous mentally deficient children are comparable to aphasic children emotionally, the mentally deficient exhibit less catastrophic type of behavior. Apparently the integrative capacities of the mentally deficient are not as seriously discrepant with the general mental level. The emotional expression and contact of the mentally deficient is essentially realistic and commensurate with his mental ability. He is cooperative and amenable accordingly. His characteristic emotional behavior is observable and useful in making a diagnosis of his auditory capacities.

His Auditory and Visual Perceptual Behavior Is Characteristic

Werner and Bowers [17] have shown that mentally deficient children vary in their perceptual capacities according to etiology. Endogenous children are superior to exogenous children in perceptual functioning. However, the mentally deficient child in general is not characterized by behavior manifesting perceptual disturbance and disintegration. Rather, his behavior suggests that he is functioning perceptually at the level of his mental capacities. Even when perceptual disturbances are manifested by perseveration, distractibility and disinhibition, his behavior does not suggest primarily an inability to integrate sensory experience meaningfully. Rather, in general, he uses sensory experience at the level of his capacity to do so. Clinical observations should emphasize his consistent use of sensory stimulation when these stimuli are concrete and simple.

Language Functioning Is Characteristic

Most mentally deficient children who are presumed to have auditory disorders in early life have little or no speech at the age at which they are brought to the diagnostician. Their receptive capacities ordinarily are adequate, but they have not been able to profit normally from their auditory environment to the extent of acquiring speech. Speech is acquired only after mental development reaches twelve to eighteen months. In contrast to the child with peripheral deafness, the mentally deficient child cannot use vision and tactile sensation in a compensatory manner and, thereby, increase his inner language. However, like the normal infant, the mentally deficient child comprehends language prior to his being able to use it verbally. This means that specific clinical observation often reveals beginning ability to comprehend words associated with the child's daily experiences. Such observations are highly significant and sometimes definitive relative to the child's auditory capacities.

SUMMARY

Some children are presumed to have peripheral deafness when their true problem is mental deficiency. Such children can be differentiated from others having auditory disorders by careful appraisal of the total problem, including the pattern of behavior. Children with mental deficiency who are presumed to be peripherally deaf have sufficient intelligence so that they do not identify themselves as being severely retarded. Therefore, idiots usually are recognized and not presumed to be deaf although they do not acquire speech. The idiot is one whose rate of mental growth is less than one-fifth of average (I.Q. 20 or below). He responds to sounds appropriately selected and administered. The imbecile is one whose rate of mental growth is between one-fifth and one-half of average (I.Q. 20 to 50). Thus if a child has a rate of mental growth which is one-third of average, he will be approximately three years of age, instead of one year, when he begins to talk. Typically such a child might be presumed to be peripherally deaf when he is between two and three years of age. The moron includes those whose rate of mental growth is one-half to seven-tenths of average (I.Q. 50 to 70). Such a child begins to speak between eighteen and twenty-four months of age and this delay may lead to the presumption of deafness. The behavior of the mentally deficient is characteristic. They manifest their inadequacy in a uniform manner with generalized inability to perform at their age level but with ability to perform when the task is appropriate to their age level. The mentally deficient child vocalizes with normal tonal quality, he vocalizes for pleasure and he uses his voice to call attention to himself. He uses gestures but only at the level of his generalized reduced capacity. He responds to simple, concrete sounds consistently but may ignore abstract sounds such as pure tones, music and conversation. His laughing, smiling and crying are not discrepant in quality from his mental age but usually are reduced in quality. He responds to other than auditory stimuli but in a limited manner consistent with his limited capacities. He attends and responds to facial expression similarly. Particularly characteristic of the mentally deficient child is his delayed motor development; he is retarded in sitting and walking and in other aspects of his development. His social awareness is consistent with his mental capacity and shows marked immaturity. His emotional development and expression likewise are retarded but he does respond emotionally and is not bizarre like the child with psychic deafness. His auditory behavior in general usually is consistent with his mental age.

BIBLIOGRAPHY

1. Bayley, Nancy: The development of motor abilities during the first three years. Society for Research in Child Development, National Research Council, Washington *1*: 1935.
2. Birch, J. W. and Matthews, J.: The hearing of mental defectives. Am. J. Ment. Deficiency *55*: 384–393, 1951.

3. Blatz, W., Bott, E. and Millichamp, D.: The development of emotion in the infant. U. of Toronto Press, Child Development Series 4: 19, 1935.

4. Doll, E. A.: The feebleminded child, in, Carmichael, L. (ed.): Manual of Child Psychology. New York, Wiley, 1946, pp. 845–885.

5. ——: Mental deficiency. Encyclopedia Britannica, 1951.

6. ——: Measurement of Social Competence. Minneapolis, Educational Test Bureau, 1953.

7. Gesell, A. et al.: The First Five Years of Life. New York, Harpers, 1940.

8. —— and Amatruda, C: Developmental Diagnosis, Ed. 2. New York, Paul B. Hoeber, 1947.

9. Hardy, W. G.: The relations between impaired hearing and psuedo-feeblemindedness. Nervous Child 7: 432, 1948.

10. Heath, S. R.: Rail-walking performance as related to mental age and etiological type among the mentally retarded. Am. J. Psychol. 55: 240, 1942.

11. Karlin, I. W. and Strazzula, M.: Speech and language problems of mentally deficient children. J. Speech & Hearing Disorders 7: 286, 1952.

12. Kennedy, L.: The speech of the feeble-minded. Proceedings of the American Society for the Study of Disorders of Speech 3: 16, 1932.

13. Kirk, S. A. and Johnson, G. O.: Educating the Retarded Child. New York, Houghton Mifflin, 1951.

14. Landis, C. and Bolles, M.: Textbook of Abnormal Psychology. New York, MacMillan, 1947.

15. Piaget, Jean: Play, Dreams and Imitation in Childhood. New York, W. W. Norton, 1951.

16. Sugar, Oscar: Congenital aphasia. J. Speech & Hearing Disorders 17: 301, 1952.

17. Werner, H. and Bowers, M.: Auditory-motor organization in two clinical types of mentally deficient children. J. Gen. Psychol. 59: 85, 1941.

PART FOUR: THE EXAMINATION— METHODS AND PROCEDURES

Chapter X

The Use of Tests

THE THREE STEPS ENTAILED IN MAKING A differential diagnosis of auditory disorders in children have been emphasized. Step one, the differential history, was discussed in Part Two. Step two, clinical observation and evaluation of behavioral symptomatology, was considered in Part Three. Step three, the examination, is discussed in Part Four. Each specialist conducts an examination of the child according to his own specialization. However, many different specialists are in a position to encounter young children with auditory disorders and each specialist has a need for techniques to evaluate these disorders. Techniques which have been found useful for this purpose are discussed in Chapter XI, but, first it is necessary to consider the problem of using tests with preschool children who have auditory disorders.

Most of the children having auditory disorders in early life are nonverbal children. The application of any tests to this group is difficult because of their age, because they lack ability to communicate verbally, and because they usually cannot comprehend language auditorially. Therefore, only a few of the standardized tests available are directly applicable to these children and most of these are tests of mental development (see Chapter XII). However, there are certain basic assumptions in the use of all tests whether or not they have been standardized. Certain tests can be used effectively with nonverbal children having auditory disorders when the assumptions of the test are understood, and when it is applied appropriately. For example, tests of auditory capacity must be suitable genetically. When common tests of auditory capacity are used it is assumed, at least tacitly, that they are appropriate to the genetic level of the child. If a child does not respond to a particular test one of the questions which must be considered is its suitability in terms of the child's maturational level. Another critical assumption of most tests is that the response is the best response that the individual can make. In terms of auditory testing this means that it is a threshold response. Stated differently, most auditory testing assumes maximum cooperation and responsiveness on the part of the child. As indicated previously, such tests are limited in their usefulness with many children requiring a differential diagnosis of auditory disorder. Testing of these children should be accomplished in such a manner that their limited ability to cooperate does not significantly reduce the level of their responses. To illustrate, although they can hear, some children lack ability to listen. Under these circumstances, if the test assumes ability to listen, the child's responses will manifest peripheral deafness which is not present. Some informal tests of auditory capacity do not assume listening ability and, therefore, are more valid for such children.

There are other considerations in the use of tests. All tests require organismic responsiveness, whether they be tests of auditory capacity, or tests of other capacities such as motor and mental abilities. Thereby, a response to an auditory stimulus is not only indicative of the child's auditory acuity but it is indicative of his capacity to use auditory sensations integratively and organismically. This inclusive concept of responsiveness is generally recognized in mental testing, and such tests are interpreted as revealing expressive intelligence primarily. Certain types of children, for example the schizophrenic, obviously have intelligence which they frequently cannot manifest on formal tests of intelligence. Likewise, some children have hearing which they cannot express, or manifest, through formal tests of hearing. The organismic aspect of test responses must be considered both in the use of tests and in the interpretation of test findings. Clinical observations, as discussed in Part Two, are essential in validating test responses. Such clinical observations are made continuously during the examination because emphasis on objective test results, without due consideration of organismic responsiveness, frequently leads to erroneous diagnoses of children with auditory disorders.

MANAGEMENT OF THE CHILD

Appropriate and skillful management of the child during the examination is an important contributing factor to the validity of test findings. Many young children presenting problems of auditory disorder are difficult to manage; they may be hyperactive, fearful, withdrawn, or aggressive. The psychological approach to the child emphasizes that there is a reason for such behavior, that he is not simply being stubborn or resistive to antagonize his parents and the diagnostician. Many of these children have had unfortunate experiences in hospitals and elsewhere. It is essential that the diagnostician make a sincere effort to understand the child's behavior and it is imperative that he not become frustrated and angry with the child. These children are exceedingly sensitive to nonverbal communication, such as attitudes of rejection, and they will be aware of the feelings of annoyance on the part of the examiner. The diagnostician should expect many of these children to present problems of behavior; he should accept this fact and conduct the examination accordingly. Complete acceptance of the child and his parents is the most consequential aspect of gaining adequate rapport for the examination. An attitude of blamefulness, or criticism, toward either the child or his parents usually results in failure and further complicates the problem for the future. All diagnosticians have responsibilities and obligations to prevent unnecessary psychological complications.

The child should be given time to become acquainted and to adjust to the testing situation. Frequently this means that he should not be rushed from his mother's lap to an examining chair and expected to proceed immediately with the examination. Rather, he should be permitted to remain with his mother for a few minutes, during which time the examiner manifests a friendly, playful manner. Giving the child an interesting toy might help him to adjust to the situation. Having the child remain with his parents for a brief period has other advantages. It affords an opportunity to observe the child's behavior in relation to his parents. Such observations, as indicated in Part Three, are directly related to the examination and to the interpretation of test findings. Some children might ignore their parents, giving them no more attention than they give to others, or they might leave their parents without normal concern. The parents' management of the child, likewise, can be observed, but there are other significant considerations. The child might vocalize to his parents, he might gesture to them, the parents might call him, stamp their feet, clap their hands, or use other ways to gain his attention. This is highly useful information diagnostically and, with other observations, provides the frame of reference for the examination.

If the child will not leave the mother, even if he will not get down from her lap, certain informal tests can be used. It is not uncommon to do both formal and informal testing in the presence of the parents; however, sometimes it is desirable to separate the child and his parents for at least part of the examination, but when fearfulness is intense such separation should be avoided. In general, the child should not be expected to make all of the compromises. The examiner, too, should adjust to the child. The techniques and procedures, and especially the manner of approach should be adjusted to the nature of the child's problem. Significant questions while examining the child include the genetic level, ability to cooperate, mental level, emotional tone, motor difficulties, and ability to listen. These, and many others, might affect the child's responsiveness. A useful discussion of the assumptions of tests and management and rapport while examining young children is given by Kent [2].

PURPOSE OF TESTS

Cronbach [1] defines a test as a "systematic procedure for comparing the behavior of two or more persons." As this definition suggests, tests are for eliciting responses, or behavior, which can be evaluated and compared with the responses of others. An important clarification is necessary in this connection. Many psychological tests, such as tests of mental ability, have been standardized, they have been given to a substantial number of individuals and average scores have been statistically determined. These scores constitute the norms. When the test is given to a particular individual, his score can be compared with the scores of others by determining his position on the norm. Such standardized psychological tests for young children are discussed in Chapter XII. In contrast to these tests, most tests of auditory capacity have not been standardized but these, too, assume comparison. Whenever such tests are used the examiner makes a comparison with the normal largely on the basis of his clinical experience. Validation of such tests is primarily through their use. Historically, this also applies to the pure tone audiometer. Moreover, most formal tests of auditory capacity in current use were devised for clinical purposes in connection with adults, including the tuning fork and audiometric tests. Only later have these tests been used for purposes of testing the auditory capacities of children. It is important that these tests have not been significantly revised, or adapted, for use with children. This implies the assumption that young children are capable of responding in like manner auditorially as compared to adults. While these tests have usefulness with some children, reliance on them to the exclusion of other validating information leads to errors of diagnosis.

There are many sources of errors in the use of tests. Kent [2] has emphasized various sources of error and the need for caution in the use of psychological tests with young children. Similar caution should be used in auditory testing. The principal purpose of the auditory test is to determine whether the child's auditory behavior is consistent with his behavior in other respects. To simply determine that he does, or does not, respond directly to a sound stimulus is inadequate diagnostically. As indicated previously, various children respond similarly to their acoustic environments and the absence of direct response to sound requires interpretation in terms of the total behavior presented by the child. The auditory test provides an opportunity to observe the child's behavior systematically, in a specific manner. Such tests are not used only to determine whether the child can give a direct response to a given stimulus. Rather, such testing includes procuring information relative to the child's ability to structure sound perceptually, to respond at the threshold of feeling, to integrate an auditory sensation, to respond consistently, and to listen attentively. The typical acuity response has been over-emphasized in diagnosis. To over-emphasize the acuity factor is to over-simplify auditory behavior and the diagnostic problem entailed. The child's responsiveness auditorially is influenced by various factors, including his acuity.

In order to evaluate and to interpret the young child's auditory capacities often it is necessary, also, to evaluate him in other respects. Such inclusive appraisal usually requires the services of more than one specialist. Evaluation of auditory, mental, social, emotional and language capacities usually is necessary. Some methods and procedures for critically appraising these areas are suggested in Chapters XI and XII.

SUMMARY

The third step in the differential diagnosis of auditory disorders in young children is the examination. Because these children are nonverbal many standardized tests are not applicable. Moreover, auditory tests alone cannot be considered as definite or adequate for making a differential diagnosis. It is necessary to include other evidence such as mental capacity, emotional status and the pattern of behavior. Auditory tests require responsiveness of the total individual. Therefore, a response to an auditory stimulus indicates not only acuity but the level at which he can utilize auditory stimuli and respond to them in an integrative manner. Thus failure to respond to an auditory stimulus does not necessarily mean inability to hear. Management of the child during testing is very important. Many children with auditory disorders are fearful, distrustful and present unusual problems of behavior. It is essential that the diagnostician accept the child and his parents and not become exasperated and angry because most of these children are highly sensitive to non-verbal communication and immediately sense the feelings of annoyance in the examiner. The child should be given time to become acquainted and to adjust to the testing situation. He might be permitted to remain on his mother's lap for a period while the examiner manifests a friendly, playful manner and observes the child's behavior.

BIBLIOGRAPHY

1. Cronbach, Lee: Essentials of Psychological Testing. New York, Harpers, 1949.
2. Kent, Grace: Mental Tests in Clinic for Children. New York, Van Nostrand, 1950.

Chapter XI

The Examination of Auditory Capacity

THE AUDITORY CAPACITIES OF YOUNG CHILDREN can be evaluated in various ways. The procedures which have been used can be classified into two types: formal and informal. Formal procedures are those which require a substantial degree of active cooperation from the child; a sound stimulus is given and the child is to give a direct indication of whether or not he heard it. Informal procedures are those which do not require active cooperation from the child and indirect responses are used as manifestations of hearing. There is an intermediary procedure, combining formal and informal techniques, which is to use calibrated or formalized tests in a sound-field manner. This method has the advantage of a more quantified type of stimulus but does not emphasize cooperative effort and the need for direct responses from the child. In the past formal procedures have been used almost exclusively. When informal procedures have been used, they have not been used systematically and they too have required direct responses from the child.

Clinical experience in the differential diagnosis of auditory disorders suggests that formal and informal procedures should be considered of equal value. Formal procedures include pure tone audiometry, tuning fork tests, speech reception tests and psychogalvanic audiometry. There are many types of informal tests but they include chiefly the sound instrument test, the sound toy test, imitation of the child's vocalizations, the voice test and the verbal comprehension test. These formal and informal methods for examining the child's auditory responsiveness are discussed in this chapter.

Informal procedures are especially useful in office practice. They do not require extensive equipment and they can be performed without the help of an assistant. In contrast some formal procedures require extensive space, equipment and staff and thereby are limited extensively to medical school or other university facilities. However, equipment and personnel requirements will vary according to the needs of individual specialists. From the point of view of differential diagnosis it is assumed that each specialist as a minimum will do his own specific examination and in addition use the informal procedures for evaluating auditory capacity. After integrating the results with those of the history and the clinical observations, appropriate referral can be made. For example, the pediatrician after doing the pediatric examination might use the history data, clinical observation of behavioral symptomatology and the informal auditory tests. If on the basis of the total findings he suspects for example psychic deafness, he might refer the child to a psychiatrist. The minimum responsibility for any specialist is an awareness that there are four types of children who respond similarly to their acoustic environments and that differential diagnosis is therefore necessary.

INFORMAL AUDITORY TESTS

The Sound Instrument Test

Ewing and Ewing [12] and Utley [26] have reported on the usefulness of selected sound producing instruments in evaluating the auditory capacities of infants and young children. Froeschels and Beebe [14] have reported on the use of Urbantschitch's whistles and tuning forks. They found that newborn infants responded to the whistles but not to the tuning forks.

The approximate frequency and intensity ranges of a typical selection of sound producing instruments were determined through the use of a sound analyzer and a sound level meter. The results were as follows for each of the instruments:

	Frequency range	Intensity range in decibels at 3 ft.
Triple bell	2800–4500	50–60
Small cricket	2400–6000	75–85
Large cricket	1700–2300	90–102
School bell	4000–6000	85–108
"A" chime	750–1200	50–85
Single bells	3000–4000	64–85
Clacker	2000–3000	50–95

Other instruments could be evaluated in the same manner and thus enlarge the battery. Such an analysis of the instruments provides the examiner with information which permits him to be more specific in his judgments although the instruments are used informally. These instruments have been used extensively with young children. The primary speech frequencies of sound are included and this battery is readily portable and flexible and can be used under variable circumstances of cooperation. Furthermore, it can be used at low genetic levels because it has been shown that normal children turn to the ringing of a bell at about five months of age. The loudness can be varied by increasing and decreasing the distance from the child. Readings should be made at various distances from the child because this permits the diagnostician to be more specific regarding the intensity which is being used.

The procedure for administering the sound instrument test varies according to the total clinical problem presented by the child. If the child is capable of a minimum of cooperative effort he is seated at a table on which has been placed an appropriate toy. The mother might be seated near by. The examiner is seated opposite or beside the child and engages him playfully with the toy. It is highly desirable that this playful activity be one in which the child can do something, such as placing rings on a peg. As the child engages himself in the playful activity the examiner produces a sound with one of the instruments. The production of the sound is not visible to the child. For example, the examiner might ring the bell under the table or behind the child's head. All movement is carefully concealed. Likewise, the child's level of attention to the game activity is noted. He is not permitted to become deeply engrossed in the foreground play activity in order that this not impede him unduly from shifting to the background auditory stimulation. The primary response given by the child consists of a cessation of the foreground activity; he momentarily ceases his play and assumes an attitude of immobilization and searching awareness. He scans the environment in an attempt to note what change has occurred and then he is assured and encouraged to again engage in his playful activity while further auditory stimulation is presented. Most often children who can cooperate and respond well in this manner are those with peripheral deafness.

When the child is hyperactive and incapable of cooperative effort the sound instrument test is presented variously. For example, if the child is attending to one object and then to another, which is characteristic of some aphasic children, the examiner might follow the child and as the child is engaged in his distractions, a sound stimulus is presented behind him. Unusually long durations of sound stimulation are necessary for such children because it is difficult for them to shift from their foreground visual sensations. In some instances it is necessary to reduce their visual field before auditory responses can be given. This can be done by having them face the wall for short intervals while the auditory stimulations are being presented.

Other procedures can be used as indicated. Children whose behavior suggests infantile autism or schizophrenia usually respond most successfully when the sounds are presented very indirectly. For example, a child might be deeply engrossed in phantasy, without apparent regard for his environment. The examiner does not attempt to gain direct contact with him. Rather, he places himself where he can observe the child and then presents sounds at varying intensities and frequencies while the sound instruments and all movements are concealed. As the sounds are presented the child might move, stop a stereotyped activity, turn his eyes, stop vocalizing or give other indirect responses. Direct responses should not be expected from such children and the examination should be conducted on this basis. Some children, notably the mentally deficient, respond most successfully when the sound is presented visually and auditorily. For example, the examiner has two of the single bells, one in each hand. While seated beside the child, he rings one bell in front of him, encouraging him to reach for it. As the child begins to reach for this bell, it is withdrawn and immediately the second bell in the other hand is rung behind him. A child who previously has not responded to background auditory stimulation might respond by this method. By presenting the sound alternately and in succession from foreground to background, the effect is to increase motivation and to keep the sound in the immediate foreground of his attention. The responses of mentally deficient and of some aphasic children can be significantly improved by this method. The characteristic response is to engage in searching behavior while the sound is presented behind them after the visual presentation has been withdrawn.

The use of sound producing instruments can be compared to tuning fork tests. Both are essentially informal and highly flexible in application and both require considerable clinical experience for maximum effectiveness. The sound instruments have a certain advantage in use with young children because tuning forks produce pure tones which are more abstract and meaningless for young children. The importance of the nature of the sound being used is discussed further in relation to pure tone audiometry.

The Sound Toy Test

Sound toys are useful in evaluating auditory capacities. The toys which have been used include a squeaking doll, growling bear, musical jack-in-the-box, quacking duck, xylophone, croaking frog, musical blocks and a ringing telephone. Sound toy tests can be used variously according to the child's behavior. Their primary value is in determining whether the child has impaired auditory acuity. The intensity level of sound toys usually is not greater than the level of ordinary conversation. If the child responds to these sound toys and if other information is corroborative, it suggests that the child's lack of speech is not due to peripheral deafness. In eliciting responses to sound toys one procedure is to simply present the toy to the child and encourage him to play with it. As he plays with it and the sound occurs unintentionally, his response is noted. Children who hear the sound usually manifest an awareness of its presence. They might show surprise, immobilization, amusement or apprehension. After the sound occurs once the child can be encouraged to produce it again by showing him how to do it intentionally. Some children enjoy producing the sounds in this manner and their response is an obvious indication of capacity to hear it. The sound toy test given in this manner is applicable to very young children. Cattell [5] has shown that the normal child responds to a similar test at approximately eleven months of age.

The sound toy test can be given in other ways. Children who lack the general ability to relate playfully with toys or with the examiner, might give imitative responses. For example, if the duck is held immediately before them and squeezed in an obvious manner by the examiner, the child might imitate the act. Usually such imitation is clearly motivated by the sound which emanates from the toy. The child might continue producing the sound over and over again without awareness that he is manifesting ability to hear. However, he might not give a listening response, integrate the sound meaningfully or show enjoyment in playing with the toy. Such responses are revealing relative to diagnosis and corroboration from clinical observation and history information might suggest that other problems than peripheral deafness should be suspected.

The sound toy test has been found useful in evaluating the auditory capacities of children presenting the behavioral syndrome of marked emotional disturbance. Such children might not respond to the sounds produced by the examiner but they will produce sounds for themselves in an autistic manner. Apparently they reject sounds emanating from the environment, especially those associated with human beings and human figures, such as dolls. However, they do not reject sounds which are not vocally produced and which they produce themselves for themselves. A toy which does not suggest animate life such as a musical block is most suitable for this purpose. The toy is placed in the child's hand and the examiner helps him to produce the sound. After starting him the child might continue to produce the sound in an autistic manner; he produces the sound only for the sake of hearing it. He does not relate the sound to the purpose of the toy, nor does the sound connote emotional contact with his environment. However, his use of the sound even for autistic purposes is revealing diagnostically. It might suggest acuity which is adequate for hearing speech even though no direct responses are made to auditory stimulation from others.

Some children respond more readily to the absence of sound rather than to its presence. The sound toy test is useful also in this connection. If two toys are identical except that one produces a sound and the other does not, the child might respond to the absence of sound in the one toy. To illustrate, two dolls or two rubber mice or two toy music boxes might be used. One of each set of toys does not produce a sound because the sound producing part of the toy has been changed so it does not function. The toy which produces the sound is given to the child and manipulated so the sound can be heard. The child might give no indication of awareness of the sound. He is then given the toy which does not produce a sound although it is identical in appearance. Care must be taken to eliminate tactile sensations, nevertheless some children immediately note the absence of sound. Apparently this test makes it possible for them to distinguish between sound and lack of sound. This procedure has been especially useful with children presumed to have auditory agnosia or emotional disturbance. The child with auditory agnosia can be expected to indicate the presence or absence of sound only. This test allows him to do so whereas he cannot respond to tests which require his indicating that he has heard. Emotionally disturbed children who have established defenses against sound might not include the immediate shift to no sound emanating from the toy so they show confusion and bewilderment indicating reaction to sound. Similar reactions have been noted in association with other tests discussed below.

The Imitation of Vocalization Test

The child should be encouraged to vocalize freely during the examination. Some children despite such encouragement remain mute and then the muteness must be evaluated symptomatically. As indicated in the discussion of behavioral symptomatology, when the child does vocalize his vocalizations can be appraised for acoustic quality. His vocalizations can be useful in other ways. As the child vocalizes in association with play, in connection with making demands or in laughing and crying the examiner can imitate him. Piaget [24] has shown that infants respond to such imitations by ceasing their vocalizations or by making other adjustments. Clinical experience has demonstrated that children who do not respond to other auditory tests frequently do respond to imitation of their own vocalizations. As the child vocalizes the diagnostician imitates him, using mild intensity. The child might not give direct responses such as looking at the examiner. His responses usually consist of cessation of vocalization, interruption of motor activity or other indirect reactions. Such reactions often can be duplicated many times. This test requires no attentive cooperation from the child. It can be used with infants and with children presenting any of the four types of auditory disorders. The child with profound peripheral deafness vocalizes projectively and in a utilitarian manner but he does not vocalize for pleasure. Imitation of his vocalizations does not cause him to react because he does not hear them, unless perhaps the examiner uses a very loud intensity. Children with partial peripheral deafness also vocalize in a characteristic manner. Imitation of their vocalizations with appropriate intensity usually causes them to give a direct response, such as looking up in a startled and scanning manner. Perhaps the greatest usefulness of this test, however, is with children who have no impairment of acuity but whose auditory function is disturbed for other reasons. It has been found highly useful with children who are delayed in genetic maturation because this test can be applied at very low genetic levels. It is useful with children presumed to be aphasic (it has been used successfully as a method of beginning language training in receptive aphasic children) because, although they might not be able to relate to other types of auditory stimulation, they can respond to imitation of their own vocalizations. This might be due to the low genetic level of the test or because it is a highly concretized and structured auditory situation. Emotionally disturbed children apparently have rejected sound primarily as it derives from other persons and from their environment. Unless they are mute they presumably have not rejected sound in connection with their own vocalizations. Thereby, when their vocalizations are imitated their defenses and equilibrium are disturbed. Their reactions are correspondingly clinically consistent and revealing. Other implications include Mowrer's [23] conception of the psychological significance of babbling. Babbling can be considered as a pleasant auditory experience associated with other persons, notably the child's parents. Emotionally disturbed children with psychic deafness might reject auditory sensations but vocalize in the manner of a much younger child. Imitation of these vocalizations apparently coincides with the level of the child's emotional acceptance of auditory experience. Furthermore, attempts are being made to help children with psychic deafness to overcome their rejection of sound by having them relate to other persons auditorially through imitation of their vocalizations. These attempts might prove helpful in further clarifying the usefulness of the imitation of vocalization test.

The Voice Tests

Simple voice tests are applicable to many children. Such tests can be used in various ways. For example, as the child is engaged mildly in a playful foreground activity the diagnostician hums at a low intensity. Children who do not respond to more formal auditory tests might respond to the examiner's humming. This test can be performed without the child's active cooperation and it is applicable to very young children. Cattell [5] has shown that normal children listen to voice at about two months of age and turn to vocalizations at about four months of age. The responses consist mainly of cessation of activity, immobilization and other direct or indirect adjustments. Voice tests also can be used to elicit imitative responses from the child. For example, the child is encouraged through praise and in the manner of playing a game to imitate the mum-mum-mum as it is produced vocally by the diagnostician. If the child imitates this sound, then bu-bu-bu is used in the same way. During this initial period the child is permitted to see the face of the examiner. After the initial training period the sounds are given alternately without the child seeing the face of the examiner with the intent that the child should imitate each sound correctly. This can be done at varying intensities and distances from the child. This test has been useful with children who are retarded genetically and with aphasic children especially. Normal children imitate vocalizations of adults beginning at approximately nine months of age [5]. A variation of this test is to use it as an auditory memory test. The examiner gives the sound once, twice or three times in succession and the child is to imitate it the correct number of times. This method is used in evaluating auditory perceptual functioning. Another variation which is useful in appraising acuity and perception is to vary the pitch. The examiner gives the sound, such as mum-mum, two or three times in succession. The first mum is given in a low pitch and the second one in a high pitch as though it is a tune. The child is to imitate the raising and lowering of the pitch and give the sound the correct number of times. A minimum degree of cooperation is required for this test but it can be applied to many hyperactive children by following them while they are moving or engaging in various activities. Delayed responses occur in some children, notably in the aphasic and autistic. The examiner must be alert to such responses because they might occur even after another activity has been begun. Moreover, some children continue producing the sound after it should be apparent that it is no longer appropriate and without awareness that other persons are hearing them; it becomes a stereotyped behavior. This occurs mainly in brain injured children but occurs also in the emotionally disturbed. Children with peripheral deafness cannot imitate the examiner's vocalizations without seeing his face. They make no distinction between mum-mum and bu-bu because in lip reading these appear as being identical.

The Verbal Comprehension Test

Some children with auditory disorders do comprehend spoken language. Children with partial peripheral deafness, aphasia, psychic deafness or mental deficiency might comprehend speech under certain conditions. A systematic evaluation of their ability to use receptive language symbolically usually is included in the examination if the child is more than eighteen months of age. Such tests of speech comprehension also are given through amplifying equipment and this method is discussed below. Often it is diagnostically helpful to give speech comprehension tests without the use of amplifying equipment. The examiner varies the intensity of his voice and adapts his procedures in other ways according to the clinical symptomatology presented by the child. For example, if the child manifests symptoms of marked anxiety and does not respond directly to auditory stimulation, the examiner might use verbal language such as "Where is mommy?" and "Show me your shoes." Clinical experience indicates that some children find it possible to respond more satisfactorily to such informal auditory situations. Autistic and schizophrenic children too might give direct or indirect responses to meaningful speech. Such responses are highly corroborative of other diagnostic information. To illustrate, a schizophrenic child who gave no direct responses to sound irrespective of intensity, frequently would slyly go to a cabinet where he knew cookies were kept when the examiner said "Get a cookie," in a natural conversational tone. Children with profound peripheral deafness do not comprehend speech but those with partial deafness will comprehend to the extent that they have been able to hear it. Aphasic children frequently comprehend isolated words or phrases inconsistently. The words which they reportedly comprehend at home sometimes can be used effectively in evaluating their hearing acuity and other receptive capacities.

Voiceless and whispered speech also can be used with success diagnostically. For example, some emotionally disturbed children respond more satisfactorily to whispered speech than to vocalized or amplified speech. A child in an anxiety state, after being given much assurance verbally and nonverbally, might even whisper a reply to a question asked in a whisper even though he ignored loud sounds previously. Likewise, voiceless speech is useful with some children who have psychic deafness. Apparently some of these children's rejections include only speech which can be heard. They might ignore or be oblivious to speech which can be heard, but when their attention is directed to the examiner's face and he speaks without voice, they might show considerable anxiety and disequilibrium psychologically. This response is not characteristic of the child with peripheral deafness who has learned to read the speaker's lips, but cautious interpretation is necessary and the total clinical syndrome must be considered.

Sound-field Tests

Tests using amplifying equipment can be applied informally in such a manner that they do not require cooperation from the child. Such tests are given by the sound-field method which means that the sounds are generated through a loud speaker into the room. This can be done while the child is seated at a table engaging himself in an activity or while he is moving about the room, if he cannot cooperate even indirectly.

Sound-field amplified tests consist mainly of two types; pure tone and social sounds. The necessary equipment includes a beat frequency oscillator, an amplifier, a loud speaker and a turntable. This equipment must be accurately matched electronically. Approximate calibration on children with normal hearing and at each age level between two and six years is highly desirable. This can be done so that the approximate intensity level at various points in the room is known. Having two or more loud speakers is an advantage because it precludes the child's being more than a few feet from the source of sound at any one time although he might be moving about the room. Moreover, switching the sounds from one speaker to another is useful as a testing procedure.

These tests are administered according to the symptomatology presented by the child. If he can be seated at a table, placed at a known distance from the speaker and mildly engaged in an activity, the test is done in this manner. As the child plays the sounds are sent through the speaker at the intensities desired and when pure tones are used, frequencies also are selected as indicated. The child might respond by looking up from his foreground activity and scanning his environment or he might respond more indirectly by momentary cessation of his activity. When pure tones are used and if the child is above three and one half years of age and finds it possible to relate well to the total situation, an approximate audiogram can be recorded. Such audiograms have been compared with the formal audiograms of children done after the child was old enough to give responses and the comparison indicated good reliability for selected children. For children who cannot relate to the testing situation, the sound-field amplified tests are used as a controlled source of sound. Very high and very low intensities can be used and furthermore, a wide variation of frequencies is available to the examiner. Many types of recorded sounds also can be used. The use of appropriate recorded materials is highly desirable as a comparison to the responses given to pure tones. Many young children respond readily to conglomerate sound although they have not responded to pure tones. This is discussed further in relation to formal audiometry. Social sounds of the type which surround the child daily seem the most appropriate for this purpose. Utley [27] has prepared records which have proved useful for such testing.

The sound-field amplified tests are an intermediary step between the more informal and more formal types of auditory testing. They are useful chiefly for children between two and six years of age. Although a minimum of electronic equipment is necessary they are useful in office practice. They can be given without the help of an assistant. When peripheral deafness is present, the degree of the hearing loss can be explored with considerable assurance and accuracy. Like all tests of auditory capacity in young children, these tests must be validated by other information.

Tests of Auditory Perception

Aphasic children frequently have disturbances of auditory perception. One of their fundamental difficulties is that they cannot listen; therefore, they cannot direct their attention selectively to an expected sound. To them the auditory environment does not consist of many individual sounds to be used as the immediate situation demands. Their auditory world is conglomerate; all sounds having equal importance and all being foreground sounds simultaneously. Special techniques frequently are necessary for testing these children. Formal audiometry cannot be used with some of them although they are considerably above six years of age. Inasmuch as they cannot differentiate between foreground and background sounds it is necessary to structure the testing situation for them. This can be done essentially in two ways. They can be tested in a sound deadened room which eliminates all background sounds; the test sounds are the only sounds present so the child cannot confuse them with background sounds. However, this procedure seems to have limitations, especially if sound-field tests are used. Many of these children seem to find it difficult to relate to a specific sound even though there is no background sound. Perhaps an auditory perceptual disturbance is alleviated only when a specific sound is appropriately related to other sounds. This hypothesis seems warranted in terms of clinical experience. Usually children with such disturbances respond more adequately when the test sounds are superimposed on controlled background sounds. For example, when the equipment used for the sound-field amplified tests is so constructed, pure tones can be sent through the speaker simultaneously with music. The music serves as a constant background onto which the test tones are superimposed. This method has been useful with some children. A less formal procedure is to use selected music (soft music with minimum percussion and variation in intensity is most satisfactory) for the background and to proceed with informal testing, such as the sound instruments and voice tests. It is apparent from clinical experience that some brain injured and aphasic children respond more adequately to tests when the sounds are given with a controlled background of sound. This procedure is being used experimentally as a training method for children with auditory perceptual disturbances. Diagnostically its primary purpose is to assist in evaluating those children who cannot respond consistently to direct auditory stimulation although they seem to be alternately and inadvertently responding to and ignoring their auditory environment. This procedure does not seem to benefit children with peripheral deafness, mental deficiency or psychic deafness.

Auditory perceptual capacities can be explored informally in other ways. For example, one of the sound producing instruments, such as the single bell, might be given to the child. The examiner has an identical sound instrument. The child is engaged in playing a game of ringing his bell in response to the examiner's. After some training the examiner rings his bell out of sight of the child. The child's response requires auditory structuring and listening. Children with partial deafness usually respond readily when appropriate intensities are used. Children who present the syndrome of brain injury and aphasia frequently cannot respond to this test consistently even though it is apparent that the intensity level substantially exceeds their threshold of audibility.

As indicated previously voice tests too can be used to evaluate auditory perception. The child's imitative responses vocally reveal certain aspects of his ability to respond perceptually. The mum-mum and bu-bu tests are applicable for this purpose. If the child can imitate such vocalizations the correct number of times and if he can imitate variations in pitch, he can be considered as having sufficient integrity of auditory perception to learn to speak. He might, however, be aphasic and incapable of normal auditory behavior in other respects.

SUPPLEMENTARY INFORMAL TESTS

The Touching Test

Informal tests of the child's ability to use other than auditory sensations are useful diagnostically. Such tests can be applied in various ways. For example, while the child is playfully engaged the examiner might casually touch him by placing his hand on the child's back in such a manner that movement is obscured. This has proved successful as a touching test. Children with peripheral deafness can be expected to note the sensation immediately and to make attempts to ascertain its significance. This is done by looking at the examiner in a quizzical way or by other appropriate reactions. Children with psychic deafness frequently ignore the sensation even when the examiner rubs his hand vigorously against the child's back. Usually when the child does react it is by moving away without direct reaction to the examiner as the source of the stimulation. Autistic children, specifically often take the examiner's hand and move it as though it were an object and without attention to the person. Aphasic children make direct attempts to eliminate the sensation by shrugging their shoulders or by other means, especially if they are engaged in a foreground situation. It is as though they are using all of their integrative capacities in the foreground visual activity and sensations coming from other sources must be eliminated. If the hand is not removed they might disintegrate and withdraw from the situation or show other signs of distractibility and disinhibition. Such reactions to the touching test provide corroborative information by indicating the child's capacity to respond to other than auditory stimulation.

The Vibration Tests

A vibration test also might be used to explore responsiveness in other ways. If a child is seated at a table with his hands on it (very young children can be placed on the table) engaging in an activity, the examiner can lightly tap a leg of the table with the palm of his hand. No movement or sound should be apparent to the child. Children having the various types of auditory disorders respond to the vibration test in essentially the same manner as they do to the touching test. Children with peripheral deafness are especially definite in their reactions to such vibratory sensations. Their use of tactile sensations in a compensatory manner was discussed in Chapter VII.

Visual Clues Test

As indicated in Part Three children having different types of auditory disorders use movement and other visual clues in a characteristically different manner. This can be observed by using movement and shadows specifically to note reaction to such visual stimulation. The informal test of attention to movement usually consists of the examiner's moving his hands casually in line with the child's peripheral vision. The shadow test consists of the examiner's causing a shadow to fall on the child or on a table before him. Children with peripheral deafness respond to such visual clues by attempts to use them as signals and as sources of information. Children with other types of auditory disorders usually ignore such visual clues or they do not react to them in an integrated manner.

RECORDING RESPONSES

In order that the evaluation of the child's responsiveness can be used by others and so that appropriate records can be kept, it is desirable to record the responses to the informal tests. A form for such recording is given below.

Informal Auditory Test Responses

Sound Instrument Test

Instrument	Mild	Moderate	Loud	Inconsistent	No response
Triple bell					
Small cricket					
Large cricket					
School bell					
"A" chime					
Single bell					
Clacker					

Sound Toy Test

Spontaneous reactions
Imitates sounds from demonstration

Imitation of Vocalization Test

Stops vocalizing
Ceases activity
Assumes listening attitude

Voice Test

Immobilizes when examiner vocalizes

Imitates examiner's vocalizations

Verbal Comprehension Test

Direct comprehension and reaction

Indirect reactions manifesting comprehension

Sound-field Test

	db range	Responses to pure tones	Responses to social sounds
Above conversational level	0–30		
Below conversational level	30–60		
Hearing on speech range	60–95		
No hearing on speech range	95–100		
Erratic and inconsistent	variable		

Auditory Perception Tests

Assumes listening attitude

Listening attitude is absent

Responses improve when background is controlled

Produces sound with bell in
response to the examiner

Repeats mum-mum or bu-bu selectively and correct number of times

Touching Test

Touching elicits scanning behavior

Rejects touching without integrative behavior

No response to being touched

Vibration Test

Vibrations elicit scanning behavior

No response to vibrations

Visual Clues Test

Movements elicit scanning behavior
Shadows elicit scanning behavior
No unusual responses to movement
No response to shadows

FORMAL TESTS OF AUDITORY CAPACITY

Formal tests of auditory capacity differ from the informal tests in several respects. Perhaps the most significant difference is the level of cooperation required from the child because direct responses to the stimuli usually are assumed. Whether the responses are voluntary or involuntary, considerable cooperative effort on the part of the child is necessary for the application of these tests. The validity and reliability of formal tests are dependent substantially on the child's effort and participation. It is noteworthy also that the formal techniques were originally devised for adults. Some adaptations have been made but the level of genetic maturation required has been considered critically only in recent years. Usually the response which is expected from the adult is expected also from the child. When validity and reliability can be ascertained the formal tests provide more specific information relative to the type and degree of the peripheral hearing loss but in the past deviate responses have been interpreted largely in terms of reduced acuity. On the basis of clinical experience and research it is apparent that these procedures are not applicable to many young children. Frequently the objectivity of the procedure has been confused with reliability and validity. With skilled application and interpretation these tests are useful with some young children. Some of the most commonly used are discussed below. Davis [8] gives a comprehensive survey of hearing tests and this discussion is suggested for those desiring background material.

The Pure Tone Audiometric Test

Various workers have devised adaptations for administering the pure tone audiometric test to young children. These adaptations consist essentially of methods for motivating the child and for simplifying the way in which he can give his responses. Bloomer [2], Westlake [28], Cotton and Hall [7], and Birch and Mathews [1] have indicated the usefulness and limitations of the pure tone test. The findings of Birch and Mathews are especially specific and pertinent. They used the pure tone test to survey a population of mentally deficient children between the ages of ten and nineteen

Table 16. — *The Age and Sex Distribution of Preschool Children Who Were Given the Pure Tone Audiometric Test*

Age	Male	Female	Total
2 yr. 1 mo. to 3 yr.	1	1	2
3 yr. 1 mo. to 3 yr. 6 mo.	4	5	9
3 yr. 7 mo. to 4 yr.	8	8	16
4 yr. 1 mo. to 4 yr. 6 mo.	2	11	13
4 yr. 7 mo. to 5 yr.	2	13	15
5 yr. 1 mo. to 5 yr. 6 mo.	3	3	6
Totals	20	41	61

years. They found that this test could be used reliably with two out of three children having mental ages of four and five years, with three out of four having mental ages between five and six years, and with seven out of eight having mental ages between six and seven years.

To investigate the genetic aspects of the pure tone test further, the writer initiated a special research study. This test was administered to sixty-one normal children between the ages of two years and one month and five years and six months. These children attended a nursery school in a suburb of a large metropolitan community. The socio-economic level was upper middle class with approximately one half of the families being in professional or managerial type of occupations. The subjects for the study were estimated to be slightly above average in ability and development. None of them presented known deviations physically or emotionally. The age and sex distribution for the total group studied is given in table 16.

After some experimentation it became apparent that the most re-

Table 17. — *The Mean Decibel Responses for Each of the Age Levels on the Pure Tone Audiometer*

Age group — 3 yr. 1 mo. to 3 yr. 6 mo.

Frequency	500	1000	2000	4000
Right ear				
No.	3	3	3	3
Mean db	12	12	13	13
S.D.	4.71	6.24	2.36	2.36
Left ear				
No.	3	3	2	2
Mean db	17	17	15	10
S.D.	6.24	6.24	5.00	0.00

Age group — 3 yr. 7 mo. to 4 yr.

Frequency	500	1000	2000	4000
Right ear				
No.	13	14	13	13
Mean db	16	9	10	12
S.D.	9.17	6.59	6.34	7.75
Left ear				
No.	11	11	11	11
Mean db	11	13	13	10
S.D.	4.31	4.94	5.79	5.22

Age group — 4 yr. 1 mo. to 4 yr. 6 mo.

Frequency	500	1000	2000	4000
Right ear				
No.	12	12	12	11
Mean db	13	8	12	12
S.D.	4.49	5.95	9.2	6.17
Left ear				
No.	9	10	9	9
Mean db	14	14	8	12
S.D.	5.22	5.66	4.36	7.45

Table 17. — *continued*

Age group — 4 yr. 7 mo. to 5 yr.

Frequency	500	1000	2000	4000
Right ear				
No.	14	15	14	14
Mean db	10	5	7	5
S.D.	3.99	3.4	4.75	5.16
Left ear				
No.	13	14	13	13
Mean db	10	10	6	5
S.D.	6.03	4.63	3.85	5.36

Age group — 5 yr. 1 mo. to 5 yr. 6 mo.

Frequency	500	1000	2000	4000
Right ear				
No.	5	5	5	5
Mean db	5	2	1	4
S.D.	3.18	2.45	2.00	6.63
Left ear				
No.	5	5	5	5
Mean db	3	5	0	4
S.D.	2.45	3.18	0.00	3.74

liable results were secured when a highly specific structured procedure was used in presenting the tones. This procedure consisted of engaging the child in playing a game of listening to the sounds made by animals. A high degree of motivation and rapport was established by talking to the child about his pets and by showing him pictures of the animals used in eliciting his responses to the tones. Because of the interests of the children, animals were identified with tones as follows: 500 cps.–dog; 1000 cps.–cat; 2000 cps.–bird; 4000 cps.–mouse. It was interesting to note that although there is no apparent similarity between the "bow-wow" of a dog and a 500 cycle tone, or between the "meow" of a cat and a 1000 cycle tone the children identified these animals with the tones more readily than objects such as an airplane. This emphasizes the importance of genetic factors because the child found it necessary to relate the sound to a concrete experience and the similarity between the sounds was unimportant. Another factor became apparent from observing the child's reactions to the tones. He used both auditory and visual experience in giving his responses. This was indicated by comments such as "the sounds are getting smaller," "I heard a little and a big sound" and "that's a real little one." Furthermore, when the child had a picture before him of the animal which was identified with the tone, his responses were given more successfully. The results of the pure tone tests for each of the age levels are given in tables 17 and 18. Only the frequencies 500, 1000, 2000 and 4000 were used in the study. All of the children at each age level could not be tested successfully. This is shown in table 19. Furthermore, the two children below three years of age could not give responses which were scorable and therefore their responses are not included in the quantitative results. The data in table 17 indicate that there is only slight difference in the responses of children between three and four and one half years of age. The mean responses cluster around 12, 13 and 14 decibels and the standard deviations are relatively uniform. From the point of view of threshold levels, there is a substantial improvement in the responses between four and one half and five years and again between five and five and one half years.

When the responses for individual ears are combined as shown in table 18, the same trend is apparent. The average threshold decreases toward the zero decibel line as the age increases. Likewise, the standard deviations become smaller as the child becomes older. This is in complete agreement with the findings of Birch and Mathews [1]. In general, research findings suggest that under very favorable circumstances normal children find it possible to respond to the pure tone test after three years of age but that these responses cannot be interpreted according to adult standards until the child is approximately five years of age. This is illustrated further by the comparisons given in figure 5. The audiograms shown in figure 5 illustrate the increasing capacity of the child to respond at threshold

Table 18. — *Average Pure Tone Thresholds for Each Age Group When the Responses for Individual Ears Were Combined*

Age group	Frequency	Mean db	Standard deviation	No. of ears
3 yr. 1 mo. to 3 yr. 6 mo.	500	14.16	6.64	6
	1000	14.16	7.21	6
	2000	14.00	7.48	5
	4000	12.00	6.36	5
3 yr. 7 mo. to 4 yr.	500	13.75	3.19	24
	1000	10.60	2.63	25
	2000	11.04	2.56	24
	4000	11.25	2.65	24
4 yr. 1 mo. to 4 yr. 6 mo.	500	13.75	3.34	20
	1000	10.45	2.56	22
	2000	10.23	3.85	21
	4000	12.00	3.08	20
4 yr. 7 mo. to 5 yr.	500	10.00	2.11	27
	1000	6.83	1.51	30
	2000	6.48	1.49	27
	4000	5.00	1.33	27
5 yr. 1 mo. to 5 yr. 6 mo.	500	4.00	1.53	10
	1000	3.50	1.45	10
	2000	0.50	0.15	10
	4000	2.77	1.57	9

Table 19. — *The Number of Children at Each Age Level Who Could Not Be Tested with the Pure Tone Audiometer*

Age group	Number in group	Number that could not be tested
2 yr. 7 mo. to 3 yr.	2	2
3 yr. 1 mo. to 3 yr. 6 mo.	9	6
3 yr. 7 mo. to 4 yr.	16	3
4 yr. 1 mo. to 4 yr. 6 mo.	13	1
4 yr. 7 mo. to 5 yr.	15	1
5 yr. 1 mo. to 5 yr. 6 mo.	6	1
Totals	61	14

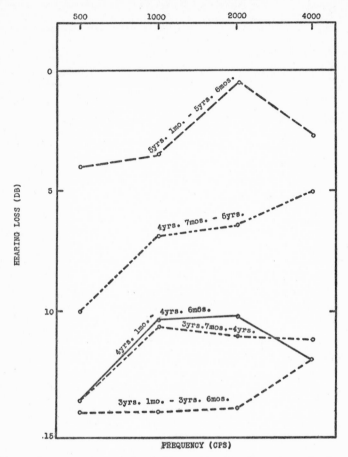

Fig. 5.—Average pure tone threshold measurements for each age level.

levels as he becomes older. This is further revealed by the data in table 19 which shows the proportion of children at each age level to whom the pure tone test could not be administered because of their inability to respond adequately. Those who could not be tested constitute a group who could not give scorable responses; they were totally unable to cope with the demands of a pure tone testing situation. It is apparent that the proportion of the total group showing such incapacity is less after four to four and one half years of age.

It must be emphasized that the results from this study are from children who have normal ability to communicate and who were normal in other respects. These results like those of Birch and Mathews [1] are useful in differential diagnosis mainly in indicating the genetic level required for responding to a pure tone audiometric test. In terms of threshold responses the indications are that the genetic level required is approximately five years. However, children having auditory disorders with their limitations in ability to cooperate, to listen and to use language, cannot be expected to give threshold responses at this age. The formal pure tone audiometric test cannot be considered useful in differential diagnosis below the age of three and one half years and extreme caution is necessary in interpreting the results from this test through the age of five years.

Some of the limitations of the pure tone audiometric test can be overcome by using the sound-field method of presenting the tones. This method reduces the demands placed on the child. However, the nature of the pure tone stimulus itself is a limiting factor irrespective of the method of presentation. Pure tones are abstract, meaningless sounds increasing the difficulty of response for all individuals irrespective of age level. It is difficult to relate the pure tone to experience; these tones cannot be concretized easily. Listening in the abstract as contrasted with listening for a concrete sound is more difficult for children than for adults. Listening in young children assumes a highly concretized and structured situation. When the pure tones were not structured and concretized, such as being identified with animals, even children above five years of age had considerably more difficulty in responding. This may be the reason many children having auditory disorders respond to vocalizations, sound toys and other types of sounds but do not respond to pure tones. However, the pure tone audiometric test can be used with some young children. When it is used the validity of the results is greater if informal methods are used corroboratively and all of the auditory responses should be further validated by the history information and by the behavioral symptomatology.

The Tuning Fork Tests

Another pure tone test used chiefly by otolaryngologists and one which preceded the audiometric is the tuning fork test. The various tests done with tuning forks will not be discussed because such discussions are available in several sources [4, 13]. Rather, this test will be considered only from the point of view of its usefulness and applicability in the differential diagnosis of auditory disorders in young children.

The nature of the auditory stimulus in the tuning fork test is the same as in the audiometric test; both are pure tones. The limitations of pure tones in use with young children have been indicated above in relation to the pure tone audiometric test. These limitations must be emphasized also with the tuning fork test although there is a significant difference between the two tests. The tuning fork test can be given in an informal manner as it is always given by the sound-field method. One of the limitations of this test in the past is the formal demands which have been made on the child. The otolaryngologist usually has followed a formalized procedure in administering the test irrespective of the age of the child. Furthermore, direct as compared to indirect responses have been required. The usefulness of the tuning fork test can be increased if it is given in the manner of the sound instrument test discussed above. The manner of presentation should be adapted to the child's ability to cooperate and indirect responses should be used in interpreting the results. The tuning fork test is highly flexible and similar to the sound instrument test when it is used more informally. The tuning fork and sound instrument tests are comparable also in that both require a high degree of clinical ingenuity and insight and both are used primarily to elicit responses from which clinical judgments can be made.

Certain inferences can be made concerning the genetic level required for responding to the tuning fork test. If this test is given in the usual formal manner it is comparable to the pure tone audiometric test. The data given in tables 17 and 18 indicate that the genetic level required for this type of threshold response is five years. Therefore, it seems reasonable to infer that threshold responses are not likely to be possible on the tuning fork test below this genetic level. Furthermore, despite intensive motivation and structuring, normal children could not respond reliably to pure tones below the age of three years. Again, by comparison the tuning fork test must be used with great caution below three years. However, clinical experience indicates that if the tuning fork test is used informally like the sound-field amplified pure tone test, it is useful down to approximately two years of age. Below two years any test using pure tones seems to be of questionable value.

The tuning fork test is useful and of diagnostic value in the differential diagnosis of auditory disorders in children. Perhaps the greatest source of error in using this test has been in the manner in which it has been applied. The child's mental and general genetic development have not been emphasized. Moreover, the test has been applied without considerate attention to the child's organismic responsiveness. An assumption in the use of the test has been that the child will respond auditorially even though he might present severe problems organismically. Like the information secured from other auditory tests, responses to the tuning forks should be validated by the history and the behavioral symptomatology.

Speech Audiometry

Considerable progress has been made in the use of speech tests for evaluating auditory capacities. Carhart [6] has presented a discussion of this work. Speech tests are used mainly in two ways; to elicit thresholds of awareness responses and imitative responses. The tests are given through electronic amplifying equipment by the live voice method or through recorded versions. The tests most widely used for purposes of speech audiometry are the Harvard Spondee Lists and the Harvard P-B Lists [8].

As indicated above the purpose of speech audiometry is to ascertain the intensity level at which the individual can comprehend speech or the level at which he becomes aware of speech sounds. If the individual had acquired speech normally, prior to sustaining auditory impairment and if he profits from amplification, then he repeats the words as they are given to him. These are imitative responses and indicate the intensity level necessary to reach his reduced threshold of acuity. This test given in this manner assumes normal language and auditory perceptual capacities and thereby it is most satisfactory for those who have peripheral deafness. It is apparent that imitative responses of this type cannot be given by most children presenting problems of differential diagnosis. Most such children have congenital disorders and therefore do not have ability to comprehend spoken language. However, speech reception tests are sometimes useful with these children to determine thresholds of awareness. This threshold is the intensity level at which the child becomes aware that auditory stimulation is present. The threshold of awareness test usually is given by the sound-field method and then is not unlike the sound-field test discussed above; the difference being only in the nature of the auditory stimulus.

From the point of view of differential diagnosis in young children speech audiometry must be used cautiously. Like most tests of auditory capacity it assumes ability to integrate sensations and to respond organismically. Children who cannot give mobilized, listening responses cannot manifest thresholds of awareness irrespective of the levels of intensity used. Therefore, many emotionally disturbed and aphasic children do not give such responses. In some instances it seems that the louder the sound the less capable the child is of giving a direct response to it. However, the use of speech audiometry in conjunction with informal auditory tests is desirable for some children. This procedure is most beneficially used with children who have peripheral deafness. A method for administering speech tests to children has been described by Keaster [20].

The Peep Show Test

Dix and Hallpike [9] originally described the test referred to as the Peep Show. This is an ingenious method for combining visual and auditory stimulation. Hirsh [19] has discussed the conditioning process entailed and compared it to that used in psychogalvanic audiometry. The test consists of training the child to press a switch when he hears the tone; only pure tones are used as stimuli. When the child presses the switch a light is turned on which illuminates pictures inside of an attractive box or doll house. The child can see the pictures by "peeping" when he learns to press the switch simultaneously with hearing the tone. This test is useful primarily in determining the extent of a previously ascertained peripheral deafness and in those children who are sufficiently matured genetically. On the basis of clinical experience and research on the use of pure tones as indicated above, the applicability of the Peep Show to children below four years of age should be questioned. Pure tone threshold tests are highly unreliable below this genetic age level even though the presentation has been simplified and responses are rewarded. Furthermore, it is apparent from clinical experience with brain injured, aphasic, emotionally disturbed and mentally deficient children that the Peep Show entails a learning and adjustment situation which is precluded in most of these children. Some aphasic children are only more distracted by the simultaneous use of visual and auditory avenues. Emotionally disturbed children usually reject visual impressions which have inter-personal meanings just as they reject auditory impressions. Therefore, the use of the illuminated pictures does not serve as a reward for these children. Furthermore, many children with brain injury and with emotional disturbance lack the amenability and cooperative effort required for this test. Young mentally deficient children too must be considered in terms of their inability to respond normally to the learning situation entailed. This test, like most formal auditory tests, assumes organismic responsiveness and integrity. While the Peep Show Test can be used with some children, its usefulness in making a differential diagnosis of auditory disorders is limited for many young children.

Psychogalvanic Audiometry

During recent years the galvanometer has been used as an instrument for determining auditory acuity. Bordley and Hardy [3],

Hardy and Bordley [17], Hardy and Pauls [18], Hirsh [19] and Doerfler [10] in particular have reported on this method. Inasmuch as this procedure is not suitable for general clinical practice it will not be considered in detail. However, because psychogalvanic audiometry is being used in various centers, a brief discussion of it and its limitations seems pertinent. Psychogalvanic skin resistance audiometry (PGSR) is done by attaching electrodes to the child and presenting a pure tone through a regular audiometer. The pure tone is followed by an electric shock. This process is referred to as conditioning. This procedure is based on the assumption that after conditioning has occurred, the child will respond to the pure tone stimulus alone in the same manner as he responded to both the pure tone and the electric shock. If this reaction were invariable and if this method could be used with all children, the problem of differential diagnosis of auditory disorders would be simplified. It is apparent that this procedure does not rely on the child's giving voluntary responses to the auditory stimulus. His responses are involuntary but because his cooperation is required this method is considered a formal type of test.

Research on the psycho-physical aspects of psychogalvanic behavior covers a period of approximately sixty years. McCleary [21] has presented a critical summary of this work. He concludes that this procedure for studying human behavior has not lived up to what was expected of it originally. In essence, this seems true also of its use as a test of auditory acuity. Further experimentation is indicated but it is clear that some children presenting problems of auditory disorders do not give the expected response. For example, some aphasic and severely emotionally disturbed children have shown marked impairment of auditory acuity by this method but close observation and use of other methods has revealed that they had normal auditory acuity. Furthermore, use of the PGSR with normal children between two and four years of age has revealed that not all of them give the expected response to this test. Hypothetically, experience with normal children of this age indicates that the usefulness of PGSR as an auditory test might be even less with children below two years of age. In general, psychogalvanic audiometry must be considered as another formal pure tone test with some of the same limitations for use with young children that are found in other tests of this type.

There are theoretical aspects of psychogalvanic behavior which remain to be clarified. These will not be considered here. Rather, the practical, clinical problems of this procedure are emphasized. The basic question requiring further study is the nature of the response and its validity. This procedure as used currently cannot be considered as valid for a substantial number of young children. Perhaps genetic factors will prove significant in this connection. Validation studies on young normal children seem essential for this purpose. Moreover, the nature of the response and its implications makes interpretation difficult. Some children respond as though they have impaired acuity when further study and observation reveals that their auditory disorders are not due to reduced acuity. Likewise, even when normal acuity is manifested on PGSR interpretation is difficult.

Other practical considerations enter into the usefulness of this test. It is unusually time-consuming, requiring an hour or more for each child. Furthermore, two examiners skilled in the procedure are necessary for administering the test successfully. In addition, the child can be tested only when he is capable of a minimum of cooperative effort. If he is highly distractible, negativistic and lacking in relationship to others, adequate responses cannot be secured. However, psychogalvanic audiometry has been found useful with some children. Its usefulness is greatest for those presenting problems of peripheral deafness and who are above three years of age. Diagnosis, however, should be made only after corroborative evidence has been secured from the history, from behavioral symptomatology and from other types of auditory tests.

Electroencephalography as a Test of Hearing Acuity

Marcus and Gibbs [22] have reported on the use of electroencephalography as a means for detecting impaired acuity in young children. This method is limited in usefulness because of the complexity of the equipment and the interpretation. Furthermore, validity has not been established on young normal children. It is evident from clinical experience that some children presumed to have marked peripheral deafness on the basis of this test have hearing acuity which is adequate for acquiring speech. This procedure is classified under formal auditory tests because in order to accomplish this test both while the child is awake and asleep, which is considered most desirable, considerable cooperative effort is required. Further research, including validation studies, is necessary before its final usefulness can be ascertained.

EVALUATION OF LANGUAGE

Evaluation of the child's language behavior is a significant aspect of the total examination. This evaluation usually is done informally. Language testing provides an opportunity for systematic observation of symbolic functioning and such observations can be made by all specialists. The child's language development is inseparable from his auditory capacities. Moreover, his language functioning is intimately related to the nature of his auditory incapacity. Thus the language evaluation provides highly relevant information in terms of differential diagnosis. One of the primary differences behaviorally between children with auditory disturbances is their use of language. For example, children with peripheral deafness develop inner language and use of gesture expressively. They develop symbolic behavior predominantly through vision but they use other sensory avenues in a compensatory manner for the development of inner language. They integrate sensory experience meaningfully although this experience lacks the impact of auditory sensation. They acquire symbolic behavior and overcome the sensori-motor level of functioning which Piaget [25] describes as being characteristic of children during the pre-language age. In contrast to children with peripheral deafness, aphasic children notably are deficient in language functioning. They are both retarded and disturbed in language behavior for two principal reasons: an inability to acquire the use of symbols and because their perceptual and conceptual disturbances preclude normal reception and integration of sensory experience. Their symbolic behavior is characteristic accordingly. Likewise, the language behavior of emotionally disturbed children with psychic deafness is differentiating diagnostically. These children typically reject language usage by not manifesting interest in it with concomitant inability to relate to the situation emotionally. Their behavior reveals intact perceptual functioning and complex symbolic behavior, but these capacities are used for autistic and phantasy purposes only. The mentally deficient child might manifest perceptual and conceptual disturbances but his performance is characterized by ability to function symbolically at a genetic level substantially below his chronological age.

The equipment used for evaluating language functioning consists of a selected battery of toy objects which is referred to as the Object Test. The objects are selected on the basis of genetic level and the child's daily experience. Clinical experience has demonstrated that objects are more suitable than pictures for language testing purposes. There are several advantages in using objects. For example, they are more concrete than pictures and concreteness is essential for testing many children with auditory disorders. Another advantage is that objects can be manipulated and related to each other. This is essential for appraising inner language in particular. Although detailed recording of the child's responses is possible and desirable, quantitative scoring has not been used. In this respect use of the object test is similar to the Object Sorting Test [15], the Eisenson [11], and the Halstead-Wepman Tests [16].

The Test of Inner Language

Inner language usually is evaluated first because other language functioning assumes a minimum of inner language. Administration of the object test should be adapted to the child. If the child's level of cooperative effort permits it is desirable to seat him at a table. However, the test can be given on the floor with the child seated on the parent's lap, or in many other positions which permit his playing with small toys. If the child is seated at a table the examiner places the objects on it one at a time. The order of presentation, the time between presentations and the number of objects presented is determined by the child's ability to integrate experientially. Objects which have not been presented or which will not be used are concealed from the child's view. Verbal instructions are not used. The examiner, however, encourages the child to play actively with the objects. Some children proceed as soon as an object has been placed before them but others require additional encouragement and demonstration. This can be done by placing two objects, such as the table and chair, before the child and showing him that he is to play with them. He is then permitted to place them in any relationship that he chooses.

Various responses to the object test situation can be observed. Some children will structure the objects in a highly meaningful and significant manner. They will place kitchen objects together appropriately indicating a kitchen. They may even place the mother figure at the stove in a working position. They might similarly structure living, dining and bedroom objects. Such activity suggests normalcy of perceptual and conceptual functioning. The child has found it possible to integrate his daily experiences meaningfully and he is capable of projecting himself actively into an imaginative play situation. Such behavior reveals that inner language is present. The child has acquired symbolic behavior; he can engage in mental trial and error processes and arrive at logical conclusions. He has internalized environmental experience and he can use ideation expressively.

Children with peripheral deafness usually reveal good inner language on the object test. Characteristically they relate to the test situation and structure the objects planfully and meaningfully. Aphasic, emotionally disturbed and mentally deficient children are notably less successful in performing with the objects. The aphasic child might manifest distractibility and disinhibition so the object presentation and the entire test situation must be controlled for him. However, even when his distractibility and disinhibition are controlled in this manner, he might show little awareness of the relationship of one object to another. He lacks ability to organize, classify and structure the problem before him. He relates to one object or even one part of an object at a time but he cannot conceive of the objects as a whole and group them logically. He attempts to integrate and to relate meaningfully to the situation but he fails because of his inability to organize his experiences. He might show little delay between sensation and response; then his attempts are characterized by sensori-motor behavior. His inner language has not developed adequately and thereby abstract functioning is lacking or is only rudimentary. Children with psychic deafness, especially schizophrenic children, ordinarily cannot relate sufficiently to the objects to perform with them. They often reject the entire situation or they grasp an object and retain it indefinitely without attempts to use it meaningfully. Nevertheless, that they have inner language usually is manifested by their bizarre behavior in other respects. Autistic children and children with anxiety states frequently reject only parts of the object test. Usually they reveal good inner language through their use of blocks and through their selected rejection of the environment. Young mentally deficient children characteristically reveal inner language but only of a highly concrete type and at a low genetic level. They do not reject the objects but relate to them and perform in an unimaginative but realistic manner.

The child's performance on the object test relative to inner language provides corroborative and supplemental information to the results from the auditory tests. If the auditory test responses have been inconsistent and otherwise suggestive of auditory disorders due to brain injury, the object test results should reveal deficiencies of inner language and a related behavioral syndrome. If the object test manifests good integrity of inner language, his performance on auditory tests should be similarly consistent.

The Test of Receptive Language

The test of receptive language capacity follows immediately after the child has performed with the objects sufficiently to manifest his inner language capacity. Receptive capacity is tested in various ways. Usually it is done first with the simultaneous use of vision and hearing. The examiner might say, "Give me the daddy," "Where is the stove?" or "Put the mommy on the bed." The instructions can be varied in difficulty according to the child's receptive capacities. During this initial test he is permitted to attend to the examiner's face as the instructions are given. The total situation is game-like and playful but not boisterous or over-stimulating. The next step consists of raising and lowering the intensity of the voice while giving instructions. This variation normally includes reducing the intensity until no voice is used and the child is dependent on vision alone (speech reading). Some children will comprehend equally well by using only vision. This indicates either that they do not hear speech or that hearing it does not increase comprehension. Increasing the intensity well above conversational level sometimes assists in differentiating those with partial deafness from the receptive aphasic. Usually increasing the intensity does not help the aphasic child and it might cause his performance to disintegrate while raising intensity might benefit those with partial peripheral deafness. The child with profound peripheral deafness does equally well irrespective of intensity variation. He is dependent on his vision only. The test then becomes an evaluation of capacity to receive language visually through speech reading.

After appraising the child's ability to receive language by using vision and hearing simultaneously and then through vision alone, his capacity to use hearing alone is evaluated. This is done by the examiner being seated beside the child to preclude visual clues but the examiner moves from one side of the child to the other to note possible advantage to either ear. A wide variation of intensity and difficulty is used. Intensity variations include very mild to loud. Variations in difficulty are achieved by altering the task. For example, a simple, concrete problem is presented by placing a table and a bed before the child. The examiner might simply say "bed" or "table" and the child's task is to identify the object. This task is made more difficult by using more objects and by giving more involved instructions such as "Put the bed by the stove." This test is useful especially for securing corroborative information relative to the differential diagnosis between peripheral deafness and aphasia. The child with partial impairment of auditory acuity might be benefited by increased intensity but if his deafness is severe he cannot give successful responses through audition. His performance is characterized by successes when vision is used and failure when hearing is used. Aphasic children occasionally do succeed when vision is used but this is not characteristic. Some are successful when very simple spoken language is used but become confused and disintegrated when average language complexity is required. Increasing the intensity is not advantageous and sometimes causes greater disintegration. Comparison of the child's ability to receive language through vision and audition simultaneously, through vision alone, and through hearing alone provides significant information regarding sensory and organismic integrity. Such information is directly related to the differential diagnosis of auditory disorders.

The Test of Expressive Language

Ability to use language expressively is evaluated last. This is done by having the child engage himself playfully with the objects if his level of cooperation permits. The test situation should be highly spontaneous and encouraging but structured according to the child's needs and not over-stimulating. As the child engages himself in play with the objects, the examiner opportunely makes comments to elicit expressive language. For example, if the child places the baby doll into the crib the examiner might say, "Where's the baby?" or "What is the baby doing?" Considerable encouragement and simplification sometimes are necessary. One of the simplest expressive functions is naming. Frequently this is the beginning point of the evaluation of expressive language. The examiner encourages the child to name the objects. Ability to name, however, should not be interpreted as ability to use language normally. Some children can name objects readily but have considerable difficulty in formulating and using even short sentences.

The basic principle of the object language test is that the child will use his language capacities most effectively in association with an activity in which he is deeply interested. The child is encouraged to play systematically and to use speech which is directly pertinent to what he is doing. This procedure has been more successful clinically than asking the child to give his name, talking about his clothes or other more formalized questioning. He uses language more freely and spontaneously when he is performing an activity playfully inasmuch as he is motivated and the language usage is at his genetic level.

Children having different types of auditory disorders perform characteristically also on this part of the examination of language capacity. For example, a child with partial peripheral deafness might use words in his expressive attempts. Speech thus used is characteristic in tonal quality and in its symbolic appropriateness. These children do not use words erratically, in a jargon manner. Moreover, because of the reciprocal relationship between reception and expression of language, whatever verbal capacity the child has is a manifestation of the extent to which he has been able to acquire speech despite his impairment of acuity. When peripheral deafness has entirely precluded acquisition of speech, the child frequently uses gestures to express himself. Such expression is then encouraged and used diagnostically. As indicated previously, the child's ability to use gestures expressively and receptively is evaluated. The object test appropriately administered gives the child an opportunity to use whatever expressive capacities he has in the manner which he chooses. In general, children with peripheral deafness perform capably with the objects and reveal integrative functioning organismically.

The aphasic child often has difficulty in using the objects meaningfully. Moreover, he might use jargon speech, inadvertently use a word correctly, or use one word to refer to any of the objects. Such utterances are of value in revealing auditory acuity, which is adequate for hearing speech. Observation of the child's performance should include noting the level of abstraction which he uses. Some children, notably those with peripheral deafness, engage in abstract imaginative play. Aphasic children might use an object playfully but without apparent awareness of its relationship to other objects. Such behavior frequently is corroborative of other information. As indicated above the child's play might be revealing also in regard to his emotional development. Some children with psychic deafness reject all of the toys, some take a toy and clutch it without attempts to use it meaningfully or even without showing cognizance of its purpose. Infantile autistic children typically reject human figures and other toys having social meanings but do not reject toys such as blocks. Listening behavior also can be observed during the evaluation of expressive language. The listening situation might be more meaningful to the child than during auditory testing and thereby further reveal his level of auditory acuity. The child's responses to the language tests should be recorded on a form such as the one given below:

Evaluation of Language

Inner

Relates objects imaginatively	Uses one object playfully at a time	Cannot relate to objects playfully

Receptive

Has visual reception	Has auditory reception	Uses vision and hearing simultaneously	Comprehends gestures	Has no language reception

Expressive

Uses phrases Uses words	Uses gesture Uses jargon	Erratic use of words Does not verbalize

SUMMARY

Auditory tests for young children may be classified as formal and informal. Formal tests require active cooperation from the child, whereas informal tests do not require active cooperation. Formal tests include pure tone audiometry, tuning forks, speech audiometry and psychogalvanic audiometry. Informal tests include sound instruments, sound toys, imitation of the child's vocalization, voice tests and the verbal comprehension test. The informal tests have certain advantages of simplicity, not requiring extensive equipment or an assistant and importantly, the active cooperation of the child is not required.

Sound Instrument Test

The child is seated at a table in front of an appropriate toy with the mother seated nearby. The examiner, seated opposite the child, engages him playfully with the toy. As the child engages himself in the activity the examiner produces a sound with a sound instrument, the characteristics of which have been determined by a sound analyzer. The production of the sound is not visible to the child. Momentary cessation of activity is the response commonly looked for; the child assumes an attitude of immobility and searching awareness and scans the environment before resuming his play. Such a response is most often obtained in children with peripheral deafness when the sound reaches their threshold. When the child is hyperactive, attending to various objects fleetingly as seen in receptive aphasics, the examiner follows him and presents the sounds for long durations, allowing time for the child to shift his attention. If the child is severely withdrawn and deeply engrossed in phantasy, the examiner, again concealing the sound instruments, produces sounds while carefully observing the child for motor movements, cessation of activity, eye movements and other indirect responses. Another method of applying the sound instrument test, especially useful with the mentally deficient and the aphasic, is to ring a bell in front of the child encouraging him to reach for it, then suddenly withdrawing it from sight while an identical bell is rung behind him. This increases attention and motivation. The sound instruments have an advantage over tuning forks in that the tones produced by tuning forks are more abstract and meaningless.

Sound Toy Test

Toys used include common ones that produce sounds such as dolls and telephones. The sounds produced do not exceed the loudness of ordinary conversation so if the child responds to them it may be assumed that his failure to learn speech is not due to peripheral deafness. The child is presented with the toy and allowed to play with it. When the sound occurs unintentionally the child who hears it manifests surprise, immobilization, amusement or apprehension. The child is then encouraged to produce the sound intentionally and if he does so, it is an indication that he hears it. The normal child of eleven months of age produces sounds with toys in this manner. This test is particularly useful for demonstrating hearing in the autistic child who apparently rejects sounds from his environment but often accepts sounds that he produces himself. Some children who do not respond to sound will respond to the absence of sound. Given two identical toys only one of which makes a sound, he will detect the difference between them.

Imitation of Vocalization Test

The child should be encouraged to vocalize during the examination because the tonal quality of his vocalizations is useful diagnostically. Furthermore, if the examiner imitates the child's laughter, crying or vocalizations in a quiet voice and notes momentary cessation of the child's crying or other activity, it suggests that the child has adequate auditory acuity. This test is particularly useful for differential diagnosis for a response may be obtained in mental deficiency, aphasia and emotional disturbance but not in peripheral deafness.

The Voice Test

While the child engages in playful activity, the examiner may hum causing momentary cessation of activity. Also, the examiner may encourage the child to imitate the sound of mum-mum-mum and bu-bu-bu. Normal children of about nine months of age will imitate such sounds. Peripherally deaf children cannot distinguish between mum-mum and bu-bu because both sounds have the same lip movements. Some children, notably the aphasic, may give delayed responses to this test and then keep repeating the sounds intermittently.

The Verbal Comprehension Test

By presenting language such as "Where is Mommy?" or "Show me your shoes" to the child at varying intensities, the comprehension or awareness of speech can be determined. Some emotionally disturbed children will respond to whispered speech although they reject spoken voice.

Sound-field Tests

These tests are useful mainly between two and six years of age. Social sounds of the type surrounding the child in daily life are most appropriate and can be obtained in recorded form. The cessation of activity responses is noted. When pure tones are used an approximate audiogram can be made for some children.

Tests of Auditory Perception

Aphasic children usually cannot listen successfully; the auditory world is conglomerate and meaningless. By constructing a uniform background of soft music and superimposing sound instruments and voice tests such children may respond more adequately, whereas, the peripherally deaf child, the mentally deficient and those with psychic deafness are not benefitted.

The Touching Test

While the child is engaged in play activity the examiner touches his back without giving visual clues. The peripherally deaf immediately note the sensation, those with psychic deafness ignore it, the aphasic attempt to eliminate it or become distracted and disinhibited.

The Vibration Test

While the child is engaged in play on the table, the table leg is tapped silently and out of view with the palm of the hand. The response has the same significance as the touching test.

The Visual Clues Test

The examiner casually moves his hands across the child's peripheral vision or causes a shadow to fall in the child's line of vision; the peripherally deaf child reacts promptly but children with other types of auditory disorders ignore these visual clues.

Formal Tests of Hearing

These tests were designed primarily for adults. Their applicability to very young children is limited. Pure tone audiometry under very favorable circumstances was responded to by normal children above three years of age but their responses were not comparable to the adult threshold until after five years of age. Therefore, pure tone audiometric tests should not be considered useful for differential diagnosis below the age of three and one-half and they must be interpreted with caution until after the age of five. Tuning fork tests have the same limitations as the audiometric test but they can be used more flexibly.

BIBLIOGRAPHY

1. Birch, J. W. and Mathews, J.: The hearing of mental defectives. Am. J. Ment. Deficiency 55: 384, 1951.
2. Bloomer, H.: A simple method for testing the hearing of small children. J. Speech Disorders 7: 311, 1942.

3. Bordley, J. and Hardy, W.: A study in objective audiometry with the use of a psychogalvanic response. Ann. Otol., Rhin. & Laryng. *58:* 751, 1949.
4. Bunch, D. C.: Clinical Audiometry. St. Louis, Mosby, 1943.
5. Cattell, Psyche: The Measurement of Intelligence of Infants and Young Children. New York, The Psychological Corporation, 1940.
6. Carhart, Raymond: Speech audiometry. Acta oto-laryngol. *40, 41:* 18, 62, 313, 1953.
7. Cotton, J. C. and Hall, J.: Administration of the 6A audiometer test to kindergarten and first grade children. Volta Rev. *41:* 291–292, 312–314, 1939.
8. Davis, H.: Hearing and Deafness. New York, Murray Hill Books, 1947.
9. Dix, M. R. and Hallpike, C. S.: The Peep Show: a new technique for pure tone audiometry in young children. Brit. M. J. *2:* 719, 1947.
10. Doerfler, L. G.: Neurophysiological clues to auditory acuity. J. Speech Disorders *13:* 227, 1948.
11. Eisenson, Jon: Examining for Aphasia. New York, Psychological Corporation, 1946.
12. Ewing, I. R. and Ewing, A. W. G.: The ascertainment of deafness in infancy and early childhood. J. Laryng. & Otol. *59:* 309, 1944.
13. Fowler, E. P. Jr.: Tests for hearing, in, Fowler, E. P. Jr. (ed.): Loose-Leaf Medicine of the Ear, New York, T. Nelson & Sons, 1939.
14. Froeschels, E. and Beebe, H.: Testing hearing of newborn infants. Arch. Otolaryng. *44:* 710, 1946.
15. Goldstein, Kurt: Language and Language Disturbances. New York, Grune & Stratton, 1948.
16. Halstead, N. C. and Wepman, J. M.: The Halstead-Wepman Aphasia Screening Test. J. Speech & Hearing Disorders *14:* 9, 1949.
17. Hardy, W. G. and Bordley, J. E.: Special techniques in testing the hearing of children. J. Speech Disorders *16:* 123, 1951.
18. —— and Pauls, M. D.: The test situation in PGSR audiometry. J. Speech and Hearing Disorders *17:* 13, 1952.
19. Hirsh, Ira: The Measurement of Hearing. New York, McGraw-Hill, 1952.
20. Keaster, J.: A quantitative method of testing the hearing of young children. J. Speech Disorders *12:* 159, 1947.
21. McCleary, R. A.: The nature of the galvanic skin response. Psychol. Bull. *47:* 97, 1950.
22. Marcus, R. E., Gibbs, E. L. and Gibbs, F. A.: Electroencephalography in the diagnosis of hearing loss in the very young child. Dis. Nerv. System *10:* 170–173, 1949.
23. Mowrer, O. H.: Learning Theory and Personality Dynamics. New York, The Ronald Press, 1950.

24. Piaget, Jean: Play, Dreams and Imitation in Childhood. New York, W. W. Norton, 1951.
25. ———: The Origins of Intelligence in Children. New York, International Universities Press, 1952.
26. Utley, Jean: Suggestive procedures for determining auditory acuity in very young acoustically handicapped children. Eye, Ear, Nose & Throat Monthly *228*: 590, 1949.
27. ———: What's Its Name? A Guide to Speech and Hearing Development. Urbana, Ill. University of Illinois Press, 1950.
28. Westlake, Harold: Hearing acuity in young children. J. Speech & Hearing Disorders. 7: 7-14, 1942.

Chapter XII

The Psychological Examination

DURING RECENT YEARS PSYCHOLOGISTS HAVE become increasingly interested in children with language and auditory disorders. However, in the past these children have been served chiefly by speech pathologists, pediatricians, otolaryngologists, child psychiatrists and neurologists. The clinical psychologist's contribution has been mainly in relation to problems of mental deficiency. The clinical psychological involvements of auditory disorders in children, nevertheless, are complex and extensive. It is not the purpose of this chapter to include a discussion of all of these involvements. Rather, only a brief discussion will be given of psychological techniques and procedures which have been found useful in the differential diagnosis of infants and young children with auditory disorders and associated language problems. Moreover, it is not the intent that all specialists will do a psychological examination but familiarity with these procedures is desirable for all who encounter these disabilities in childhood. Inasmuch as the clinical psychologist and the child psychiatrist are primarily responsible for the diagnostic determination of psychological factors, the techniques discussed will be used chiefly by these specialists but some neurologists, speech pathologists, audiologists, pediatricians and otolaryngologists might use them according to their interests, experience and training. More extensive discussions of the use of psychological tests with infants and young children are given by Kent [25] and Watson [47].

There is essentially a two-fold purpose in the psychological examination of children with auditory disorders. The first is to ascertain whether a discrepancy exists between psychological development and auditory functioning. For example, some children are presumed to have auditory disorders when their basic problem is mental deficiency and others are considered peripherally deaf when their problem is aphasia. In the case of the mentally deficient child the clinical psychologist's task is to ascertain whether the auditory incapacity is attributable to the mental retardation. If the child's problem cannot be accounted for on the basis of the unitary causal factor of mental deficiency, then multiple involvements must be pursued. In the case of an aphasic child the psychological determination consists primarily of ascertaining whether the auditory incapacity is a manifestation of symbolic or perceptual incapacities. Another example is the emotionally disturbed child whose auditory disorder is attributable to psychological factors. If discrepancies exist between psychological development and auditory functioning, then the possibility of other factors such as peripheral deafness is greatly increased.

The second major purpose of the psychological examination is to study the child's behavior in terms of the syndromes of peripheral deafness, psychic deafness, brain injury and mental deficiency. The psychology of these various groups of children with auditory disorders differs significantly. The clinical psychologist and child psychiatrist should evaluate these differences because they are specialists in making definitive observations of behavioral symptomatology as discussed in Part Three. Frequently it is necessary to use specific procedures to elicit such behavioral patterns. It is in this way especially that the psychological examination provides highly pertinent information diagnostically. For example, if peripheral deafness is present the psychological findings should reveal a behavioral syndrome consistent with organic adjustments on the basis of sensory deprivation. In this manner the psychological findings should corroborate a presumptive diagnosis or suggest other diagnostic possibilities.

Standardized procedures frequently cannot be applied to infants and young children presenting problems of auditory disorder. As indicated in Chapter XI many of these children cannot engage in cooperative effort. Furthermore, most standardized psychological tests assume normal verbal capacities and these children are essentially lacking in the comprehension and use of verbal language. However, certain tests can be used. Whenever possible they are given in a standard manner and scored quantitatively. When this is not possible these tests are administered according to the child's level of cooperation and the results are used qualitatively. There are other reasons for using tests in a qualitative rather than a quantitative manner with these children. The nature of their problem frequently precludes normative comparison with the average. For example, the brain injured aphasic child might fail simple test items and succeed on more difficult ones. What is simple and what is difficult for him is not only a function of genetic maturation but it is dependent on the nature of his problem. What is simple for the normal child might be difficult for brain injured children because of the way the task is presented. Moreover, the aphasic child might solve the problem but only by a circuitous mental process. Thus, although he scores correctly his performance is deviate. Children with psychic deafness, likewise, do not perform according to normative standards. Their inability to relate adequately to the test situation often makes normative comparison precarious or impossible. Undue emphasis on quantitative test results with such children leads to erroneous diagnosis and classification.

The areas usually included for specific appraisal in the psychological examination are social maturity, mental development, motor functioning and emotional development. Although evaluation of these various aspects of behavior usually proceeds simultaneously, each area is discussed separately.

EXAMINATION OF SOCIAL MATURITY

Development of social competence is a fundamental aspect of the maturation of all children. Social maturity, therefore, is significantly related to the differential diagnosis of children with auditory disorders. Doll [12] has done the major work in defining the area of social maturity and has provided the basic means for its measurement. This measuring instrument is the Vineland Social Maturity Scale [13]. This Scale is a standardized developmental schedule extending from birth to adulthood. It measures the gradually increasing capacity of the individual to care for himself and to assist with the care of others. It measures the extent to which the individual achieves independence, or stated differently, the extent to which he remains dependent and requires assistance from others. It is unique in that it measures how an individual uses his capacities rather than the extent of his capacities. Watson [47] has discussed the use of this Scale as a clinical diagnostic instrument. An extensive discussion of theoretical, research and clinical applications is given by Doll.

A distinct advantage of the Social Maturity Scale as a diagnostic instrument for children with auditory disorders is that participation of the individual being evaluated is unnecessary. The Scale is administered with the aid of an informant and therefore the examiner secures the required information from someone who is intimately associated with the child, usually his parents. This procedure not only overcomes any inability on the part of the child to cooperate but it circumvents his language disability. The information is secured by the interview method. The examiner secures the necessary information concerning the child and scores him on a series of specific items. This procedure should not be confused with a rating scale in which the informant makes the judgment and does the scoring. When the Scale is used for examining children with auditory disorders it is usually administered in conjunction with taking the differential history. Social maturation is divided into six categories: (1) self-help, which is divided into three sub-categories called self-help general, self-help eating, and self-help dressing; (2) locomotion; (3) occupation; (4) communication; (5) self-direction; (6) socialization. The development of social maturity in early life consists of learning to care for oneself, during adolescence it consists mainly of developing ability to direct oneself, and in adulthood it consists of assuming responsibility for the care of others. Scores derived from administering the Scale are social quotients and social ages, which are comparable to mental ages and intelligence quotients. For maximum results in the use of the Social Maturity Scale specific training and experience are necessary. To illustrate more concretely the nature of this Scale, four items and the scoring criteria from the two to three year range are given below:

35. (Self-help)   Asks to go to toilet.
      General   By actions or speech expresses to someone desire to go to toilet and rarely has daytime toilet "accidents." May be assisted at toilet.

38. (Self-help)   Eats with fork.
      Eating   Uses fork without much spilling for eating solid food which does not require cutting.

42. (Self-help)   Puts on coat or dress unassisted.
      Dressing   Puts on own coat, dress or overcoat without help, but need not button.

44. (Commun-   Relates experiences
      ication)   Gives simple accounts of experiences or tells stories (unprompted) with sequential and coherent content and relevant detail. Vocabulary and language forms not so important as the continuity of the account.

Studies of the effect of peripheral deafness on social maturity include those of Bradway [9], Myklebust and Burchard [33], Streng and Kirk [44], Avery [4] and Treacy [46]. Avery, and Streng and Kirk used different scoring procedures than the other workers making the differences in their results more apparent than real. In general there is agreement that children with peripheral deafness are below the normal in social maturity. This is to be expected particularly in view of their deficiencies in communication. An analysis of the social competence of the children seen for differential diagnosis of auditory disorders and on whom a diagnosis had been established is given in table 20. These findings show that the children least retarded in social competence are those with peripheral deafness, followed by those with psychic deafness, then the aphasic and the mentally deficient. These findings are in agreement with those given in tables 10 through 15. A further comparison between the groups is given in table 21. There was a significant difference

Table 20. — *The Mean Social Quotients for Each of the Groups of Children Having Auditory Disorders*

	Peripheral deafness	Aphasia	Psychic deafness	Mentally deficient
No.	79	58	27	29
Mean	91.84	74.21	78.26	56.86
S.D.	19.36	19.01	25.88	22.87

Table 21. — *Comparison Between Each of the Groups in Mean Social Quotients*

	Peripheral deafness	Aphasia	Psychic deafness	Mentally deficient
No.	79	58	27	29
Mean	91.84	74.21	78.26	56.86
S.D.	19.36	19.01	25.88	22.87
t		5.32	2.50	7.33
Req.t		2.65 †	2.04 *	2.73 †

	Aphasia	Psychic deafness	Mentally deficient
No.	58	27	29
Mean	74.21	78.26	56.86
S.D.	19.01	25.88	22.87
t		0.73	3.52
Req.t		2.04 *	2.73 †

	Psychic deafness	Mentally deficient
No.	27	29
Mean	78.26	56.86
S.D.	25.88	22.87
t		3.27
Req.t		2.76 †

* for 5% level of significance.
† for 1% level of significance.

between those children having peripheral deafness and all of the other groups; the difference being the greatest when they were compared with the aphasic and the mentally deficient. Furthermore, significant differences were found between the aphasic and the mentally deficient and between the emotionally disturbed and the mentally deficient. Differences between the emotionally disturbed and the aphasic were not significant. These findings are in agreement with clinical experience and substantiate the diagnostic procedures which were used. The evaluation of social maturity provides information which is useful in the differential diagnosis of auditory disorders in young children because the groups can be compared in their development of social competence. Children presenting different types of auditory disorders in general manifest different kinds and degrees of incapacity in social competence. This is to be expected because the social maturity evaluation considers the child as a unitary functioning organism and the different etiologies of the auditory disorders make different organismic adjustments necessary. The sensory deprivation of peripheral deafness, while necessitating organismic adjustment, is not as debilitating in its effects as marked emotional disturbance, mental deficiency or brain injury. This is further revealed in a study by Fuller [15] who made an intensive analysis of the variations in social maturity of the children having different types of auditory disorders. This analysis included a sample of the children from whom the data in tables 20 and 21 were derived. Fuller used sub-group classifications and considered the total social quotients but also analyzed the performances in terms of the six categories (self-help, locomotion, communication, socialization, self-direction and occupation) measured on the Vineland Social Maturity Scale. This analysis corroborated the concept of organismic behavioral differences between the groups of children presenting problems of auditory disorders. The Social Maturity Scale measures the child's ability to inter-act with and to control his environment. Such behavior requires integrative behavior. The social maturity data revealed that children with peripheral deafness function integratively despite their sensory limitation. These children were superior to the others on all items except those entailing verbalization; children with psychic deafness, aphasia and mental deficiency verbalize more than those with peripheral deafness. The emotionally disturbed comparatively reject their environment and thereby do not inter-act with it or control it. These children not only were notably inferior on the category of socialization but also were deficient in general in social competence. The aphasic cannot integrate their environmental experience as meaningfully as those with peripheral deafness. However, they were superior to the emotionally disturbed and the mentally deficient in socialization and were inferior to the emotionally disturbed on locomotion. The mentally deficient showed the most generalized incapacities in the development of social maturity. This analysis manifests the relative intactness of the social maturity of children with peripheral deafness as compared to those with other types of auditory disorders. Such use of the Vineland Social Maturity Scale is unusually profitable from the point of view of differential diagnosis. It furnishes a systematic and standardized procedure for comparing the developmental behavior of these children. The evaluation of social maturity constitutes an important part of the psychological examination.

EXAMINATION OF MENTAL CAPACITY

The examination of the mental capacity of infants and young children is difficult even when handicaps are not present but it is more difficult when the child presents a problem of auditory disorder. Therefore, the results of the mental examination often must be stated in approximate terms. Statements such as "these results suggest that this child is mentally deficient" or "these results reveal that this child's mental level is within normal limits" frequently are used to describe a child's performance. The value of such findings, even though approximate, should not be underestimated. The primary purpose of the psychometric examination is to ascertain whether a discrepancy exists between mental development and auditory behavior. Another way of stating the purpose of this evaluation is to determine whether the mental level is adequate for acquiring language. The presumption is that if mental level and language behavior are not discrepant, other factors such as deafness are not influential. A diagnosis of peripheral deafness, psychic deafness or aphasia can be made with assurance only after ascertaining that intellectual potential is adequate for acquiring language. If the psychometric evaluation makes such statements possible, it has contributed significantly to the final diagnosis.

In view of the complexity of the total diagnostic problem in connection with young children with auditory disorders, it is understandable that some confusion surrounds the determination of intelligence. Hardy [20] has suggested caution in the use of psychometric techniques with children having peripheral deafness. However, caution also must be used in other respects. Aphasic children and children with psychic deafness are readily confused with the mentally deficient [30]. Usually such confusions derive primarily from undue emphasis on the mental test performance alone. Just as the auditory test results require corroboration from other sources, the mental test results too must be interpreted in light of the total clinical syndrome. Furthermore, children having different types of auditory disorders perform characteristically on tests of intelligence and the qualitative aspects of their performances are significant and useful diagnostically. As in testing auditory capacity, what the child does is revealing but frequently what he does not do and the manner in which he does not do it are also revealing clinically.

Tests of Mental Capacity

The Cattell Test for Infants and Young Children: The most useful mental tests for children presenting problems of auditory disorder are those requiring a minimum of language and which provide maximum opportunity for observing the child's behavior. For very young children the Cattell Test [11] fulfills these requirements. This test covers the age range of two to thirty months. A discussion of the reliability, validity and general clinical usefulness of this test is given by Watson [47]. Cattell states that the reliability of this test is greater after the child reaches eighteen months of age. A distinct advantage of these tests is that there is no time limit and no definite order of presentation. These factors add to the flexibility of administration which is required for many children. Another advantage of these tests is the inclusion of developmental aspects of auditory behavior. For example, the items "attends to voice" and "babbles" occur at the two month level. The item "turns to voice" occurs at four months, and "turns to bell" at five months. Combining two syllables such as "ma-ma" and "ba-ba" occurs at eight months. Ringing a bell in imitation of the examiner, adjusting to gesture and imitation of vocalization occur at nine months. After twelve months and to thirty months items are included which measure the child's progress in language acquisition. It is apparent that this test has diagnostic implications for auditory disorders in early life. These infant tests of mental development can be administered to many children presenting problems of auditory disorder but administration and interpretation requires special training in clinical psychology.

The Ontario School Ability Examination: Another test which can be used in evaluating the intelligence of young children with auditory disorders is the Ontario School Ability Examination [2]. This test covers the age range of two years to adulthood. It is a performance test in that verbal directions and responses are not required. The block building and geometric designs test are especially useful for children below six years of age. This test was assimilated for the purpose of examining school age children with peripheral deafness. Although findings for such children are available, the standardization and norms must be considered as tentative. The standardization group consisted of two hundred and eighty-eight children at the Ontario School for the Deaf. This test also has the disadvantage of not having been used extensively with normal children. However, selected items are revealing regarding the child's level and quality of mental functioning.

The Nebraska Test of Learning Aptitude for Young Deaf Chil-

dren: This test, like the Ontario, was devised for the specific purpose of examining young children with peripheral deafness and was standardized on such children [*24*]. Comparable norms for normal children are not available. The standardization group consisted of four hundred and sixty-six children selected on the basis of age (four to ten years) from six residential schools for the deaf. By extrapolation the norms have been extended to include children from three to eleven and one-half years of age. Learning ages and learning quotients are used instead of mental ages and intelligence quotients. Kirk and Perry [*26*], and MacPherson and Lane [*28*] have compared the scores obtained on this test with those obtained on tests of intelligence. According to these studies learning scores on the Nebraska Test are comparable to mental ages and intelligence quotients. Abbreviated scales for three to seven and eight to eleven years have been provided. Items which have been found especially useful in the differential diagnosis of mental deficiency, brain injury and peripheral deafness are the pictorial associations, block patterns, memory for digits and pictorial identification. This test can be administered to many children presenting problems of auditory disorder as it is a performance test and does not require verbalization in administration or response. Inasmuch as norms for normal children are not available, direct comparison with the normal cannot be made but comparison with the standardization group provides inferential evidence for normalcy of mental growth.

The Geometric Design Drawing Test: The Stanford Binet [*45*], the Ontario School Ability Examination and other tests have included the drawing of geometric designs. The circle, cross, square and diamond have a long history of usefulness and standardization through the Stanford Binet. Other designs and an extended range have been provided by Starr [*42*]. Geometric designs which have proved to be unusually applicable to children with auditory disorders in order of presentation are: lines, circle, cross, square, triangle, diamond. The usual manner of administering this test to these children is to draw the figure on a plain sheet of paper while the child is observing and then indicate that he is to draw one like it. Levels of performance and interpretation are based primarily on the norms for the Stanford Binet.

The Draw a Man Test: The Goodenough Draw a Man Test is useful with some children above four years of age [*19*]. This test has a long history of research and clinical significance. It has been used with peripherally deaf children of school age [*32*] and although these studies are not all in agreement, these children are not significantly retarded in intelligence as measured by this test. Drawings of human figures also have been used as a projective test of personality [*29*] and it is helpful in analyzing perceptual and conceptual disturbances in aphasic children.

Administration of the Draw a Man Test to children with auditory disorders presents certain difficulties inasmuch as verbal instruction cannot be used. The instructions can be made clear to many children by placing the paper and pencil before him and encouraging him to draw spontaneously. Another sheet of paper is then placed before the child and he is encouraged to make a picture of a man. As the examiner gives the instructions by speaking and gesticulation, he simultaneously might point to a carefully selected male doll figure or in some instances to the picture of a man; the use of a picture instead of the doll figure is more difficult for some children. The doll figure or picture is held some distance from the child and it is exposed briefly only to illustrate what the examiner is asking the child to do. Care must be taken not to give the child the impression that he is to draw the particular man used for demonstrating the problem. This procedure is used only when speech reading and auditory comprehension cannot be used. It has been found helpful in giving the Goodenough Test to many children and this test has value in the examination of mental capacity.

Tests which can be used with children above five years of age: Standard tests of intelligence which are useful for children with auditory disorders above five years of age are the Grace Arthur Point Scale of Performance Tests [*3*], the Leiter International Performance Test [*27*] and the Wechsler Intelligence Scale for Children [*48*]. It is not common to use all of the items in any one of these test batteries but selected items from these various tests can be used according to the child's level of cooperation and the problem which he presents. The Grace Arthur and Leiter tests have been used with school age children having peripheral deafness [8,33]. These studies provide background information for the use of these tests with young children presenting problems of auditory disorder.

Interpretation of Mental Test Findings

A considerable amount of research and clinical experience has been reported which is directly applicable to the interpretation of mental test results. The work of Birch and Birch [8], Heider and Heider [23], Myklebust and Burchard [33], Oléron [35], and Myklebust and Brutten [32] on the mental functioning of children with peripheral deafness is especially pertinent to this group of children. The work of Goldstein [18], Benton [7], and particularly that of Strauss and Lehtinen [43] has been found helpful in interpreting the results for the children having brain injury. Studies by Watson [47], and Rapaport [38] have provided background information for evaluation of mental test results from emotionally disturbed children. Doll's [14] contribution includes work both on brain injury and the mentally deficient. As these references suggest, there is extensive literature and experience which is related to the interpretation of mental test results from children who have auditory disorders. It is not the purpose to review this literature or to discuss the theoretical aspects, but rather to suggest clinical applications and interpretations of the mental test results.

Children presenting problems in the differential diagnosis of auditory disorders differ in their behavior on mental tests just as they differ in their reactions to any other formalized test situation. The child with peripheral deafness is the most amenable to formal mental testing. With appropriate skillful management several tests usually can be given. It is rare, however, to give complete batteries of tests to any child presenting a problem of auditory disorder. Specific tests are selected from the batteries discussed above and the selections are based on the particular diagnostic problem presented by the child. Frequently a few tests, such as the drawing of geometric designs, the Cattell formboard or the block tower from the Ontario can be given to children having the symptomatology of brain injury or mental deficiency. With the aphasic, however, the administration of such tests requires certain adaption and flexibility. For example, time limits usually cannot be applied. More important, perhaps, is the manner in which the test is given. The presentation must include structuring of the testing situation. This can be illustrated by the geometric design drawing test. Only one design should be given on each plain sheet of paper. If one design is on the paper as the child proceeds to the next, he is distracted by the design which already has been drawn. Even the water mark on the plain sheet of paper frequently has been found distracting; the child proceeds to trace the water mark rather than draw the design. Such responses are revealing diagnostically and should be considered as part of the total results of the testing. In general, these responses suggest visual perceptual disturbances and often such children have sufficient intelligence to draw the design if the structuring of the task makes it possible for them to comprehend and to proceed with it. There are many other such manifestations which are meaningful to the experienced examiner. Some children when given a large crayon (for easy grasping) and when a plain sheet of paper is placed before them, immediately proceed to draw lines as a border around the outer edge of the paper. These lines assist them in structuring the surface of the paper making their visual field and task more manageable. Others use the edge of the paper as a means of structuring it and draw the figures in corners or at the outer edges of the paper. Most of the children presenting the symptomatology of brain injury with aphasia use such devices for accomplishing the tests and observation of this behavior is unusually significant in understanding their learning problems and their daily behavior. Such children who have a minimum of verbal capacity commonly use other means to assist them in accomplishing tasks which are required of them. For example, when presented with the circle and urged to make one like it, they hesitate, then say "ball" and proceed to make the circle; when given the cross, some say "airplane" and then proceed to draw it. The same phenomena can be observed in young normal children but the undueness and compulsiveness of it in aphasic children is unusual and diagnostically significant. It seems that their reduction in ability to function abstractly makes it necessary for them to call the figure something; to concretize it before they can proceed with the drawing. This need to concretize has been observed also in children with congenital peripheral deafness [32]. However, the manifestation of concreteness in young peripherally deaf children is significantly different. They do not manifest the need for structuring of the situation. They proceed with the solution as long as the essentials of the task are visual and remain before them and therefore they perform normally on block design tests and tests of similarities involving matching. Their limitations become apparent in problems involving analogy, conceptualization, inference and reasoning and these limitations are attributable to the lack of auditory experience and deficiencies of internalization because of the inability to use verbal language; generalized deficiencies of abstract ability are not apparent.

Other mental test responses which are helpful in the differential diagnosis of aphasia and peripheral deafness particularly are those involving block building. The three block tower is found on the Stanford Binet, Gesell, Cattell, Ontario and Hiskey Tests. Varying presentations have been used. For example, in the Hiskey a demonstration tower is not built by the examiner. Instead the child is shown a picture of the tower (similar presentation is used for all of the block design tests on the Hiskey) and asked to make one like it. This item falls at the three year level on the Hiskey and building a tower from demonstration falls at the two year level on the Stanford Binet and the Ontario. This indicates that building a tower from a design is more difficult than building it from an actual model. This is in agreement with clinical experience although the differences in these tests are considerably greater for some children. The designs on the Hiskey Block Designs Tests are drawn in perspective and emphasize visual perceptual abilities. Therefore, frequently aphasic children fail these tests but pass them when models are used, such as on the Ontario. These marked differences of performance are not common with children who have peripheral deafness.

Another test on which similar differences can be demonstrated is the Healy Picture Completion I. Some aphasic children, who find the many figures on this test distracting, complete it successfully when the background is structured for them. This can be done by using a cardboard to obscure all of the figures except those involved in each solution. If such structuring is of no benefit to the child, it is unlikely that a visual perceptual disturbance is impeding the use of his intelligence. Children with peripheral deafness typically do not require assistance in structuring this test.

Mental test results are unusually difficult to secure from children with psychic deafness. Either their marked anxiety or their generalized rejection of the environment makes the application of such tests tenuous or impossible. Estimates and inferences of mental level frequently must be made on the basis of history, genetic development, behavioral symptomatology and language involvements. When mental tests can be used, usually they are of the formboard type. Some children, especially those with autistic symptomatology, perform well on formboards sometimes showing superior ability. One of the dangers in examining the emotionally disturbed child psychometrically is to conclude that because he cannot relate to the situation and because he is bizarre, he is inferior in intellectual capacity. This is unfortunate because the problems of lack of intelligence and inability to use intelligence are widely different therapeutically and in general scientific implication. Whenever possible confusion of these problems should be avoided. The experienced psychologist can make many pertinent and valid observations regarding mental capacity even though standardized tests of intelligence cannot be applied directly. The inapplicability of a test is not tantamount to failure on the test and thereby concluding that the child is mentally deficient is unwarranted. This same caution is essential for all children presenting problems in the differential diagnosis of auditory disorders but is most consequential for the aphasic and those with psychic deafness.

The identification of the mentally deficient through psychological examination likewise presents a complex problem. Such a diagnosis, like the diagnosis of the auditory disorder itself, should be made only when the history, behavioral symptomatology and test results are reciprocally corroborative. The importance of genetic factors is indicated by tables 10 through 15. Mental tests usually can be applied in a standard manner and these results show substantial internal consistency.

A Suggested Battery of Mental Tests for Use with Children Below Six Years of Age Who Present Problems of Auditory Disorder

Certain mental tests have been found through clinical experience to be especially suitable for young children with auditory disorders. A list of these tests and the age range covered by each is given below:

Test	Age range	Selected from
Scribbling in imitation	16 months	Cattell
Scribbling spontaneously	18 months	Cattell
Copying circle	3 years	Binet
Copying cross	$3\frac{1}{2}$ years	Binet
Copying square	5 years	Binet
Copying triangle	6 years	Ontario
Copying diamond	7 years	Binet
Block building	2 to 8 years	Ontario
Block patterns	3 to 11 years	Hiskey
Pictorial associations	3 to $11\frac{1}{2}$ years	Hiskey
Pictorial identification	3 to $7\frac{1}{2}$ years	Hiskey
Three hole formboard	16 to 20 months	Cattell
Three hole formboard	2 to $3\frac{1}{2}$ years	Binet
Manikin	5 to 6 years	Grace Arthur
Healy picture completion I	5 to 14 years	Grace Arthur
Kohs block design	5 to 15 years	Grace Arthur
Sequin formboard	5 to 14 years	Grace Arthur
Draw a man	3 to 13 years	Goodenough

Developmental items which are especially pertinent below one year of age

Attends to voice and babbles	2 months	Cattell
Turns to voice	4 months	Cattell
Turns to bell	5 months	Cattell
Combines syllables	8 months	Cattell
Rings bell in imitation	9 months	Cattell
Adjusts to gesture and imitates	9 months	Cattell

EXAMINATION OF MOTOR CAPACITY

Examination of motor capacity provides significant information for the diagnostician of auditory disorders in young children. Children with peripheral deafness might have balance deficiencies due to concomitant vestibular impairments [31]. Aphasic children frequently have generalized psychomotor incoordination resulting from damage to the central nervous system. Autistic children usually are robust and give no indication of motor disturbance. Schizophrenic children engage in stereotyped motor activities and manifest a reduction of spontaneity motorically but their motor functioning does not suggest neurological disorder and it is of good quality when it can be elicited. Mentally deficient children manifest retardation of motor development in general. Data concerning the developmental aspects of the motor capacities of the various types of children are given in tables 10 and 12. Motor tests provide an opportunity for the diagnostician to secure corroborative information because a diagnosis of aphasia or of psychic deafness especially, can be made with greater assurance when the examination of motor capacity reveals the expected motor behavior. The child's motor behavior should be consistent with his syndrome. If the motor functioning is in disagreement with the basic syndrome, it suggests multiple involvement such as neurological injury superimposed on sensory impairment or emotional disturbance.

Motor testing usually is done informally. Clinical observation, parental report and special tests are used. The Vineland Social Maturity Scale [13] provides a schedule for pertinent aspects of motor development. Moreover, motor tests which can be used have been devised by Bayley [6], Oseretsky [37], Doll [13] and Heath [22]. The test devised by Bayley covers the age range of one to fifty months. The Oseretsky Test, which has been adapted by Cassell [10] and by Sloan [41], extends from four to sixteen years. The Heath Railwalking Test extends from six years to adulthood but it can be used clinically with children down to four years of age. Inasmuch as formal tests often cannot be applied, a schedule of motor development which can be used with most children is given below.

Schedule of Motor Development

Test item	Expected age of occurrence
(items from Bayley)	(month)
Holds head erect and steady	2.9
Sits with support	3.5
Sits unsupported	7.5
Pulls to standing position	10.5
Walks with help	11.6
Stands alone	12.5
Walks alone	13.0
Stands on right or left foot with help	19.9
Tries to stand on walking board	22.5
Walks with one foot on walking board	27.6
Stands momentarily on right or left foot without assistance	29.3
Walks on tip-toe	30.1
Stands on walking board with both feet	31.0
Walks on a line (10 ft.) in general direction and stepping on line	31.3
Walks on board with two or more alternating steps	38.0
Hops on right foot two or three hops	49.3
Walks downstairs alternating foot forward	50.0
(items from Oseretsky)	(year)
Stands with one foot before the other with eyes closed	4
Touches the nose with forefinger with eyes closed	4
Makes circles with forefinger, arms extended outright from sides	4
Balances on tip-toe	5
Hops 15 feet on one foot	5
Rolls a small piece of thin paper into a ball by using the fingers of one hand only	5
Balances on one foot for ten seconds	6
Throws a ball at a target five feet away	6
Jumps over a rope (20 cm. high)	6

The items have been selected from the sources indicated. This schedule of motor activities can be used without verbal instruction. Usually the examiner demonstrates in a playful manner what the child is to do and as the child performs the motor tasks, the examiner checks his level of performance. When the child is incapable of such cooperation the examiner observes his spontaneous motor activity and evaluates it as much as possible in terms of the expected levels.

Tests of Laterality

Laterality refers to the preferential use of one side over the other. The most common manifestation of laterality is handedness. However, preference or dominance also can be noted in the legs and eyes. Usually a right sided individual is right handed, right legged and right eyed. If the right hand and the left leg are dominant or vice versa, the individual is referred to as having a mixed dominance. Laterality is considered to be due primarily to the dominance of one hemisphere of the brain over the other. In the right sided individual the left hemisphere is dominant and for the left sided individual it is the opposite [21]. This relationship between cerebral dominance and laterality has been emphasized in connection with language disorders in young children. Orton [36], Barger [5], Selzer [40], Nice [34] and Gesell [17] have emphasized the importance of cerebral dominance in relation to laterality and language functioning. Clinical experience reveals a high incidence of confused and incomplete dominance in children presenting problems of auditory disorder. These laterality disturbances are especially common in children presenting the syndrome of brain injury with concomitant subtle, pervasive motor incoordination. Hand preference can be noted in normal children between eight and twelve months of age [16]. Between eighteen and twenty-four months preference for one hand becomes established. This maturational aspect of laterality serves as a background for interpreting test results for young children.

Handedness tests: The child's hand preference can be examined in various ways. Harris [21] has described a number of tests which can be used with children. The throwing test has been found especially useful with children having auditory disorders. The examiner engages the child playfully in throwing a rubber ball. The child is given an opportunity to throw the ball approximately five times. The hand used in throwing is noted, including observation of ambidexterity. Corroborative evidence is secured by observing the child as he engages in playing with blocks, drawing or in any other activity in which preferential use of hands is commonly manifested.

Preferred leg test: This test usually is given immediately after the throwing test for handedness. The ball is placed on the floor and the examiner kicks it so it rolls toward the child. The examiner demonstrates to the child that he is to kick the ball back again; the game is for the child and the examiner to kick the ball back and forth to each other. The ball is kicked to the child in such a manner that he must choose the leg he prefers to use. This is done for approximately five times and the dominance or incomplete dominance is noted.

The Railwalking Test

Heath [22] has devised a railwalking test which is useful in examining motor capacities. This test has been used with school age children having peripheral deafness [31]. This study shows the usefulness of the test in revealing vestibular deficiencies with concomitant motor disturbance. Seashore [39] has used a similar test to measure the development of balance in normal children. As shown in the schedule of motor development on page 308, the normal child tries to stand on a walking board at twenty-two months and walks with one foot on the board at twenty-seven months. He stands on the walking board with both feet at thirty-one months and walks on the board with two or more alternating steps at thirty-eight months. The first rail of the railwalking test devised by Heath can be used to determine these levels of performance for children below three years of age. Heath has administered this test to children between six and fourteen years of age. The results on the basis of age and sex are given in table 22. These findings are useful as a guide for interpreting the performance of a child clinically. When this test is used for differential diagnosis of children between four and six years of age, marked differences often can be observed.

Table 22. — *The Mean and Median Scores for Each Age Level on the Heath Railwalking Test* *

Age	Males				Females			
	No.	Median	Mean	S.D.	No.	Median	Mean	S.D.
6	30	36	40.0	18.5	36	40	44.4	22.0
7	36	43	45.6	21.8	52	42	49.0	19.7
8	38	53	59.0	27.8	33	55	57.2	24.4
9	44	55	62.2	32.9	54	56	59.0	28.8
10	36	79	82.3	31.5	44	78	76.7	26.7
11	48	91	88.6	30.2	47	82	82.3	33.2
12	44	106	99.0	23.8	38	92	95.3	26.4
13	41	112	106.1	32.1	50	92	93.0	26.0
14	53	115	115.4	27.5	56	101	99.9	32.9

* Data supplied by S. Roy Heath, Jr.

Interpretation of Motor Test Findings

The motor test results are an important part of the psychological examination. These results should be in agreement with the syndrome presented by the child. For example, if the child has perceptual disturbances and needs structuring on the mental tests, he would be expected to show some retardation in motor development genetically, some delay or confusion in laterality and evidences of generalized incoordination. Below two years of age the history of motor development interpreted on the basis of the Schedule of Motor Development given above and as indicated by the locomotion category on the Vineland Social Maturity Scale together with the examiner's observations serve as the evaluation of motor capacity.

As indicated by the findings given in tables 10 through 13 the motor behavior of the various types of children having auditory disorders can be contrasted. The most evident motor problem of children with peripheral deafness is disturbance of balance [31]. However, not all of these children have balance difficulties because this is limited essentially to those who have reduced functioning of the semi-circular canals. The semi-circular canals are the primary balancing mechanism and therefore when these have been destroyed, balance is impaired. This can be shown by such tests as standing on one foot or by the railwalking test. Marked disturbances of balance with good integrity of generalized coordination is highly suggestive of semi-circular canal destruction with implications for etiologies of such diseases as meningitis. Such children are referred to the otolaryngologist for caloric and other types of study. Children having peripheral deafness as a result of diseases such as rubella often have more generalized incoordinations and balance is not specifically deficient. Such children present problems indicating mild inclusive damage to the central nervous system with resultant disturbance of motor capacity. Nevertheless, children with peripheral deafness do not as a group present obvious deficiencies in motor functioning. As indicated by table 12, they are the most capable motorically of any of the children seen for differential diagnosis of auditory disorders.

Aphasic children characteristically have problems of generalized incoordination and frequently these problems are manifested by their gait and grasp as well as by more specific motor tests. However, these motor symptoms are not apparent to specialists who are inexperienced in their detection. Furthermore, considerable incoordination may be observable even though neurological findings are negative. Therefore, the general neurological implications of some of the motor test findings are not always clear but progress is being made in coordinating these findings with those of the neurologist. The work of Orton [36] and of Gesell [16] is especially pertinent in this connection.

Children with psychic deafness usually do not manifest generalized incapacity to coordinate. Autistic children often are robust and excellent in motor behavior. Schizophrenic children might be inconsistent, at times revealing good integrity of motor functioning and at other times showing rigidity, poor balance, hesitancy or awkwardness. Stereotyped motor activities are common. It is their ability to perform excellently at times that most often differentiates them from the aphasic and from the mentally deficient. Children having auditory disorders as a result of their mental deficiency present problems of generalized retardation in motor development. This is indicated by the findings in tables 10 and 12. In early life these children are more delayed than disturbed motorically. Careful appraisal of their genetic development is the most significant indicator of the nature of their problem.

Laterality tests, such as throwing and kicking tests, can be administered to many of the children in need of differential diagnosis of auditory disorder. With proper encouragement most of these children will perform such tests. Even the emotionally disturbed frequently will throw or kick a ball although they might do so automatically and without regard for the examiner as a playmate or person. When laterality is delayed or when it is mixed, it suggests neurological involvements with implications for a complete study neurologically. Inasmuch as laterality is presumed to be at least partially endogenous, left sidedness without inconsistencies should not be considered suggestive of motor disturbance. When laterality is not mixed and is well established, it is corroborative evidence for sensory or emotional factors being present because disturbances of laterality are more common in the aphasic and the mentally deficient.

EVALUATION OF EMOTIONAL ADJUSTMENT

Formal psychological tests cannot be used for evaluating the child's emotional adjustment. Inasmuch as the child does not speak and usually does not comprehend speech, tests such as the Rorschach [1] cannot be applied and even spontaneous discussion or interviewing are precluded. Therefore, evaluation of emotional adjustment must be achieved primarily by clinical observation such as has been discussed under Behavioral Symptomatology in Part Three. Additional information is secured from the history and especially from analysis of performance on the Vineland Social Maturity Scale as suggested above. A list of behavioral symptoms has been found helpful for systematically observing the child's behavior.

Such a list is given below. It is not intended to be exhaustive but only to summarize the types of behavior which have been discussed in Part Three. Use of such a list has the advantage of focusing observations in specific areas and it serves as a written record of these observations.

List of Symptoms for Evaluation
of Emotional Adjustment

Symptom	Evaluation			
	yes	no	sometimes	formerly

I. Relationships with people:

    Relates to others
    Laughs and smiles responsively
    Rejects people's faces
    Fearful of strangers
    Fearful of leaving parent
    Ignores people generally
    Amenable to suggestion

II. Relationship to toys:

    Uses toys playfully
    Uses blocks only
    Plays imaginatively
    Grasps toy meaninglessly
    Plays cooperatively with others
    Associates toys realistically

III. Personal relationship:

    Is oblivious and withdrawn
    Pulls hair or ears
    Rocks in stereotyped way
    Bangs head
    Cries, sheds tears
    Is willfully negativistic
    Is fretful, anxious
    Highly distractable
    Aimless, hyperactive
    Reticent and shy
    Extremely meticulous
    Demanding of cleanliness
    Appears happy, contented

The importance of behavioral symptomatology has been discussed in Part Three and will not be reiterated here. Interpretation of these symptoms follows the pattern of the findings for other areas. The child with peripheral deafness is in contact with his environment and uses it experientially. He is not bizarre, oblivious or disintegrated. He is normally reticent, shy and playful in attitude when his confidence has been gained. Aphasic children are distractible, hyperactive, lacking in ability to play but make attempts to inter-act with their environment. Children with anxiety states are fretful, fearful, anxious and cling to their parents. Schizophrenic and autistic children are oblivious, withdrawn, engage in phantasy, show no overt fear, seem to willfully ignore others, make no distinction between parents or strangers and show general bizarreness, generalized immaturity and phlegmaticness although they might be fretful and generally be in a state of unhappiness. Interpretation of the behavioral symptoms must be made cautiously and in light of the total findings.

SUMMARY

The primary purpose of the psychological examination is to determine whether a discrepancy exists between the child's psychological capacities and his auditory functioning. The psychologist also uses specific tests for eliciting behavior which characterizes each of the four types of children with auditory disorders. The areas covered by the psychological examination include especially social maturity, mental development, motor capacity and emotional adjustment. The Vineland Social Maturity Scale is applicable to all of the children because it is administered through an informant rather than to the child. Of the four groups of children having auditory disorders the peripherally deaf are the nearest normal, followed by those with psychic deafness, then the aphasic and finally the mentally deficient.

Mental Capacity

Only non-verbal tests are applicable to young children with auditory disorders because of their inability to communicate. Tests which have been found useful for determining mental capacity include the Cattell Test for Infants and Young Children, The Ontario School Ability Examination, The Nebraska Test of Learning Aptitude for Young Deaf Children, The Geometric Design Test and The Draw a Man Test. Adaptations of the standard administration must be used for some children, especially techniques for structuring the task. The peripherally deaf child performs most successfully on the mental tests as compared to children who have psychic deafness, aphasia or who are mentally deficient.

Motor Capacity

Children with auditory disorders differ in motor development genetically and in motor coordination. The peripherally deaf and those with psychic deafness are most like the normal child in motor functioning and development. The mentally deficient are significantly retarded motorically and the aphasic have generalized incoordination. These differences often are apparent to clinicians who are trained to observe them but motor tests provide further evidence. Items from the Bayley norms for normal children and from the Oseretsky are highly useful for motor testing.

Emotional Adjustment

There are no tests of emotional adjustment which are directly applicable to young children with auditory disorders. However, a check list of behavior symptoms can be used to supplement clinical observations. These behavior symptoms should cover the child's relationship to other people, toys and to himself. Psychological tests, like auditory tests require corroboration from the history and from the child's behavior.

BIBLIOGRAPHY

1. Ames, L. B. et al.: Child Rorschach Responses. New York, Paul B. Hoeber, 1952.

2. Amoss, Harry: Ontario School Ability Examination. Toronto, The Ryerson Press, 1936.

3. Arthur, Grace: A Point Scale of Performance Tests. New York, The Commonwealth Fund, 1930.

4. Avery, C.: A study of preschool acoustically handicapped children. Unpublished M.A. thesis, Northwestern University, 1947.

5. Barger, W. C.: An experimental approach to aphasia and nonreading children. Am. J. Orthopsychiat. 23: 158, 1953.

6. Bayley, Nancy: The Development of Motor Abilities During the First Three Years. Washington, Society for Research in Child Development, National Research Council, #1, 1935.

7. Benton, A. L. and Collins, N. T.: Visual retention test performance in children. Arch. Neurol. & Psychiat. 62: 610, 1949.

8. Birch, J. and Birch, J.: The Leiter International Performance Scale as an aid in the psychological study of deaf children. Am. Ann. Deaf 96: 502, 1951.

9. Bradway, K.: The social competence of deaf children. Am. Ann. Deaf 82: 122, 1937.

10. Cassell, R. H.: The Vineland Adaptation of the Oseretsky Tests. Vineland, The Training School. Mon. Supplement #1, 1950.

11. Cattell, Psyche: The Measurement of Intelligence of Infants and Young Children. New York, The Psychological Corporation, 1940.

12. Doll, E. A.: The Measurement of Social Competence. Minneapolis, The Educational Test Bureau, 1953.

13. ——: Vineland Social Maturity Scale. Minneapolis, Educational Test Bureau, 1947.

14. ——: The feebleminded child, in, Carmichael, L. (ed.): Manual of Child Psychology. New York, Wiley, 1946, pp. 845–885.

15. Fuller, Carl: A study of the social maturity profiles of selected communication impaired children. Unpublished research project, Northwestern University, 1952.

16. Gesell, Arnold et al.: The First Five Years of Life. New York, Harpers, 1940.

17. —— and Amatruda, C. S.: Developmental Diagnosis. New York, Paul B. Hoeber, 1948.

18. Goldstein, Kurt: Language and Language Disturbances. New York, Grune & Stratton, 1948.

19. Goodenough, F. L.: Measurement of Intelligence by Drawings. Chicago, World Book Co., 1926.

20. Hardy, W. G.: The relations between impaired hearing and pseudo-feeble-mindedness. Nerv. Child 7: 432, 1948.

21. Harris, A. J.: Harris Tests of Lateral Dominance. New York, The Psychological Corporation, 1947.

22. Heath, S. R.: Railwalking performance as related to mental age and etiological type among the mentally retarded. Am. J. Psychol. 55: 240, 1942.

23. Heider, F. and Heider, G.: Studies in the psychology of the deaf. Psychol. Monogr. No. I, 1940.

24. Hiskey, M. S.: Nebraska Test of Learning Aptitude for Young Deaf Children. New York, Psychological Corporation, 1914.

25. Kent, Grace: Mental Tests in Clinics for Children. New York, Van Nostrand, 1950.

26. Kirk, S. and Perry, June: A comparative study of the Ontario and Nebraska Tests for the deaf. Am. Ann. Deaf 93: 315, 1948.

27. Leiter, R. G.: The Leiter International Performance Scale. Santa Barbara, Calif., Santa Barbara State College Press, 1940.

28. MacPherson, M. and Lane, H.: A comparison of deaf and hearing on the Hiskey Test and on performance scales. Am. Ann. Deaf 93: 178, 1948.

29. Machover, Karen: Personality Projection in the Drawing of the Human Figure: A Method of Personality Investigation. Springfield, Ill., C. C Thomas, 1949.

30. Myklebust, H. R.: The relationship between clinical psychology and audiology. J. Speech & Hearing Disorders 14: 98, 1949.

31. ——: Significance of etiology in motor performance of deaf children with special reference to meningitis. Am. J. Psychol. 59: 249, 1946.

32. —— and Brutten, M.: A study of the visual perception of deaf children. Acta oto-laryng., Suppl. 105, 1953.

33. —— and Burchard, E. M. L.: A study of the effects of congenital and adventitious deafness on the intelligence, personality and social maturity of school children. J. Ed. Psychol. 36: 321, 1945.

34. Nice, M. M.: Ambidexterity and delayed speech development. Ped. Sem. 25: 141, 1918.

35. Oléron, Pierre: Conceptual thinking of the deaf. Am. Ann. Deaf 98: 304, 1953.

36. Orton, S. T.: Reading, Writing and Speech Problems in Children. New York, W. W. Norton, 1937.

37. Oseretsky, N.: The Oseretsky Tests of Motor Proficiency. Minneapolis, Educational Test Bureau, 1946.

38. Rapaport, D. et al.: Diagnostic Psychological Testing. New York, Year Book Publishers, 1945.

39. Seashore, H. G.: The development of a beam walking test and its use in measuring development of balance in children. Am. Assoc. for Health, Phys. Ed. and Recreation, Research Quarterly *18:* 246, 1947.
40. Selzer, C. A.: Lateral dominance and visual fusion. Cambridge, Harvard Mon. in Ed., Harvard University Press, 1933, vol. 12.
41. Sloan, W.: The Lincoln Adaptation of the Oseretsky Test. Lincoln, Ill., State School and Colony, 1950.
42. Starr, Anna: The Rutgers Drawing Test. Vineland, The Training School Bulletin *49:* 45, 1952.
43. Strauss, A. and Lehtinen, L.: Psychopathology and Education of the Brain-Injured Child. New York, Grune & Stratton, 1947.
44. Streng, A. and Kirk, S.: The social competence of deaf and hard of hearing children in a public day school. Am. Ann. Deaf *83:* 244, 1938.
45. Terman, L. M. and Merrill, M. A.: Measuring Intelligence. New York, Houghton Mifflin, 1937.
46. Treacy, L.: A study of social maturity in relation to factors of intelligence in acoustically handicapped children. Unpublished M.A. thesis, Northwestern University, 1952.
47. Watson, Robert: The Clinical Method in Psychology. New York, Harpers, 1951.
48. Wechsler, David: Wechsler Intelligence Scale for Children. New York, The Psychological Corporation, 1949.

PART FIVE: ILLUSTRATIVE CASES AND RECOMMENDATIONS

Chapter XIII

Case Studies

ONE OF THE WAYS IN WHICH TO ASCERTAIN the effectiveness of diagnostic procedures is to continue contact with specific children over a period of time. This seems advisable also because diagnoses for some children must be tentative and verification can be accomplished only through follow-up study. Clinical experience suggests that many children should be seen at least on two occasions. The interval between examinations varies according to the urgency of the problem, age of the child and other factors. However, three or not more than six month intervals seem most suitable for young children. In the interval between examinations it is helpful to have the parents make monthly reports in terms of specific aspects and expected development. For example, suggestions might include that they imitate the child's vocalizations and play with him auditorially in other ways. The parents then might report on the child's auditory responsiveness and development in other respects. Such reports are entered in the child's record for appraisal and evaluation according to the diagnosis which has been made. This information is especially useful when the child is seen again.

Another reason for seeing some children at least on two occasions is that in the interim information can be secured from other specialists. For example, the parents might be advised to consult a neurologist, psychiatrist, pediatrician or otolaryngologist and these findings should be available when the child is seen again. The case studies presented in this chapter illustrate the need for such cooperative effort and the value of the follow-up study. These cases also indicate the importance of caution and the need to evaluate the child as a total functioning organism rather than only in terms of his auditory acuity.

The following case studies have been selected chiefly on the basis of type of auditory disorder. Due to the research nature of the diagnostic center from which they were selected, some of these children have been seen periodically over a period of four years. Some have had extensive follow-up study in order to ascertain the validity of the diagnosis which had been made. The form of the case presentation is according to the three steps entailed in making a differential diagnosis as discussed throughout this manual; the history, behavioral symptomatology and test findings. The interdependence of these steps in the diagnostic process is emphasized. It should not be inferred that all children present the complexity of diagnostic involvements illustrated by these cases. Many children can be diagnosed with assurance of correctness without involved study and follow-up. These cases were selected partially because they revealed the many factors entailed in the diagnosis of auditory disorders in young children. The names used in the case studies are fictitious.

ILLUSTRATIVE CASES OF PERIPHERAL DEAFNESS

Case One

Billy was first seen by a pediatrician who requested further differential diagnosis of the auditory disorder. The pediatrician had found Billy to be in excellent health but he could not elicit response to sound. Billy was seen for further evaluation at the children's center for auditory disorders when he was eleven months of age. His case is presented because it illustrates how readily uncomplicated peripheral deafness can be diagnosed in some children at a very early age. Moreover, it illustrates the consistency of the history findings, the behavioral symptomatology and the test findings.

Summary of history data: Billy was the second of two pregnancies, his older sister being normal. His mother had peripheral deafness apparently congenital in nature. No other deafness had occurred in either of the parents' families. The pregnancy was uneventful and of nine months duration. Labor continued for ten hours and the birth weight was seven pounds and twelve ounces. Billy's development was excellent immediately following birth; he took nourishment well and regained his birth weight normally. He had not contracted any childhood illnesses. Genetic development was normal as he sat alone at seven months and walked at fourteen months. The parents reported good responsiveness to people, visual alertness and general contentedness. There was no history of unusual fretfulness, rocking, head banging or otherwise symptomatic behavior of emotional disturbance. Likewise, the parents reported good spontaneous integrative behavior in social situations and in play. The report of auditory responsiveness was simply that he had never been observed to respond to auditory stimulation. Vocalizations occurred but babbling and vocalizing for pleasure had not been observed.

Behavioral symptomatology: Billy was an attractive robust child. He pulled himself upright and walked slightly by holding onto a chair. He was alert and happy in general, showing vigorous likes and dislikes with shyness and apprehension of unfamiliar people and surroundings. He played well with toys but continuously gave up attention to objects for responsiveness to people. Laughing and smiling occurred appropriately and always in response to visual contact with others. The tonal quality of the laughter and of other vocalizations seemed suggestive of peripheral deafness but the heartiness of these expressions made interpretation difficult. Scanning visual behavior was frequent and accompanied both vibratory sensations and changes in the visual field. He showed no distractibility or disinhibition suggestive of perceptual disturbances but he occupied himself in a sustained manner and kept in close contact with his environment visually. He functioned integratively, using changes in his environment to appraise him of its satisfactoriness.

Test responses: Billy scored plus on all of the Cattell items below twelve months except those involving use of his voice and hearing. On the items from the Bayley schedule of motor development he scored between eleven and twelve months. On the Social Maturity Scale he earned a quotient of 89 with failures only in the communication area. His behavior and adjustment were considered excellent. On the sound instrument tests he responded only to very loud sounds (large cricket and clacker). These were interpreted as essentially responses at the threshold for feeling. In view of completely consistent findings from the history, behavioral symptomatology and tests a diagnosis of severe bilateral nerve deafness was made; the etiology was classified as presumptively endogenous. Billy is still under two years of age. A second evaluation revealed no new symptoms or additional evidence. Recommendations were made for training and management on the basis of peripheral deafness without complications. His progress has been excellent.

Comments on techniques and procedures used: This case illustrates the use of parental reports, other history data and behavioral symptomatology as corroborative evidence in the diagnosis. Moreover, it indicates the consistency of responses on all types of tests (mental, motor, social maturity and auditory) for children with peripheral deafness. All test data revealed integrity of the organism except for the sensory deprivation.

Case Two

John was brought to an otolaryngologist when he was eighteen months of age. He had been adopted at two months and his adoptive parents had been concerned about his hearing from the time he was six months of age because he did not awaken to noises when they entered his room. A pediatrician suggested the examination by an otolaryngologist who reported no apparent pathology of the ears but he requested a further study, especially a psychological evaluation, before making a diagnosis. Response to the tuning forks was suggestive of peripheral deafness but emotional involvements were suspected.

Summary of history data: Inasmuch as John was adopted, little information concerning the pregnancy and birth was available at the time of the first examination at the children's center for auditory disorders. Later the adoptive agency was requested to furnish this information. The natural mother was approximately thirty years and the father forty years of age. The mother had cataracts on both eyes and peripheral deafness reportedly due to scarlet fever at seven years of age. Delivery was by outlet forceps after eight and one half hours of labor. There were no complications and the delivering physician reported "a normal, healthy baby." John was a first born child and birth weight was six pounds and ten ounces. He has had no childhood illnesses. He sat alone at seven months and walked at fifteen months. The parents observed that his coordination was good. He was not a management problem but sometimes seemed somewhat unresponsive to them. His attention could be attracted by touching or by vibratory sensation. He used gestures such as pointing in attempts to make his wants known. He sobbed and shed tears when crying. He kept contact with his parents by looking into their faces. The parents had noticed no direct responses to sound but on occasion his behavior was confusing and suggested that he had heard environmental sounds other than speech. He made no attempts to imitate speech sounds. Vocalizations occurred frequently and were loud but were not for pleasure and were not used projectively to control others. Toilet training was progressing.

Behavioral symptomatology: John was a healthy appearing boy who engaged in activities readily but who was moderately passive toward those around him. He was not distractible or disinhibited. He walked with good coordination and his movements were intentional and purposeful. He used simple gestures which frequently were accompanied by vocalization. These vocalizations seemed to be beginning attempts to use his voice to attract those around him; they were not the vocalizations of pleasure associated with play. John used his vision for evaluating the social circumstances of his environment but this behavior seemed less obvious than is apparent in most children with peripheral deafness. It was apparent also that he was using tactile sensation as a warning sense in a compensatory manner. The tonal quality of his vocalizations was slightly suggestive of peripheral deafness but they were more varied in intensity and more continuous than expected. There was no use of speech, jargon or echolalia and no comprehension of speech could be observed. John was slightly passive in attitude and would sit, engrossing himself in an activity for longer periods than seemed desirable and these activities were somewhat stereotyped.

Test responses: John's genetic development and his observed motor behavior indicated normal motor capacity. He fell slightly below the 19 month level on the Bayley schedule of motor development. His performance on the Cattell Infant Scale was satisfactory and within the expected level with the exception of those items requiring normal auditory functioning. A social quotient of 80 (failure essentially on communication items) corroborated these findings of normal intelligence. His performance motorically and intellectually was indicative of peripheral deafness. Responses to the auditory tests were not conclusive. There was some inconsistency and some apparent willfulness in his lack of response and, moreover, it was difficult to elicit responses. However, there was evidence of hearing through use of the Sound Toy test, the Imitation of Vocalization or Voice tests. Responses were elicited by the sound instruments but there was no apparent reaction to sound-field tests, including pure tones. Although the history and behavioral symptomatology did not contradict a diagnosis of peripheral deafness, in view of the inconclusiveness of the auditory responses the diagnosis was deferred with a tentative classification of peripheral deafness with a superimposed involvement of mild emotional withdrawal. This examination, however, had clarified the clinical problem in certain respects. It was apparent that John's lack of speech and auditory disorder was not due to mental deficiency or aphasia because the history, behavioral symptomatology and test responses were consistent in revealing symbolic and integrative behavior within normal

limits. Therefore, the clinical problem which remained was to further evaluate the relationships between peripheral and psychic deafness. Recommendations to the parents included mainly suggestions
for development of spontaneity and use of sounds in a playful
manner.

John has been seen five times for further study over a period of
eighteen months; he is now three years of age. After the second
evaluation it became apparent that peripheral deafness was present
but emotional involvements continued to obscure this basic problem. When John was around two years of age the emotional
problem in the home was considerable; stereotyped motor activity
such as twirling and sleeplessness were common. Through the
assistance of the pediatrician and the otolaryngologist, an electroencephalographic study was made. This showed no abnormality
and no response to auditory stimulation. Psychogalvanic audiometry
also was attempted at this time. John's poor cooperation made
conditioning difficult but after repeated attempts it was concluded
that this method showed only slight ability to respond at maximum
levels of intensity. When John was between two and three years
of age the parents were counseled frequently regarding his training and management. They had a great deal of anxiety regarding
him and there were evidences that their attitudes were reflecting
to John. As he became better adjusted he responded more directly
and consistently to sound tests and manifested benefit from the
use of amplification in auditory training. It is now evident that he
has a moderately severe peripheral deafness (60 to 70 db on the
speech range). He has responded well to tutoring and has entered a
day school for the deaf.

Comments on techniques and procedures used: This case illustrates
the difficulty of ascertaining the relative influence of impaired
acuity and superimposed emotional factors. While impaired acuity
was present the extent was not as great as indicated by the electroencephalogram or psychogalvanic audiometry. Moreover, this case
reveals the increased difficulty of diagnosis when behavioral symptomatology is mixed. This boy's behavior included symptoms of

peripheral deafness and of emotional disturbance of the passive, withdrawal type. Final diagnosis could be made only through follow-up study and alleviation of the superimposed emotional factors.

ILLUSTRATIVE CASE OF RECEPTIVE APHASIA

Case Three

Ann was under the care of a pediatrician who requested a study and observation from the point of view of differential diagnosis. The pediatrician was primarily concerned about peripheral deafness but there were related problems of impaired vision with a possibility of mental deficiency. An otological examination had been performed and the otologist too was concerned about the multiple symptoms. Ann was first seen for further differential evaluation when she was three years and six months of age.

Summary of history data: Ann was the youngest of three children, the two older being normal in all respects. The parents were between thirty and thirty-five years of age, well educated and insightful. The mother had rubella during the first three months of pregnancy. Duration of pregnancy was nine months. False labor pains occurred a week before delivery but labor at the time of delivery was not unusual. Birth weight was five pounds and ten ounces and this weight was regained normally.

The parents reported that Ann was slower than their other children in genetic development. She sat alone at approximately eight months and walked at eighteen months. The parents were concerned about peripheral deafness and reported Ann's auditory responses as inconsistent but that she usually responded to sounds of moderate intensity. Often, however, when she was engrossed in an activity, she was inattentive even to loud sounds. Ann used only a few gestures which were highly concrete and she had no other expressive language. She vocalized rather freely in a jargon manner. Her inability to comprehend and her hyperactivity and randomness made home management difficult but bizarreness was not reported.

Behavioral symptomatology: Ann was an extremely distracted and disinhibited child. She continuously made attempts to relate to her environment but her distractibility precluded sustained attention at any time. She vocalized randomly but the tonal quality of these utterances was indefinite. She did not relate visually to adults present but she did not reject human contact and relationship. When demands were pressed her random motor behavior increased to the extent of requiring control and restraint. She did not cry but whined and showed otherwise poor emotional expression. No rocking, head banging or other indications of withdrawal were manifested. Her behavior was characterized by disinhibition and disintegration; she seemed typical of children who cannot organize sensations experientially because of perceptual disturbance. Her behavior was suggestive of central nervous system damage with aphasia.

Test responses: Ann's ability to cooperate with the examiner was very poor. She made fleeting attempts to give sustained attention but disinhibition and distractibility interfered. However, through restraint and intensive structuring of the testing situation (reducing incoming stimuli as much as possible to those of the specifically immediate situation), the Binet Formboard was administered. Ann completed this test successfully at the two year level and showed some ability at the three and one half year level. She could not do geometric design drawing at this time.

Sound-field amplified tests, sound instruments, sound toy tests, imitation of vocalizations and voice tests were used to evaluate auditory capacity. Ann's disinhibition made interpretation difficult but because her responses seemed to fall at the conversational level of intensity and because of the behavioral symptomatology, it was concluded that she probably had adequate acuity for hearing speech. The language evaluation revealed a deficiency of inner language considerably greater than could be attributed to peripheral deafness alone. The Social Maturity evaluation revealed a social age of two years and five months; a retardation of one year and seven months. Analysis of her social competence showed failure mainly in the areas of communication and motor function. In view of her total problem the social score was considered inferentially to indicate potential within normal limits. The tentative diagnosis included that the lack of speech could not be attributed to mental deficiency, peripheral deafness or psychic deafness; a classification was made of receptive aphasia with the possibility of a mild peripheral loss of auditory acuity superimposed; etiology was considered to be rubella. Recommendations were made for speech and language training and for re-evaluations to be made periodically.

Ann is now seven and one half years of age. She has been intensively re-evaluated once a year during the past four years. She has continued under the care of a pediatrician with occasional assistance from other specialists, but the principal program has been one of language training. This training was done originally by a private tutor but during the past two years Ann also has been attending a private day school. Her progress has been good. Only the most recent test results will be given.

Manikin	5 years
Kohs	5 years
Geometric designs	6 years
Draw a man	7 years
Hiskey block patterns	$7\frac{1}{2}$ years

Auditory comprehension continues to be the most difficult problem and the symbolic nature of this problem is obvious. The symbolic disorder is limited to aphasia because reading and writing are progressing satisfactorily. Ann prefers sounds to be louder than average which is not uncommon in these children. Informal auditory testing does not preclude a mild impairment of auditory acuity. Ann continues to be unable to structure the auditory field sufficiently to respond to standard pure tone audiometry. Her speech development expressively has been good. She has no difficulty making herself understood although articulation is not average for her age. Interestingly Ann also continues to show poor responses auditorially when she is preoccupied or otherwise does not expect sounds. This is rather typical in such children and manifests difficulty in combining the visual and auditory processes in a supplementary manner. Piaget found these processes to be combined by the third month in normal children. Such integration seems much delayed in some aphasic children. Ann's responsiveness and behavior manifest better auditory acuity than she can use readily when the auditory field is not structured. It is apparent that her basic difficulty is a combination of receptive aphasia and auditory perceptual disturbance. This has been revealed further by the use of amplification which does not benefit her except through providing a more structured auditory field. This seems to be the basis for her preference of having sounds louder, especially if the situation is somewhat perplexing and complex. Her motor coordination is improved but scores on motor tests cluster around five years. Social maturity falls at the six and one half year level. Prognosis for eventual adjustment is good.

Comments on techniques and procedures used: This case illustrates one of the most difficult problems of differential diagnosis between peripheral deafness, receptive aphasia and mental deficiency. The original presumptions included both peripheral deafness and mental deficiency. Literal quantitative interpretation of mental and formal auditory tests would have resulted in a diagnosis of mental deficiency with peripheral deafness. The history data and behavioral symptomatology, however, did not corroborate such a diagnosis. Furthermore, the informal auditory tests revealed substantial capacity to hear and were in disagreement with a diagnosis of moderate or severe peripheral deafness. It seems possible that a number of children like Ann are classified for training in schools for the deaf or for the mentally deficient. Although such classifications might not be harmful in some instances, it is becoming increasingly clear that aphasic children require a program that differs widely from that ordinarily provided for children with peripheral deafness or mental deficiency.

This case illustrates another experiential observation which has been gained from training aphasic children. This observation is that unless substantial recovery and progress has occurred by seven years of age, the prognosis is less favorable. Apparently spontaneous recovery and development is less likely to exceed normal maturational progress after seven years. The rate of development seems to be more stabilized after this time and the mental age can be taken as more indicative of the child's actual potential.

ILLUSTRATIVE CASE OF PREDOMINANTLY EXPRESSIVE APHASIA

Case Four

Bobby was first seen by an otolaryngologist when he was two years of age. The parents were concerned about his lack of speech. The otolaryngologist found infected tonsils and an adenoid mass causing a postnasal obstruction. He concluded further that the child could hear noises but not conversation. The diagnosis given was deafness due to recurrent respiratory infections. A tonsillectomy and adenoidectomy was performed two months later. Approximately six months after this the otolaryngologist requested further evaluation because speech development continued to be seriously retarded.

Summary of history data: Bobby was seen at the center for auditory disorders in children when he was two years and ten months of age. His parents were professional people with deep concern about him but without handicapping anxiety. Bobby was the fourth pregnancy; the siblings were without defects. The parents stated frankly that although Bobby had no speech, they were confident that he had a great deal of hearing and doubted that his lack of speech could be attributed to peripheral deafness. The pregnancy was uneventful and of nine months duration. Labor was precipitous, being of only two hours duration. There was no evidence of injury at the time of birth. Birth weight was six pounds and there was no difficulty in swallowing or feeding immediately after birth. The illness history was negative. Bobby sat alone at eight months and walked at fourteen months. He was retarded in feeding and in acquiring toilet habits as compared to his siblings. He had a preference for the right hand and the parents had not observed unusual awkwardness or incoordination motorically. They reported that he had always been responsive to people, was playful and in general was a happy contented boy. The history of auditory behavior revealed responses to many environmental sounds including speech. He did not babble and only rarely produced meaningful sounds in play, such as "choo-choo" while engaged with a toy train. Moreover, he used very few gestures and these had occurred only recently. He used vocalizations projectively. Interestingly in view of the previous diagnosis of peripheral deafness, he comprehended speech rather readily. He made no attempts to imitate speech but used "mom" to refer to many objects and wants. He was not echolalic and used no jargon. He was expressive in laughing, crying and smiling and these expressions manifested good emotional tone.

Behavioral symptomatology: Bobby was a friendly boy who presented no unusual behavior symptoms with the exception of his lack of verbal ability. He was normally shy, inhibited, playful and manifested good relationship to his environment. He responded to simple verbal commands and engaged himself integratively and imaginatively with toys, crayons and other objects. His behavior was unlike that of children with peripheral or psychic deafness and was not typical of receptive aphasics or the mentally deficient. The clinical impression was distinctly one of predominantly expressive aphasia.

Test responses: Bobby's chronological age was thirty-four months and his performance on the Cattell ranged from twenty-seven to thirty months, while on the block building test from the Ontario he fell at three years. His performance was well integrated except for the geometric designs on which he fell at eighteen months. His score and behavior on this test suggested a visual perceptual disturbance which was not apparent behaviorally but became evident in the test situation. Such findings are not uncommon in children with expressive aphasia. The mental test findings indicated intelligence falling within normal limits with a perceptual disturbance in the visual area. The Social Maturity evaluation corroborated the mental test findings; his social quotient was 92 with failures limited to items involving verbalization. Bobby's motor ability fell at thirty months but his grasping ability was noticeably inferior. However, general coordination seemed unaffected. He performed excellently on the Object Language Test indicating intact inner speech and good receptive language capacity. All auditory tests corroborated the language and speech tests. He not only heard well but interpreted symbolically and integrated auditory experience in a satisfactory manner. His only deficiency was in speech; he could not imitate even simple vocalizations when they were given through the auditory area alone. When he was permitted to observe the examiner in a mirror, he could imitate some sounds such as "mum-mum" and when vision and hearing were used intensely and simultaneously some imitation was possible. The history data, the behavioral symptomatology and the test findings were reciprocally corroborative; therefore, a diagnosis was made of aphasia, predominantly expressive. The most probable etiology was determined to be injury at the time of birth due to precipitous delivery. Recommendations were made for immediate training and such training has been in progress for six months. The eventual outcome in terms of verbal language is not known but adjustment and progress are good. Receptive language is judged to be normal.

Comments on techniques and procedures used: This case is presented to illustrate errors in diagnosis which result chiefly from undue reliance on the assumption that lack of speech can be directly attributed to peripheral deafness. The parental report and the child's auditory response to speech and other sounds were minimized by the otolaryngologist because of this traditional assumption. This case, moreover, illustrates the characteristic behavioral differences between expressive and receptive aphasics; the expressives are well preserved organismically. The use of speech comprehension as the primary means for evaluating auditory capacity is common in such children. When speech is comprehended (evaluated systematically through the Object Language Test) at conversational level, the lack of speech cannot be attributed to deficiencies in acuity. This case seems to have intact receptive functioning; such wide discrepancies between receptive and expressive language functions is not uncommon in young aphasic children. Intensive neurological study has not been accomplished at this time but such findings sometimes are negative on this type of child.

ILLUSTRATIVE CASES OF PSYCHIC DEAFNESS

Case Five

Parents' report of the problem: Paul was first seen for a differential diagnosis when he was two years and ten months of age. However, his father is a physician and some diagnostic work had been achieved prior to this time. Paul had been enrolled in a nursery school program for children with peripheral deafness. The teacher suspected that his problem was not simple peripheral deafness and advised the parents to proceed with additional diagnostic work. The problem as described by the teacher and Paul's parents was that he seemed so immature. He had not responded to toilet training. The teacher's report included, "Paul does not pay attention to anyone; he usually sits in the doorway and rocks himself. He plays with his own hands or his shadow on the wall. He glances at the toys I give him but he will not play with them. He has an obsession to put his fingers into small holes in the wall, in the corner or any crack he can find." The parents reported that Paul would not look at them and that they could not play with him or get him to relate to them in other ways.

Summary of history data: Paul was a full term infant with an uneventful birth. He was a healthy child in all respects. There was no evidence of injury at birth. The genetic history too suggested normal integrity and potential. He sat alone at six months of age and walked alone at fifteen months. He has been oblivious to his environment from very early life. Due to the father being in military service the home lacked stability during Paul's first year of life.

The parents stated that he was not picked up and fondled but that he was handled only when his care required it. He seemed not to hear, never responding directly to sound. He has never spoken and he vocalizes only rarely and without intent to attract attention. He is not distractible or disinhibited. He has always been bizarre; engaging in stereotyped activities such as clinging to an object, refusing to relinquish it even while eating.

Behavioral symptomatology: Paul engaged in rocking behavior almost continuously. Whether seated on the examiner's lap or on a small chair, he kept rocking himself from side to side throwing his head vigorously. While seated at a table he began kicking, hitting the calves of his legs against the table. While it was apparent that this activity was moderately painful and not a play activity, Paul showed no awareness of pain. He was continuously abstracted and oblivious, being pre-occupied at various times in putting his fingers into a tear in a ball or putting blocks and other toys into his mouth. At no time did he relate to or directly show awareness of the persons present. He ignored his parents and his teacher as well as the examiner. Inner speech seemed well developed. At times without provocation he would raise his arms indicating he wished to be carried, or he would take the hand of an adult and lead him to the door. This behavior was deliberate but without showing emotional contact with others and without looking at them or regarding them in the usual manner. He did not gesture and vocalization was essentially lacking. There was no smiling, laughing or crying. He made no attempt to compensate for inability to hear. Direct social perceptual awareness was lacking. Use of his hands, his gait and other motor functioning did not suggest problems of incoordination. However, his motor activities like his other activities were at times unusual. At no time did his behavior suggest simple peripheral deafness.

Test responses: The parents had become concerned about Paul's unusualness when he was between eight and ten months of age. They suspected that his problem was peripheral deafness. When he was eleven months of age he was examined by various specialists.

An electroencephalogram was made at this time and the report of this test stated, "The electroencephalogram was normal. Paul appeared to respond to sounds at the estimated level of 80 decibels." On the basis of the electroencephalogram and formal auditory tests, some diagnosticians concluded that Paul was a child with peripheral deafness without complicating factors.

The parents then proceeded to get training for Paul on the basis of peripheral deafness. This training continued intermittently until he was seen for differential diagnosis at the age of two years and ten months. Informal auditory tests revealed considerable ability to hear. Ability to cooperate was lacking and responses were mainly indirect. He was given the single bell to play with and he immediately put it into his mouth. It was taken from him and jingled in a playful manner. He became distressed and tried to retrieve it. The examiner walked away, putting the bell into his pocket without allowing Paul to see what he was doing. The examiner, after changing his position and out of Paul's line of vision, jingled the bell while it was still in his pocket. The level of intensity was very mild. As this process was repeated a few times, Paul left his chair, went to the examiner and located the bell. At no time had he seen associated movements. It must be emphasized that Paul did not show awareness of the examiner as a person during this testing. When he was not given the bell he again became distressed in a whining manner. On the basis of this and other similar responses, and on the basis of history and behavioral symptomatology it was suggested that Paul should not be considered as peripherally deaf. Rather, a program for a severely emotionally disturbed child was suggested. On the basis of his normal genetic development motorically, his inner language and complex behavioral functioning, he was not considered mentally deficient. Recommendations for management were given to the parents and to the teacher. It was suggested that Paul should be seen again in three to six months.

In view of the conflicting diagnoses regarding Paul, the parents found it difficult not to think of him as having peripheral deafness. As a result they did not return for further appraisal until ten months later. Paul was then three years and eight months of age. He had been trained as a peripherally deaf child during the interim. He was becoming increasingly difficult to manage in the home and he had shown no response to his school training; he did not respond to auditory or tactual training and he showed no response to speech reading instruction. The examination revealed findings consistent with those of the examination done ten months previously. Various indirect responses to sounds, including conversational speech, could be elicited. The behavioral symptomatology was now entirely suggestive of childhood schizophrenia. Increased bizarreness was obvious.

Due to the severity of Paul's problem and because the nursery school no longer found it possible to manage him, it was suggested that the parents bring Paul to the children's center for diagnostic training regularly. He was worked with for a period of two hours twice a week for the ensuing year. During this time psychotherapeutic procedures only were used and the parents were counseled regularly. It was possible to demonstrate conclusively that Paul's hearing was entirely adequate for purposes of hearing speech. Frequent indirect responses included manifestations of some comprehension of speech. The psychiatrist who had previously considered the problem to be peripheral deafness or brain injury now concurred on a diagnosis of childhood schizophrenia.

After a year of this type of therapy it seemed that Paul could be worked with more intensively. Residential psychiatric treatment was suggested. Such treatment has been in progress for approximately one year. Paul is now almost six years of age. His marked emotional disturbance is still apparent but noteworthy progress has been made. He does not speak but he responds auditorially in many situations. He relates to the therapist and to other children with increasing success. What his eventual adjustment will be is not known.

Comments on techniques and procedures used: It is apparent that the diagnosis of peripheral deafness made at eleven months of age was in error. This suggests that the validity of the electroencephalographic method of hearing testing should be questioned. Further-more, it is apparent that all tests, and especially formal tests, cannot be interpreted literally. They should be validated by history in-formation and by behavioral symptomatology. Another observation which seems pertinent is that when behavior is bizarre it is an un-warranted over-simplification to classify the child as simply having peripheral deafness. Even if such deafness is present the child's needs cannot be adequately met on this basis. The question of audi-tory acuity should be left open until psychiatric and psychological aspects have been clarified.

Case Six

Henry was first seen for differential diagnosis when he was four years and six months of age. He was referred for further study of his auditory disorder by an otolaryngologist. This specialist had seen Henry over a period of approximately one year and had secured examinations from several other specialists. For example, he had requested that a psychogalvanic audiometric study be made. This study indicated "a bilateral nerve type of impairment" with losses for the speech frequencies ranging from 60 to 100 decibels. A diagnosis of peripheral deafness was made and a school for the deaf was recommended.

Henry was entered in a school for the deaf and remained there for a period of one year. During this time he was studied by the staff of the school. The psychologist found his functional mental level to be "below two years." Evaluation of his auditory capacities by sound-field tests, informal sound toy tests and speech tests re-vealed that he had sufficient hearing for the development of speech. The principal of the school for the deaf recommended that he not be continued with children who had peripheral deafness inasmuch as his hearing was normal and he had not profited substantially from a year of such training.

Henry was then examined by a neurologist who found "no evi-dence of neurological disorder." Two electroencephalograms and one pneumoencephalogram had been done with consistently negative results. The otolaryngologist then suggested further evaluation of Henry's lack of awareness and other unusual symptoms.

Summary of history data: Henry is the youngest of three children. The mother's pregnancy proceeded normally without illnesses or other complications. Delivery was by forceps but there was no evidence of injury at the time of birth. Henry has had no childhood diseases but between one and two years of age he had several attacks of otitis media. During this time head banging also occurred. Sitting and walking were only slightly retarded. Toilet training was not established. The parents reported that Henry sometimes behaved as though he had understood what was said but he did not respond directly to any sounds and that he had never used verbal language. However, he occasionally hummed short melodies in an inadvertent manner. He had not used his hearing projectively. He had been oblivious to his environment in general but frequently took the hand of a parent and tried to use it as though it were a tool. He had not made face to face contact with parents except on occasions when he seemed to be defying them provocatively. "Teasing" and other willfully provocative behavior had been common. The parents stated frankly that their original concern had been in terms of hearing and language development but that they now realized that this was only part of a more generalized problem.

Behavioral symptomatology: Henry is an attractive boy who is physically well developed and appears in excellent health. He is withdrawn, preoccupied and generally out of contact with his environment. However, he gives definite evidence of being superficially aware of people and happenings in his environment. He is not completely oblivious. He refuses eye and face to face contact except when he is momentarily provocative. For example, when asked to give a ball to the examiner, he threw the ball to the floor and fleetingly looked at the examiner in a mischievously defying manner. He roamed around the examining room without apparent intent or purpose but with well executed motor movements. His movements were occasionally accompanied by spontaneous vocalizations which were acoustically normal in quality. He showed resistance at times but he did not laugh, cry or smile; social responses were extremely rare and when they occurred they were momentary and superficial. He did not manifest hyperdistractibility or hyperactivity. On the contrary his general behavior showed good perceptual competence. He revealed no compensatory behavior by undue use of vision or tactile sensations. His behavior was characterized by detachment, phantasy activity and withdrawal.

Test responses: Because of Henry's inability to relate to the examiner and to formal test situations, only informal procedures were used. He responded well to these tests. His movements, manipulation of objects and other random activity ceased consistently when sounds were produced at very mild intensities by the sound instruments. He responded similarly to the sound toy test. Furthermore, some comprehension of speech was readily established. For example, as he engaged in stereotyped manipulation of toys, the examiner said "no" in a soft whisper and each time Henry interrupted his activity. Other indirect but definite responses were elicited to such statements as "where's Mommy," "show me the ball" and "sit down." The only psychological tests which could be applied were those involving blocks and formboards and these could not be given in a standard manner. However, on the basis of his genetic development, the complexity of his behavior and his general excellence of perceptual and motor functioning, a diagnosis of mental deficiency seemed unwarranted. His social competence as measured by the Social Maturity Scale was two years. In view of the history information, the behavioral symptomatology and the test responses Henry was diagnosed as severely emotionally disturbed with symptomatology most like that of infantile autism. Hearing acuity was concluded to be entirely adequate for hearing conversational speech and his poor use of his hearing was considered consistent with the total syndrome which he presented. Residential psychiatric treatment was recommended and Henry now has been under such treatment for 18 months. The attending psychiatrist reports considerable improvement in general behavior. Henry consistently understands simple spoken commands and integrity of auditory capacities is no longer questioned. Furthermore, words are spoken occasionally and this speech is well articulated and excellent in tonal quality; like other children of this type, his speech seems unduly precise. The prognosis is guarded; improvement in emotional adjustment is anticipated but the eventual outcome can be determined only by further treatment and observation.

Comments on techniques and procedures used: As suggested in the comments of the procedures used with case five, all tests of auditory capacity should be validated by the history information and by the total syndrome presented by the child. This case emphasizes the importance of caution in interpreting psychogalvanic audiometric responses literally. It also illustrates the need for psychological and psychiatric evaluation of some children. Furthermore, this case is characteristic of children with psychic deafness of this type who are entered in schools for the deaf and his lack of benefit from such training is typical. Only through deliberate, painstaking effort and cooperation between specialists can a differential diagnosis be accomplished before such erroneous placement is made and before further damage to the child occurs.

ILLUSTRATIVE CASE OF MENTAL DEFICIENCY

Case Seven

David was first seen for evaluation of his auditory capacity when he was three years and one month of age. His parents, who had a background of college education, requested the evaluation because they wanted to know "the reason for his not talking and if there were a loss of hearing." David had presented many health and management problems so much diagnostic work had been achieved prior to the examination of auditory capacity.

Summary of history data: Pregnancy was normal but of nine and one-half months duration. Delivery was considered normal but labor was difficult and only of two and one-half hours duration. Birth weight was seven pounds and the initial weight was regained satisfactorily. However, due to blueness x-rays were made on the fourth day of life; these showed no defects in the lungs or throat. Colds, respiratory infection and bronchitis have been recurrent from the age of six months. The first convulsion occurred at six months of age and these have recurred at intervals of several weeks to several months. David has received constant medication including thyroid and drug therapy. He was retarded in all aspects of genetic development. He sat alone at one year and walked at nineteen months. The parents have observed marked clumsiness and poor balance. He has shown no response to toilet training. At two years of age the beginning of speech imitation was observed in such vocalizations as da-da and ma-ma. Vocalizations were deficient prior to two years and babbling was not observed until approximately eighteen months. Self help in eating and dressing were substantially retarded. David was attending a guidance center nursery school for brief periods during the afternoon where the approach was to help children overcome emotional factors which might be inhibiting his speech. The parents reported responses to sounds but these were limited largely to highly specific situations. For example, he sometimes gave evidence of hearing the telephone but other louder sounds might be ignored. Some response to vocalizations were noted but he showed no comprehension of speech. He was aware of people; looked at them but showed little awareness of social situations. He cried and shed tears but emotional expression was not strong; he was distractible to the extent that this was a major complaint of the parents.

Behavioral symptomatology: David's behavior deviated significantly in several respects. Social awareness was highly deficient but it was not obliviousness of the type seen in many children with psychic deafness. Random, aimless motor movements were common and these showed gross incoordination. In general his behavior was characterized by immaturity and retardation. He seemed perceptually disturbed both visually and auditorially because of unusual distractibility in both areas but his explorative attempts to relate to his environment were grossly deficient. Compensatory use of vision or other senses was not apparent. Negativism, whining and fretting occurred frequently and indicated general organismic incapacity to relate to the situation. He made no attempts to use speech or gesture, but he vocalized and the tonal quality of these vocalizations did not suggest an inability to monitor auditorially. The behavioral syndrome was one of generalized retardation and in contrast to that characteristically observed in children with peripheral or psychic deafness, or with aphasia.

Test responses: Due to David's immaturity and distractibility the application of standard tests was difficult. However, after several attempts he completed the Binet Formboard forward but failed it reversed. Other mental tests which were attempted included the geometric designs, block building and items from the Cattell. His responses indicated a functional mental level of twelve to fourteen months (C. A. thirty-seven months). Perceptual deficiencies were indicated but structuring of the task did not improve the performance. It was concluded that intellectual development was seriously retarded. This was substantiated in various ways by the Social Maturity evaluation because his social quotient was 55 with failure on items in all areas. Motor functioning was at the thirteen month level on the Bayley schedule of motor development. Auditory capacity was evaluated by amplified sound-field tests, sound instruments, speech, voice and imitation of vocalization tests. Response to pure tone sound-field tests was inconsistent and erratic. No response was made to speech, to gesture or to speech and gesture used simultaneously. He imitated simple vocalizations given at mild intensities and responded to sounds from the sound instruments at the conversational level of intensity. The history, behavioral symptomatology and test responses indicated that the basic problem was mental deficiency and that this was the cause of his lack of speech. David was diagnosed as mentally deficient and tentatively classified as imbecile level; his auditory acuity was considered normal and aphasia was judged not to be present because there was no discrepancy between language level and intellectual capacity.

The most probable etiology was determined as anoxia due to damage sustained at birth. Recommendations emphasized the need for training and management as a mentally retarded child, not as a child with emotional disturbance, peripheral deafness or aphasia. The importance of continued medication for seizure control was stressed and a neurological examination was suggested. Several electroencephalograms now have been performed with inconsistent results but with indications of diffuse brain injury.

David was seen again when he was four years and eight months of age; one year and seven months after the initial examination. His seizures were under control by drug therapy. Both comprehension and use of speech revealed intact auditory acuity. He understood simple spoken language and used a few words symbolically and appropriately. This was in agreement with the findings of mental tests which placed his level of intelligence at two years with an intelligence quotient of 44; the social quotient was 49. He was using language at the expected level in view of his mental age. Motor incoordination was obvious with poor grasp, poor gait and general awkwardness being evident. David is attending a day school for retarded children and making progress in accordance with expectations. His rate of mental growth seems stabilized although perceptual involvements continue to be apparent. He has made between one-third and one-half of normal progress in mental growth which indicates that his mental level at maturity probably will not exceed seven years, the highest level of imbecility.

Comments on techniques and procedures used: This case illustrates the importance of mental level in the evaluation of language and auditory capacities. The principle problem from the point of view of differential diagnosis was to ascertain whether peripheral deafness or aphasia were present because psychic deafness was not presumed despite the emphasis on emotional involvements when he was first seen. The history immediately suggested mental deficiency because of the generalized retardation. Behavioral symptomatology and test findings were in agreement with this suggestion. Formal tests of auditory acuity can be used with confidence only rarely with these children. All auditory tests require corroboration from the history, the behavioral syndrome and the psychological, social maturity, motor and language test results.

ILLUSTRATIVE CASE OF AUDITORY AGNOSIA

Case Eight

Jan was first studied from the point of view of differential diagnosis when she was five years and four months of age. Prior to this she had been under the care of an otologist who reported that his audiometric and tuning fork tests were inconsistent and inconclusive. He stated further that he could not corroborate the parents' report that Jan heard faint sounds at times. Jan now has been studied over a period of four years and the findings are extensive. Only a brief resume of these and her progress can be given.

Summary of history data: The pregnancy was uneventful except for a flow of blood during the fifth month. Duration of labor was long, thirty-two hours. Forceps were not used; no injury was noted at the time of delivery. Birth weight was five pounds and seven ounces. The illness history was negative. Jan was retarded in holding her head erect, in sitting and in walking; she sat alone at eight months and walked at seventeen months. The parents began seeking assistance at eighteen months because they were concerned about the lack of speech. They reported that Jan seemed to hear sounds of a door being closed, the snap of fingers, but at times she did not respond to any sounds, even those that were very loud. She used gestures with considerable adequacy. She was not difficult to manage in the home; she ate and slept well. She vocalized a great deal but they were without meaning and occurred only in a random manner. She did not use hearing or vocalizations projectively and her vocalizations were not used for pleasure in association with specific activities. She was responsive to people and enjoyed contact with them. However, mild disinhibition and distractibility prevented such contacts from being satisfactory. Her balance had been poor and she had seemed awkward and incoordinated. Improvement had been noted in this respect.

Behavioral symptomatology: Jan was highly distractible, disinhibited and perseverative. She gave only momentary attention to objects or people. She vocalized in an inadvertent, compulsive manner almost continuously. These vocalizations were unlike those of children with peripheral deafness in tonal quality, lack of purpose and other psychological aspects. She was hyperactive and her movements too were essentially without purpose except as she revealed an awareness of the environment and attempts to control it. The motor movements were not well executed; awkwardness, stumbling and poor coordination were apparent. She used gestures with good symbolic content but in a disintegrated manner. She seemed to function on a visual basis and some compensatory use of vision was noted. No use of hearing could be observed. Social perception was unusually good when attention could be sustained. Laughter occurred and it was appropriately used but not frequent and it did not reveal psychological integrity. At this time the vocalizations and laughter seemed different from the normal. There was a distinct lack of inflection, marked disturbances of pitch, suggesting an inability to monitor auditorially, but the vocal quality in general seemed different from that resulting from peripheral deafness.

Test responses: It was possible to administer several types of tests to Jan because she was amenable despite her limited ability to attend. Her attempts at drawing a circle, cross and square were unsuccessful although she drew circles which were poor in quality and size. She seemed unable to structure these tasks perceptually. She responded to gestures and seemed to comprehend but could not perform on mental tests above the two year level. It was evident clinically that intellectual capacity was above this level. This was verified by a social maturity quotient of 80 and a social age of four years; one year and four months retarded. Performance on motor tests was markedly inferior. She failed the test of standing on one foot, could not walk with one foot on the rail and showed awkwardness of gait, grasp and grip. Her motor performance in general fell at the two to two and one half year level. The suggestion of her motor involvements was that they were central in origin; they did not seem typical of the motor problems associated with vestibular destruction alone. Jan gave no responses to pure tone tests through

formal audiometry or through amplified sound-field tests. Her responses to sound instruments and sound toys were unusual and provocative. She responded to the discontinuance of the sound much
more readily than to its initial presentation. In other words, when
the examiner ceased producing the sound, she engaged in scanning
behavior in an attempt to ascertain what had been occurring in
the environment. She gave similar responses to the vocalization test;
when the examiner ceased his vocalizing, she with some consistency
made cessation of activity and scanning responses. Furthermore, she
gave a few mildly imitative responses to the vocalization of mmm-
mmm. On the basis of the history, the behavioral symptomatology
and the test responses, it was concluded that despite Jan's inability
to perform on pure tone tests, she could not be considered as a child
with peripheral deafness. Moreover, she was not considered characteristic of children with psychic deafness and although intellectual
capacity was questioned, she did not seem to be mentally deficient.
It was concluded that a tentative diagnosis of mixed expressive-receptive aphasia should be made. Further study revealed the essential
error in this classification because as Jan developed and follow-up
examinations were made, the more extensive nature of her central
auditory disorder became apparent.

Jan has been re-examined at approximately six month intervals.
The parents were given suggestions for training and management
and became competent observers of auditory behavior, furnishing
excellent data to be used with each succeeding examination. After
the second examination it became more apparent that Jan was
capable of much more hearing from the point of view of acuity
than she ordinarily manifested and after the third contact she was
tentatively classified as an auditory agnosia. Referral was made to
a neurologist who made a diagnosis of "cerebral dysrhythmia" and
prescribed drug therapy which had immediate beneficial effects
in Jan's attention and general behavior. The neurologist continued
his study of Jan and performed an electroencephalogram which was
negative. He has not changed his diagnosis after several examinations but indicated that the speech and hearing deficiency was due

to an aphasia although no response to sound was noticed during the electroencephalogram.

When Jan was approximately six and one half years of age it was recommended that she enter a day class for children with peripheral deafness. This recommendation was an admitted compromise in an attempt to procure the most suitable type of instruction available. However, because prognosis for development of auditory comprehension in agnosics seems to be poor, classifiying these children with those who are peripherally deaf may not be a seriously limiting factor in their development. Frequent reports have been received from Jan's teacher and these too have been useful in clarifying the nature of her auditory disorder. Jan continued to make progress in all respects with the exception of auditory comprehension. For example, one of the re-examinations occurred when she was seven years and four months of age and after she had been attending school for one year. She was markedly improved in visual perceptual functioning as illustrated by a score of nine years on the Healy Picture Completion I without assistance in structuring the task. Rare, intermittent responses were made to pure tones of high intensity. Responses to sound instruments were definite and it was apparent that marked impairment of auditory acuity could not be present. Motor coordination remained inferior but noticeable improvement was present. Gesticulation was highly symbolic expressively and was accompanied by meaningless vocalizations. She had no speech and no comprehension of speech. In this respect she differed significantly from children with peripheral deafness. Jan showed no benefit from training in speech reading or speech; her symbolic capacity receptively seemed to be limited to comprehending the gestures of others.

Jan is now nine years and seven months of age and she has been under intensive study for four years. She has continued schooling in the class for children with peripheral deafness for three years. At a recent examination (C.A. nine yrs. one mo.) her score on the Draw a Man Test was seven years and nine months, IQ 85; her score on the Kohs Block Design was eight years; the score on the

Healy Picture Completion I was between eleven and twelve years. Her behavior was much more integrated and she was capable of good cooperative effort. However, she gave no responses to formal audiometry at maximum intensity. In view of her inability in this respect, her sustained ability to cooperate and her age, psychogalvanic audiometry was attempted. Her responses indicated normal hearing on the speech range. Motor abilities were improved. Her social quotient was 86. In view of the total findings the diagnosis of auditory agnosia, made on the third contact, seems to have been sustained. Jan has hearing but she cannot interpret any sound.

Comments on techniques and procedures used: This case illustrates one of the complex problems of differential diagnosis of auditory disorders in young children. Clinical experience suggests that this type of auditory problem may be seen with some frequency in cerebral palsied children. This case suggests the importance of the nature of the sound used for testing and the inadequacy of the concept of intensity alone as a measure of auditory capacities in children. Moreover, inasmuch as response to psychogalvanic audiometry indicated acuity within normal limits, it raises the question of interpretation of these results. Presence of normal responses on this test does not necessarily mean normal integrity of auditory function. Experience suggests that this case will not be able to profit from such ability to respond auditorially. This does not minimize the importance of the differential diagnosis between peripheral deafness and auditory agnosia. Agnosic children are brain injured and should be trained differently according to the nature of their specific learning problems, which are more extensive than those of children with peripheral deafness. Experience with this case and a few others similar to her, suggests that the prognosis is poor for development of auditory comprehension in these children.

Chapter XIV

Summary and Recommendations for Training

THIS MANUAL IS A DISCUSSION OF THE DIAG-
nostic process entailed in making a differential diagnosis of auditory
disorders in infants and young children. The procedures which have
been discussed include three basic steps: taking a differential history, observing the behavioral symptomatology and administering
suitable tests. These procedures are based on the assumption that
auditory disorders occur on varying etiological bases and etiology
causes specific and systematic changes in organismic adjustment.
After the specialist recognizes the organismic adjustment which
accompanies the primary types of auditory disorders he hypothesizes the diagnostic classification of each child and proceeds to
determine whether the hypothesis can be substantiated. Complete
substantiation includes consistent patterns of results from the history, behavioral symptomatology and test findings. A brief resume
of these patterns is given in table 23. This resume is intended to
serve as a guide only because a differential diagnosis cannot be
made except after intensive study of every individual child.

Inasmuch as the nature of the auditory disorder in each of the
groups of peripheral deafness, aphasia, psychic deafness and mental
deficiency is widely different, their needs, too, are basically different. Therefore, recommendations for training, to be most effective, must be based on the total nature of the disorder, not only on
the lack of response to sound. For example, although children with
psychic deafness may overtly manifest little response to sound, to
recommend the use of a hearing aid is to misconceive the child's
problem and oversimplify his needs. It is not the purpose of this
manual to include a discussion of the training needs of children
having auditory disorders. However, a brief general guide indicat-

ing the type of recommendations made for each group is given in this chapter.

A general recommendation for all groups includes the management of the parents. All specialists have responsibility for reducing parental anxieties. Encouragement can be given to all parents irrespective of the nature of their child's problem. This is done by assisting them to feel less blameful, giving them assurance that they can cope with their child's handicap, that there are individuals, schools and agencies available that can help them with various aspects of the problem. Furthermore, there is an apparent relationship between established etiology and acceptance of the problem on the part of the parent. Whenever possible the cause should be ascertained and then discussed with the parent in a friendly, objective manner. This is an important factor in fostering parental acceptance and preventing prolonged searching for a more favorable diagnosis. Moreover, placing undue responsibility on the parent for doing specialized training with their child seems unwise. Many parents become unusually zealous in their training attempts, apparently, because they find it difficult to accept the child's problem, and their training becomes an effort to eliminate the problem rather than helping the child to learn to live with it. Parents should be encouraged to participate in the training program but this participation should emphasize the child's total problem, including his unusual needs for affection and acceptance.

RECOMMENDATIONS FOR CHILDREN WITH PERIPHERAL DEAFNESS

Even if the child has profound peripheral deafness the parents should be informed that their child can be taught to speak. This may be done chiefly by the visual-tactile method, or through the use of hearing aids if residual capacity to hear is sufficient. The opportune time for beginning any training depends on the child's total involvements and capacities. Parental guidance should be given immediately at the time of the diagnosis. Specific training measures

Table 23. — *The Characteristic Performance of Each Type on the Areas Evaluated in Making a Differential Diagnosis*

Type of disorder	History	Behavioral symptomatology	Test findings					
			Auditory responses	Mental capacity	Social maturity	Motor capacity	Language functioning	Emotional adjustment
Peripheral Deafness	Indicates alertness in general and often consistent response to loud sounds. Not bizarre or seriously retarded genetically	Not bizarre. Compensatory use of other sensory avenues. Integrated and use environmental clues well	Consistent and integrated. Good listening behavior. Use hearing projectively. Give scanning responses.	Cluster around average level. Little scatter. Integrated and consistent in performance on tests.	Good except for communication area. Average social quotient of approximately 90.	Good but balance may be disturbed. No generalized incoordination or retardation.	Good inner language. Good gesture. Use voice projectively. Behave symbolically.	Good responsiveness to people through vision. Social perception and contact with environment is good.
Aphasia	Indicates some retardation in development. Confusion regarding hearing. Lack of shyness but not bizarre.	Disinhibited, hyperactive and forced responsiveness. Not use other sensory avenues in compensatory way.	Inconsistent, erratic, cannot listen. Disturbed in auditory perception. Not use hearing projectively.	Inconsistent and much scatter. Perceptual disturbances improve with structuring.	Retarded in all areas but especially in communication, socialization and motor areas. Average social quotient of approximately 75.	Slightly delayed in sitting and walking. Generalized incoordination.	Poor inner language. Little or no use of gesture. Not use voice projectively. May unexpectedly use a word. May be echolalic.	Emotional expression lacks intensity. Try to relate to people. Are not oblivious or bizarre.

Psychic Deafness	Began using speech, then stopped. Many anxieties. Willfulness in rejection of environment. Withdrawn and in world of their own.	Bizarre, no compensatory use of senses. Not relate to people. Poor social perception. No projective use of hearing or voice and no gesture.	Seem to willfully reject sound, give indirect responses. No projective use of hearing. Not disturbed in auditory perception. May show fear of sound.	Not perceptually disturbed. May do well on formboards. Reject the test situation in total or in part. Behavior suggests good mental ability.	Deficient in all areas but notably in socialization. Average social quotient of approximately 80.	Stereotyped activity. Rigidity and random movements. Only slight retardation in sitting and walking.	Good inner language but used only for phantasy. No use of gesture and do not use voice projectively. May be mute.	Withdrawn in own world. Lacking in relationship to people. Stereotyped and bizarre.
Mental Deficiency	Retardation in all development is most characteristic in history.	Responsive but in low genetic and concrete manner. Not bizarre.	Respond directly or indirectly to tests which are suitable genetically. Use hearing projectively.	Marked retardation in general.	Marked generalized retardation in all areas. Average social quotient of approximately 55.	Generalized retardation with incoordination. Marked delay in sitting and walking.	Language is deficient but not seriously discrepant with mental age. Retarded in all phases of language development.	Passive, phlegmatic, infantile and deficient in animation.

can be begun for many of these children at approximately two years of age. The specialist making the diagnosis should assist the parents in securing trained educators to help them in planning and inaugurating this training program. There are several agencies in each state, and often several in an individual community, that can be of assistance with the program for children with peripheral deafness. These include state departments of public welfare, state departments of education, county and city public school systems, and a number of private agencies and schools. It has been found helpful to have lists made in advance covering various suggestions that can be made. This list of suggestions can be given to the parent at the time of the initial discussion following the diagnosis. It should include suggestions for contacting appropriate parents' groups and suggestions for pertinent reading materials [3].

RECOMMENDATIONS FOR APHASIC CHILDREN

The aphasic child is one of the most difficult for whom the specialist must make recommendations. Society, in general, has not provided for these children. With the exception of a few private schools, no specific programs have been developed for them. This is one of the most urgent needs in the field of special education. It seems probable currently that most of these children are included in the group referred to as mentally handicapped; however, it is evident that some are classified with those having peripheral deafness.

From the point of view of the specialist making a differential diagnosis of aphasia, one of the most helpful recommendations is to give the parents suggestions on home management [2]. The aphasic child often is difficult to live with, especially when he is misunderstood. A basic suggestion is that he requires assistance in integrating himself, which means that he requires patient, calm handling. Overstimulation is his greatest problem; therefore, the parents are advised to reduce stimulation. He is given only one toy at a time, he is not exposed to large groups, and if taken to the grocery store he is protected from the conglomerate stimulation of the environment; many parents report that shopping with their child is one of their most difficult experiences. A specific room in the home should be set aside for the child when possible. This room should be free from obvious distractions and the child's stimulation controlled by the parent by giving him appropriate blocks, sound toys and other objects. This type of handling is referred to as the "reduction of stimuli" method. Somewhat dramatic results can be achieved by this method when it is expeditiously applied. Children who are hyperactive and disintegrated to an extreme degree might become amenable when their environment and total stimulation is carefully controlled. This is an essential step in their initial training. All specialists can make such recommendations to the parents of these children.

Language training for aphasic children usually is done by a speech correctionist. A program sometimes can be arranged through the public school system, sometimes through a private tutor. Often assistance for these children can be secured through a university speech and hearing center. All specialists should actively encourage more experimentally oriented training programs for aphasic children because only through such emphasis can the needs and potentials of these children be realized.

RECOMMENDATIONS FOR CHILDREN WITH PSYCHIC DEAFNESS

Children with psychic deafness present a challenging problem. Only slight progress has been made in the development of specific programs for these children. Their primary need is for psychotherapy; therefore, recommendations for a psychotherapeutic program should be paramount. However, the psychotherapy often must be non-verbal in nature and such programs are difficult to secure. It remains for child psychiatry and clinical psychology to emphasize the development of non-verbal psychotherapeutic techniques. This does not imply that programs for children with psychic deafness cannot be secured. Many psychiatrists and psychologists are in position to assist with the planning and direction of such programs. A number of private and public schools provide residential treatment which is necessary for some children. The parents should be encouraged to explore all possibilities; they should not, except in rare instances, be led to believe that they can solve such a difficult problem without the help of an appropriate specialist.

RECOMMENDATIONS FOR THE MENTALLY DEFICIENT

Many communities have well developed programs for the mentally handicapped. Moreover, as they do for children with peripheral deafness, states have public programs and schools which serve many people. Private and public schools, also, have made provision for these children. It is the specialist's responsibility to be familiar with these programs and to make recommendations which are suitable for each child. Usually training facilities for the pre-school mentally deficient child are available in urban, metropolitan areas through parents who have organized for this purpose. These parents' associations for the mentally retarded should be recommended whenever possible. Recommendations should include both immediate and long term aspects. Realistic but helpful suggestions should include management of the child in terms of his mental level and according to the mental level expected at maturity [1].

BIBLIOGRAPHY

1. Levinson, Abraham: The Mentally Retarded Child. New York, John Day, 1952.
2. Lewis, R., Strauss, S. and Lehtinen, L.: The Other Child—The Brain-Injured Child. New York, Grune & Stratton, 1951.
3. Myklebust, H. R.: Your Deaf Child. Springfield, Ill., C. C Thomas, 1950.

Index of Authors

Index of Subjects

of mental capacity, 297 ff.
of motor capacity, 307 ff.
of motor tests, 307 ff.
purposes of, 290 f.
of social maturity, 292 ff.
standardized procedures for, 291 f.
suggested mental tests for, 306
See also Tests
Psychological tests. See Tests
Psychopathology of hearing. See Auditory disorders
Pure tone audiometry. See Tests

RECEPTIVE LANGUAGE
disorders of, diagram of, 14
function of, 12 f.
See also Language
Rubella, 57

SOCIAL MATURITY, 292 ff.
mean scores for groups, 295
See also Tests
Speech, 2, 3
audiometry, 271 f.
verbal comprehension test, 253 ff.
See also Tests
Speech pathologist, role of, in differential diagnosis, 26 f.
Symbolic behavior, defined, 10
Symbolic disorders. See Aphasia; Language; Language function
Symptomatology. See Behavioral symptomatology

TACTILE SENSATION, 169 f., 205 f.
Test(s)
administration of, 239 f.
in aphasia, 162 ff.
assumptions and use in, 237 ff.
of auditory perception, 256 ff.
child management in, 239 f.
electroencephalography, 275 f.

of expressive language, 281 f.
formal, auditory, 262 ff.
imitation of vocalization, 250 ff.
informal, 323 ff.
auditory, 245 ff.
of inner language, 277 ff.
of laterality, 309 f.
of mental capacity, 297 ff.
Cattell, 298 f.
geometric design, 300 f.
Goodenough, 301
Nebraska, 299 f.
Ontario, 299
of mental deficiency, 220 ff., 224 f.
of motor capacity, 307 ff.
of non-verbal communication, 105 ff.
object language, 277 ff.
peep show, 272 f.
of peripheral deafness, 111 ff.
of psychic deafness, 195 f.
psychogalvanic audiometry, 273 ff.
psychological, 291 ff.
pure tone audiometry, 262 ff.
limitations of, 265
responses of normal children to, 262 ff.
purpose of, 240 ff.
railwalking, 310
of receptive language, 280 f.
record form for, 260 ff.
of social maturity, 292 ff.
sound-field, 255 f.
sound instrument, 245 ff.
sound toy, 248 ff.
of speech audiometry, 271 f.
suggested mental, 306
touching, 158 f.
tuning fork, 270 f.
verbal comprehension, 253 ff.
voice, 252 f.
Toilet training, 82 ff.
mean age for groups studied, 83 ff.